Outcomes and Therapeutic Management of Thyroid Carcinoma

Outcomes and Therapeutic Management of Thyroid Carcinoma

Editors

Giovanni Conzo
Renato Patrone

MDPI • Basel • Beijing • Wuhan • Barcelona • Belgrade • Manchester • Tokyo • Cluj • Tianjin

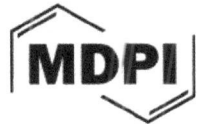

Editors
Giovanni Conzo
Oncologic and Bariatric
Surgery University of
Campania "Luigi Vanvitelli"
Italy

Renato Patrone
University of Federico II of Naples
Istituto Nazionale
Tumori-IRCCS-Fondazione G.
Pascale
Italy

Editorial Office
MDPI
St. Alban-Anlage 66
4052 Basel, Switzerland

This is a reprint of articles from the Special Issue published online in the open access journal *Journal of Clinical Medicine* (ISSN 2077-0383) (available at: https://www.mdpi.com/journal/jcm/special_issues/Outcomes_Management_Thyroid_Carcinoma).

For citation purposes, cite each article independently as indicated on the article page online and as indicated below:

LastName, A.A.; LastName, B.B.; LastName, C.C. Article Title. *Journal Name* **Year**, *Volume Number*, Page Range.

ISBN 978-3-0365-6263-6 (Hbk)
ISBN 978-3-0365-6264-3 (PDF)

© 2023 by the authors. Articles in this book are Open Access and distributed under the Creative Commons Attribution (CC BY) license, which allows users to download, copy and build upon published articles, as long as the author and publisher are properly credited, which ensures maximum dissemination and a wider impact of our publications.
The book as a whole is distributed by MDPI under the terms and conditions of the Creative Commons license CC BY-NC-ND.

Contents

About the Editors vii

Annamaria D'Amore, Renato Patrone, Ludovico Docimo, Giovanni Conzo and Celestino Pio Lombardi
Thyroid Cancer: Toward Surgical Evolution
Reprinted from: *J. Clin. Med.* 2021, 10, 3582, doi:10.3390/jcm10163582 1

Renato Patrone, Nunzio Velotti, Stefania Masone, Alessandra Conzo, Luigi Flagiello, Chiara Cacciatore, et al.
Management of Low-Risk Thyroid Cancers: Is Active Surveillance a Valid Option? A Systematic Review of the Literature
Reprinted from: *J. Clin. Med.* 2021, 10, 3569, doi:10.3390/jcm10163569 5

Andrea Polistena, Monia Ranalli, Stefano Avenia, Roberta Lucchini, Alessandro Sanguinetti, Sergio Galasse, et al.
The Role of IONM in Reducing the Occurrence of Shoulder Syndrome Following Lateral Neck Dissection for Thyroid Cancer
Reprinted from: *J. Clin. Med.* 2021, 10, 4246, doi:10.3390/jcm10184246 13

Chiara Offi, Claudia Misso, Giovanni Antonelli, Maria Grazia Esposito, Umberto Brancaccio and Stefano Spiezia
Laser Ablation Treatment of Recurrent Lymph Node Metastases from Papillary Thyroid Carcinoma
Reprinted from: *J. Clin. Med.* 2021, 10, 5295, doi:10.3390/jcm10225295 27

Giorgio Grani, Gianluca Cera, Giovanni Conzo, Valeria Del Gatto, Cira Rosaria Tiziana di Gioia, Marianna Maranghi, et al.
Preoperative Ultrasonography in the Evaluation of Suspected Familial Non-Medullary Thyroid Cancer: Are We Able to Predict Multifocality and Extrathyroidal Extension?
Reprinted from: *J. Clin. Med.* 2021, 10, 5277, doi:10.3390/jcm10225277 35

Joohyun Woo, Hyeonkyeong Kim and Hyungju Kwon
Impact of Multifocality on the Recurrence of Papillary Thyroid Carcinoma
Reprinted from: *J. Clin. Med.* 2021, 10, 5144, doi:10.3390/jcm10215144 43

Martina Mandarano, Marco Andolfi, Renato Colella, Massimo Monacelli, Andrea Polistena, Sonia Moretti, et al.
Impact of Epithelial–Mesenchymal Immunophenotype on Local Aggressiveness in Papillary Thyroid Carcinoma Invading the Airway
Reprinted from: *J. Clin. Med.* 2021, 10, 4351, doi:10.3390/jcm10194351 51

Giuliano Perigli, Fabio Cianchi, Francesco Giudici, Edda Russo, Giulia Fiorenza, Luisa Petrone, et al.
Thyroidectomy for Cancer: The Surgeon and the Parathyroid Glands Sparing
Reprinted from: *J. Clin. Med.* 2021, 10, 4323, doi:10.3390/jcm10194323 63

Francesca Privitera, Rossella Gioco, Ileana Fazio, Alessio Volpicelli, Maria Teresa Cannizzaro, Salvatore Costa, et al.
Risk Factors for Low Levels of Parathyroid Hormone after Surgery for Thyroid Cancer: A Single Center Study
Reprinted from: *J. Clin. Med.* 2021, 10, 4113, doi:10.3390/jcm10184113 75

Enke Baldini, Chiara Tuccilli, Daniele Pironi, Antonio Catania, Francesco Tartaglia, Filippo Maria Di Matteo, et al.
Expression and Clinical Utility of Transcription Factors Involved in Epithelial–Mesenchymal Transition during Thyroid Cancer Progression
Reprinted from: *J. Clin. Med.* **2021**, *10*, 4076, doi:10.3390/jcm10184076 87

Salvatore Buscemi, Giuseppe Di Buono, Rocco D'Andrea, Claudio Ricci, Laura Alberici, Lorenzo Querci, et al.
Perioperative Management of Pheochromocytoma: From a Dogmatic to a Tailored Approach
Reprinted from: *J. Clin. Med.* **2021**, *10*, 3759, doi:10.3390/jcm10163759 107

Liviu Hîțu, Paul-Andrei Ștefan and Doina Piciu
Total Tumor Diameter and Unilateral Multifocality as Independent Predictor Factors for Metastatic Papillary Thyroid Microcarcinoma
Reprinted from: *J. Clin. Med.* **2021**, *10*, 3707, doi:10.3390/jcm10163707 115

Giuseppa Graceffa, Giuseppina Orlando, Gianfranco Cocorullo, Sergio Mazzola, Irene Vitale, Maria Pia Proclamà, et al.
Predictors of Central Compartment Involvement in Patients with Positive Lateral Cervical Lymph Nodes According to Clinical and/or Ultrasound Evaluation
Reprinted from: *J. Clin. Med.* **2021**, *10*, 3407, doi:10.3390/jcm10153407 125

Alessandro Longheu, Gian Luigi Canu, Federico Cappellacci, Enrico Erdas, Fabio Medas and Pietro Giorgio Calò
Tall Cell Variant versus Conventional Papillary Thyroid Carcinoma: A Retrospective Analysis in 351 Consecutive Patients
Reprinted from: *J. Clin. Med.* **2021**, *10*, 70, doi:10.3390/jcm10010070 135

Maria Irene Bellini, Marco Biffoni, Renato Patrone, Maria Carola Borcea, Maria Ludovica Costanzo, Tiziana Garritano, et al.
Poorly Differentiated Thyroid Carcinoma: Single Centre Experience and Review of the Literature
Reprinted from: *J. Clin. Med.* **2021**, *10*, 5258, doi:10.3390/jcm10225258 145

Salvatore Sorrenti, Vincenzo Dolcetti, Daniele Fresilli, Giovanni Del Gaudio, Patrizia Pacini, Pintong Huang, et al.
The Role of CEUS in the Evaluation of Thyroid Cancer: From Diagnosis to Local Staging
Reprinted from: *J. Clin. Med.* **2021**, *10*, 4559, doi:10.3390/jcm10194559 153

Stefania Masone, Nunzio Velotti, Silvia Savastano, Emanuele Filice, Rossana Serao, Antonio Vitiello, et al.
Morbid Obesity and Thyroid Cancer Rate. A Review of Literature
Reprinted from: *J. Clin. Med.* **2021**, *10*, 1894, doi:10.3390/jcm10091894 167

About the Editors

Giovanni Conzo

Giovanni Conzo was born in Naples on 29-12-1963. He began his career in 1990 as an assistant surgeon at the Institute of Surgical Semeiotics, Second University of Naples, directed by Prof. Antonino Caraco and is now a specialist in General Surgery (July 1993) and Thoracic Surgery (October 2001). He is currently an Associate Professor of Surgery-MED18 and a Consultant Surgeon at the Division of General, Oncological, Mininvasive, and Obesity Surgery—School of Medicine and Surgery, University of Campania "Luigi Vanvitelli". He is responsible for the IPAS of Pancreatic Surgery of the AOU "L. Vanvitelli" of Naples. He is an Endocrine Surgeon of the European Board for NeuroEndocrine Tumours (ENETYS). He accomplished his surgical training at the Second University of Naples. He later attended several training periods at international referral centers for Upper GI, HPB, and liver transplantation surgery as well as for laparoscopic surgery.

He leads his research largely in the field of digestive pathology and endocrinology, as well as minimally invasive surgery. He has been involved in several national and international meetings either as a speaker or moderator and was also the promoter of countless conferences and training sessions in the field of endocrine and minimally invasive surgery. He is involved in different academic duties at the Campania University: he runs general surgery teaching sessions at the Degree course in Medicine and Surgery at the Specialization Course in General Surgery and Endocrine Surgery and he is also a teacher of the Degree course in Nursing and PhD in Nephrology.

His scientific work is based on over 360 papers published in national and international journals, books, monographs, and chapters printed on national surgical books. His I.F. is > 400 with an H-index of 34 with more than 3000 citations (SCOPUS 12/2022). Conzo's surgical experience is based upon over 7000 interventions, including more than 3000 as the first operator, with a large number of them in Endocrine and Oncological Surgery and minimally invasive surgery in elective and urgency surgery. He is a member of the Italian Society of Surgery, Italian Society of Endoscopic Surgery, Neapolitan Society of Surgery (Vice President), European Association of Endoscopic Surgery, Italian Society of Colon Proctology, Executive Council of the UEC, and Executive Council of the Italian Society of University Surgeons, Italian Society of Endocrine Surgery (Vice President), and Board of National Assistant Professors of Surgery-Med 18 (Chairman). In June 2017, he cofounded the Società Italiana Unitaria di Endocrino-Chirurgia (SIEUC) and became the National Secretary. In 2017, he founded Campania Pancreas—a collaborative group and electronic platform for the prevention, diagnosis, and treatment of pancreatic cancer in the Campania Region. In 2018, he was named Delegato Regionale of Campania Region in Italian Society of Surgery (SIC). In 2021, he become President of Italian Society of Gastrointestinal Pathology (SIPAD).

Renato Patrone

Renato Patrone was born in 1986 in Naples, Italy. After graduation as a Medical Doctor in 2012, he dedicated his professional career to Surgery and he is now a specialist in General Surgery, with a sub-speciality in oncological surgery. During the first year of his career, the interest in endocrine surgery was preeminent but, gradually, oncological surgery has become the main surgical activity of his clinical practice. At the same time, he contributes a lot of research, publications, and congress activities. Presently, he works at the National Cancer Institute of Naples, the biggest oncological and research hospital of southern Italy—IRCCS Pascale INT. His research activity has been implemented with the PhD XXXVI cycle in INFORMATION AND COMMUNICATION TECHNOLOGY FOR HEALTH—Robotic 4 Health. His H-index is 16 and he is author of more than 50 research articles published in peer-reviewed journals. In 2018, he was named as the Young Regional delegate for the SIUEC and, in 2021, he accomplished the Advanced Laparoscopic School. Dr. Patrone is a member of numerous Italian and international scientific societies (Italian Society of Surgery—SIC, Neapolitan Society of Surgery—SNaC, Italian Society of Endocrine Surgery—SIUEC, European Society of Surgical Oncology—ESSO, European/African/Middle-Eastern Hepato-Pancreato-Biliary Association—E-AHPBA, and the l'International Hepato-Pancreato-Biliary Association—IHPBA).

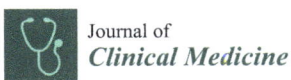

Editorial
Thyroid Cancer: Toward Surgical Evolution

Annamaria D'Amore [1], Renato Patrone [2,*], Ludovico Docimo [3], Giovanni Conzo [3] and Celestino Pio Lombardi [1]

[1] Department of Gastroenterologic, Endocrine-Metabolic and Nephro-Urologic Sciences. Endocrine Surgery Division, Fondazione Policlinico Universitario A. Gemelli IRCCS, 00168 Rome, Italy; annamaria.damore@policlinicogemelli.it (A.D.); cplombardi@libero.it (C.P.L.)
[2] PhD ICHT, University of Naples Federico II, 80131 Naples, Italy
[3] Department of Cardiothoracic Sciences, University of Campania "Luigi Vanvitelli", Division of General and Oncologic Surgery, Via Pansini 5, 80131 Napoli, Italy; ludovico.docimo@unicampania.it (L.D.); giovanni.conzo@unicampania.it (G.C.)
* Correspondence: dott.patrone@gmail.com; Tel.: +39-3491327226

Citation: D'Amore, A.; Patrone, R.; Docimo, L.; Conzo, G.; Lombardi, C.P. Thyroid Cancer: Toward Surgical Evolution. *J. Clin. Med.* **2021**, *10*, 3582. https://doi.org/10.3390/jcm10163582

Received: 9 August 2021
Accepted: 10 August 2021
Published: 14 August 2021

Publisher's Note: MDPI stays neutral with regard to jurisdictional claims in published maps and institutional affiliations.

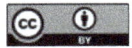

Copyright: © 2021 by the authors. Licensee MDPI, Basel, Switzerland. This article is an open access article distributed under the terms and conditions of the Creative Commons Attribution (CC BY) license (https://creativecommons.org/licenses/by/4.0/).

It has been more than five years since the American Thyroid Association (ATA) and the Italian consensus on thyroid cancer was published [1,2]. It revaluated and retrospectively analyzed the results of thyroid cancer treatment and the outcomes in terms of disease-free survival and recurrence rate. Both suggested a more conservative approach for low/intermediate-risk well-differentiated thyroid cancers (DTCs), rehabilitating hemithyroidectomy as the surgical approach of choice. It is well known that DTCs represent the most common of all thyroid cancers [3]. Moreover, in recent decades, we have assisted in a continual and constant increase in the number of new diagnoses. It is quite clear that overdiagnosis and the incredible spread of neck ultrasound using thyroid nodule detection as well as fine-needle aspiration of a nodule of less than centimeter in dimension justifies this enormous number of new thyroid cancer diagnoses we have to manage daily. It is strongly evident that, usually, DTCs carry very good prognosis (10-year survival rate more than 90%) with a low rate of death, whereas, by contrast, persistent or recurrent disease is more common than the others. Furthermore, the 8th edition of the American Committee on Cancer and Union Internationale Contre le Cancer (AJCC/UICC) reviewed the DTC staging system: a larger part of tumors are now downstage to I or II because of the absence of distant metastases, even if it is smaller than 4 cm associated with microscopic extension to perithyroidal soft tissues and, in the case of lymph-node metastases, in the central and lateral compartments [4]. This new consideration leads to the identification of a small proportion of DTC patients, approximately 5–10%, who are at risk of death because of their cancer and their stage (usually III or IV) [5]. After these considerations, it is understandable that the recent guidelines push towards a new therapeutic approach to DTCs with low/intermediate risk. The previous almost paradigmatic indication of an absolute, complete, and more aggressive approach pressed physicians and endocrine surgeons in the past to prefer the typical "one-size-fits-all" mode and to suggest total thyroidectomy associated with central neck dissection, and radio iodine remnant ablation in the majority of patients. Presently, evidence suggests a new idea for surgery: a conservative approach for all DTCs with a preoperative low/intermediate risk, no evidence of lymph-node metastasis or other signs of aggressive presentation of the hilum and no other conditions that upgrade risk. The risk of thyroid cancer recurrence is common and moderately both in low and intermediate DTCs, but it is not influenced by an early surgical approach [6]. It is evaluated by international database reports and clarified in the literature that the recurrence rate between hemithyroidectomy and total thyroidectomy is similar and seems not to affect prognosis [7]. Moreover, a new surgical operation in the case of contralateral recurrence does not impact survival [8]. Even if the American and Italian guidelines are definitive towards this new concept of conservative and repeatable surgery, daily routines involving physicians and surgeons do not yet follow that line. Overdiagnosis and possible overtreatment is still prevalent in real-life cohorts in Italy, and no significant changes have been recorded in recent years. The rate of lobectomies is growing, but the procedure still represents a minority of all performed surgeries [9–12]. However, such an approach needs a solid multidisciplinary group to decide and propose strategy, to manage follow-up and establish new indications for treatment. Patients need to be well identified, all clinical features must be known and analyzed, and surgical approaches must be well explained and accepted by patients. Moreover, a wider knowledge of minimally invasive surgical techniques for thyroid diseases needs to be massively widespread, as well as the possibility for patients to refer to an endocrine center performing such surgery. Actual surgery for low and intermediate DTCs must be well fitted for every patient. In our experience, according to the guidelines and in contrast with the Italian trends, we are constantly contributing to an increased number of hemithyroidectomy performed for DTCs, which in recent months represented about 20% of all interventions for thyroid disease, compared to 5% in the last decade, with a large number of patients at follow-up stage. In this group, thyroidectomy was necessary in about 25% of cases because of evidence at final histology of extensive disease in contrast with preoperative features (histological variant, extra thyroidal disease, and/or multifocality and/or lymph-node metastases). We have a time constraint for follow-up, and a small number of cases require total thyroidectomy to produce dynamic and statistical evidence, so we are confident that a larger number of colleagues will follow this approach to implement and strengthen this guideline consensus.

Author Contributions: Conceptualization, C.P.L., R.P., L.D., G.C. and A.D.; writing—original draft preparation C.P.L. and A.D.; writing—review and editing, R.P. and G.C.; supervision, L.D. and G.C. All authors have read and agreed to the published version of the manuscript.

Conflicts of Interest: The authors declare no conflict of interest.

References

1. Haugen, B.R.; Alexander, E.K.; Bible, K.C.; Doherty, G.M.; Mandel, S.J.; Nikiforov, Y.E.; Pacini, F.; Randolph, G.W.; Sawka, A.M.; Schlumberger, M.; et al. 2015 American Thyroid Association Management Guidelines for Adult Patients with Thyroid Nodules and Differentiated Thyroid Cancer: The American Thyroid Association Guidelines Task Force on Thyroid Nodules and Differentiated Thyroid Cancer. *Thyroid* **2016**, *26*, 1–133. [CrossRef] [PubMed]
2. Pacini, F.; Basolo, F.; Bellantone, R.; Boni, G.; Cannizzaro, M.A.; De Palma, M.; Durante, C.; Elisei, R.; Fadda, G.; Frasoldati, A.; et al. Italian consensus on diagnosis and treatment of differentiated thyroid cancer: Joint statements of six Italian societies. *J. Endocrinol. Investig.* **2018**, *41*, 849–876. [CrossRef] [PubMed]
3. Lamartina, L.; Grani, G.; Durante, C.; Borget, I.; Filetti, S.; Schlumberger, M. Follow-up of differentiated thyroid cancer–what should (and what should not) be done. *Nat. Rev. Endocrinol.* **2018**, *14*, 538–551. [CrossRef] [PubMed]
4. *AJCC Cancer Staging Form Supplement AJCC Cancer Staging Manual*, 8th ed.; Springer: Berlin/Heidelberg, Germany, 2017.
5. Tuttle, R.M.; Haugen, B.; Perrier, N.D. Updated American joint committee on cancer/tumor-node-metastasis staging system for differentiated and anaplastic thyroid cancer (Eighth Edition): What changed and why? *Thyroid* **2017**, *27*, 751–756. [CrossRef] [PubMed]
6. Kim, M.J.; Lee, M.C.; Lee, G.H.; Choi, H.S.; Cho, S.W.; Kim, S.J.; Lee, K.E.; Park, Y.J.; Park, D.J. Extent of surgery did not affect recurrence during 7-years follow-up in papillary thyroid cancer sized 1-4 cm: Preliminary results. *Clin. Endocrinol.* **2017**, *87*, 80–86. [CrossRef] [PubMed]
7. Lamartina, L.; Leboulleux, S.; Terroir, M.; Hartl, D.; Schlumberger, M. An update on the management of low-risk differentiated thyroid cancer. *Endocr. Relat. Cancer* **2019**, *26*, R597–R610. [CrossRef] [PubMed]
8. Park, J.H.; Yoon, J.H. Lobectomy in patients with differentiated thyroid cancer: Indications and follow-up. *Endocr. Relat. Cancer* **2019**, *26*, R381–R393. [CrossRef] [PubMed]
9. Lamartina, L.; Durante, C.; Lucisano, G.; Grani, G.; Bellantone, R.; Lombardi, C.P.; Pontecorvi, A.; Arvat, E.; Felicetti, F.; Zatelli, M.C.; et al. Are Evidence-Based Guidelines Reflected in Clinical Practice? An Analysis of Prospectively Collected Data of the Italian Thyroid Cancer Observatory. *Thyroid* **2017**, *27*, 1490–1497. [CrossRef] [PubMed]
10. Grani, G.; Zatelli, M.C.; Alfò, M.; Montesano, T.; Torlontano, M.; Morelli, S.; Deandrea, M.; Antonelli, A.; Francese, C.; Ceresini, G.; et al. Real-World Performance of the American Thyroid Association Risk Estimates in Predicting 1-Year Differentiated Thyroid Cancer Outcomes: A Prospective Multicenter Study of 2000 Patients. *Thyroid* **2021**, *31*, 264–271. [CrossRef] [PubMed]

11. Parmeggiani, D.; Gambardella, C.; Patrone, R.; Polistena, A.; De Falco, M.; Ruggiero, R.; Cirocchi, R.; Sanguinetti, A.; Cuccurullo, V.; Accardo, M.; et al. Radioguided thyroidectomy for follicular tumors: Multicentric experience. *Int. J. Surg.* **2017**, *41* (Suppl. 1), S75–S81. [CrossRef] [PubMed]
12. Medas, F.; Ansaldo, G.L.; Avenia, N.; Basili, G.; Boniardi, M.; Bononi, M.; Bove, A.; Carcoforo, P.; Casari, A.; Cavallaro, G.; et al. The THYCOVIT (Thyroid Surgery during COVID-19 pandemic in Italy) study: Results from a nationwide, multicentric, case-controlled study. *Updates Surg.* **2021**, *16*, 1–9. [CrossRef]

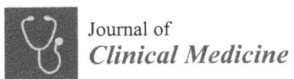

Review

Management of Low-Risk Thyroid Cancers: Is Active Surveillance a Valid Option? A Systematic Review of the Literature

Renato Patrone [1,*], Nunzio Velotti [2], Stefania Masone [3], Alessandra Conzo [4], Luigi Flagiello [4], Chiara Cacciatore [4], Marco Filardo [5], Vincenza Granata [6], Francesco Izzo [7], Domenico Testa [8], Stefano Avenia [9], Alessandro Sanguinetti [10], Andrea Polistena [11] and Giovanni Conzo [4]

1. PhD ICHT, 80131 Naples, Italy
2. Department of Advanced Biomedical Sciences, University of Naples "Federico II", 80131 Naples, Italy; nunzio.velotti@gmail.com
3. Department of Clinical Medicine and Surgery, University of Naples "Federico II", 80131 Naples, Italy; stefania.masone@unina.it
4. Department of Cardiothoracic Sciences, University of Campania "Luigi Vanvitelli", Division of General and Oncologic Surgery, Via Pansini 5, 80131 Napoli, Italy; aleconzo@hotmail.it (A.C.); luigiflagiello.93@gmail.com (L.F.); cacciatore.chiara@virgilio.it (C.C.); giovanni.conzo@unicampania.it (G.C.)
5. Division of Endocrine Surgery, Department of Oncological and Gastrointestinal Surgical Science, University of Study of Padova, Via Giustiniani 2, 35128 Padua, Italy; marcofinly43@gmail.com
6. Radiodiodiagnostic Unit, "Istituto Nazionale Tumori IRCCS Fondazione Pascale-IRCCS di Napoli", 80131 Naples, Italy; v.granata@istitutotumori.na.it
7. Hepatobiliary Surgical Oncology Unit, "Istituto Nazionale Tumori IRCCS Fondazione Pascale-IRCCS di Napoli", 80131 Naples, Italy; f.izzo@istitutotumori.na.it
8. Otolaryngology-Head and Neck Surgery Unit, Department of Cardiothoracic Sciences, University of Campania "Luigi Vanvitelli", 80100 Naples, Italy; domenico.testa@unicampania.it
9. Scuola di Specializzazione in Chirurgia Generale, Università degli Studi di Perugia, 06123 Perugia, Italy; s.aveni@gmail.com
10. 1SC Chirurgia Generale e Specialità Chirurgiche, Azienda Ospedaliera S. Maria, 05100 Terni, Italy; a.sanguinetti@aospterni.it
11. UOC Chirurgia Generale e Laparoscopica, Dipartimento di Chirurgia Pietro Valdoni, Sapienza Università di Roma, Policlinico Umberto I, 00185 Roma, Italy; apolis74@yahoo.it
* Correspondence: dott.patrone@gmail.com; Tel.: +39-3491327226

Citation: Patrone, R.; Velotti, N.; Masone, S.; Conzo, A.; Flagiello, L.; Cacciatore, C.; Filardo, M.; Granata, V.; Izzo, F.; Testa, D.; et al. Management of Low-Risk Thyroid Cancers: Is Active Surveillance a Valid Option? A Systematic Review of the Literature. *J. Clin. Med.* **2021**, *10*, 3569. https://doi.org/10.3390/jcm10163569

Academic Editor: Pierpaolo Trimboli

Received: 2 July 2021
Accepted: 10 August 2021
Published: 13 August 2021

Publisher's Note: MDPI stays neutral with regard to jurisdictional claims in published maps and institutional affiliations.

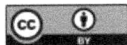

Copyright: © 2021 by the authors. Licensee MDPI, Basel, Switzerland. This article is an open access article distributed under the terms and conditions of the Creative Commons Attribution (CC BY) license (https://creativecommons.org/licenses/by/4.0/).

Abstract: Thyroid cancer is the most common endocrine malignancy, representing 2.9% of all new cancers in the United States. It has an excellent prognosis, with a five-year relative survival rate of 98.3%. Differentiated Thyroid Carcinomas (DTCs) are the most diagnosed thyroid tumors and are characterized by a slow growth rate and indolent course. For years, the only approach to treatment was thyroidectomy. Active surveillance (AS) has recently emerged as an alternative approach; it involves regular observation aimed at recognizing the minority of patients who will clinically progress and would likely benefit from rescue surgery. To better clarify the indications for active surveillance for low-risk thyroid cancers, we reviewed the current management of low-risk DTCs with a systematic search performed according to a PRISMA flowchart in electronic databases (PubMed, Web of Science, Scopus, and EMBASE) for studies published before May 2021. Fourteen publications were included for final analysis, with a total number of 4830 patients under AS. A total of 451/4830 (9.4%) patients experienced an increase in maximum diameter by >3 mm; 609/4830 (12.6%) patients underwent delayed surgery after AS; metastatic spread to cervical lymph nodes was present in 88/4213 (2.1%) patients; 4/3589 (0.1%) patients had metastatic disease outside of cervical lymph nodes. Finally, no subject had a documented mortality due to thyroid cancer during AS. Currently, the American Thyroid Association guidelines do not support AS as the first-line treatment in patients with PMC; however, they consider AS to be an effective alternative, particularly in patients with high surgical risk or poor life expectancy due to comorbid conditions. Thus, AS could be an alternative to immediate surgery for patients with very-low-risk tumors showing no cytologic evidence of aggressive disease, for high-risk surgical candidates, for those with concurrent comorbidities requiring urgent intervention, and for patients with a relatively short life expectancy.

Keywords: thyroid cancer; active surveillance; thyroid surgery

1. Introduction

Thyroid cancer is the most common endocrine malignancy, representing 2.9% of all new cancers in the United States (US). It has an excellent prognosis, with a five-year relative survival rate of 98.3%, and has a higher frequency in females than males, with ratio of 3:1 [1]. Differentiated thyroid cancer (DTC) represents 90% of all thyroid malignancies and includes three main types: papillary thyroid cancer (PTC), the most common type, comprising 85% of all DTC; follicular thyroid cancer (FTC); and the rare subtype, Hürthle (oncocytic) cell thyroid cancer (2–5%) [2].

In the last ten years, the incidence of DTC has dramatically increased. This tendency is mainly as a result of the diffusion of imaging systems, the use of ultrasound-guided Fine Needle Aspirations Cytology (FNAC), and improvements in histological evaluations [3,4].

Actually, papillary microcarcinomas (PMCs) represents the most diagnosed thyroid tumors, with a 35% incidence of occult papillary thyroid microcarcinomas in autopsy studies [5]. The increased diagnosis of these malignancies, associated with a low risk of recurrence and death, has led to the need for redefining of the multimodal therapeutic approach to avoid potential overtreatments. With regard to treatment, historically, the only option was surgery. In the last few years, active surveillance (AS) has been established as an alternative approach; it is aimed at identifying patients who would likely benefit from rescue surgery [6].

Considering the data in the literature and the available evidence, we reviewed the current management of low-risk DTC, and PMCs in particular, to better clarify the indications for active surveillance for low-risk thyroid cancers.

2. Materials and Methods

According to the PRISMA flowchart (Preferred Reporting Items for Systematic reviews and Meta-Analyses), a systematic search was performed of electronic databases (PubMed, Web of Science, Scopus, and EMBASE). We used medical subject headings (MeSH) and free-text words, using the following search terms in all possible combinations: "differentiated thyroid cancer", "micro papillary cancer", "management", and "active surveillance". The last search was performed in May 2021. Attention was focused on the following primary outcomes: growth of the primary tumor, metastatic disease (lymph node or extra nodal), tumor recurrence after delayed thyroid surgery (DTS), and thyroid-cancer-related mortality. The secondary outcomes selected were decreased volume of primary tumor (>3 mm), overall mortality, and incidence of/indication for thyroidectomy.

The retrospective application of the surveillance criteria to patients surgically treated for thyroid nodules was not one of inclusion criteria for the studies reporting on AS of low-risk PTC; AS was limited to employment of surveillance strategies. Low-risk PTC was defined as T1a or T1b, N0, M0 disease. The search strategy was limited to articles written in the English language; moreover, papers on animal studies, review articles, editorials, and case series were excluded.

R.P. and G.C., two independent authors, analyzed all the papers, selected the suitable manuscripts, and performed the data extraction independently. All duplicate studies were removed. Two other authors (N.V. and S.M.) then checked the eligibility of the studies selected. Discrepancies were resolved by consensus.

3. Results

We identified a total of 2976 articles, of which 87 articles were selected for full text review. After full text review, 14 studies were included for the final analysis. The results are summarized in the PRISMA flowchart (Figure 1) [7–20].

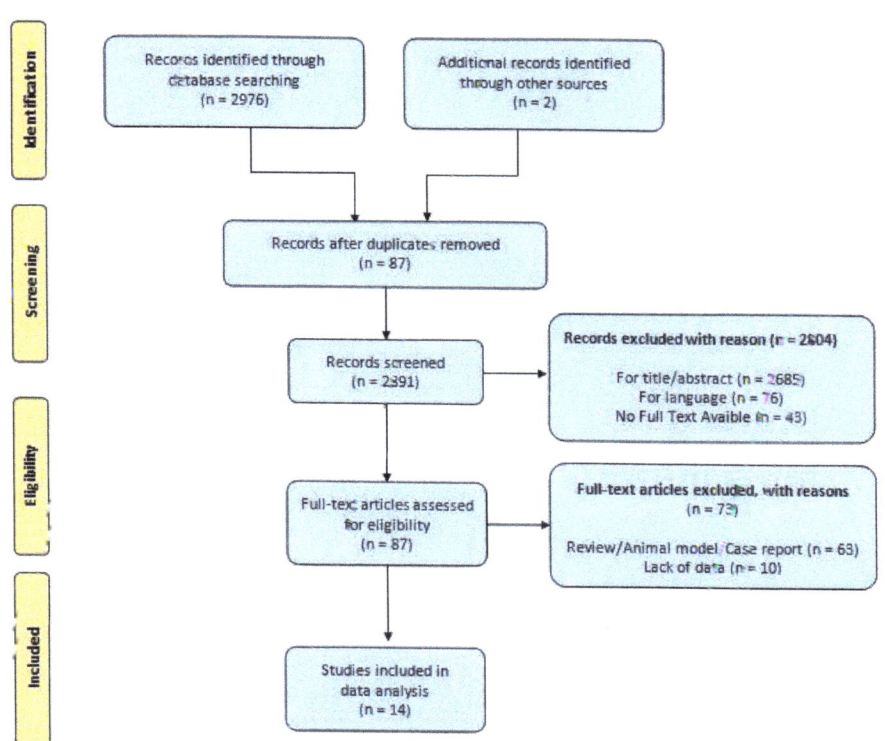

Figure 1. PRISMA flowchart.

The authors used the Newcastle-Ottawa Scale (NOS) to certify the quality of each included study. A maximum of nine stars was assigned to each study (Table 1).

Table 1. Newcastle-Ottawa Scale (NOS).

References	Selection				Comparability	Outcome Assessment		
	1	2	3	4	1	1	2	3
Gorshtein, 2021	*	*	*	*	**	*	*	
Rozenbaum, 2021	*		*	*	*	*	*	
Hu, 2021	*	*	*	*	**	*	*	*
Rosario, 2019	*	*	*	*	**	*	*	*
Oh, 2019	*	*	*	*	**	*	*	
Kim, 2018	*		*	*	*	*	*	*
Fukuoka, 2016	*	*	*	*	*	*		
Ito, 2014	*	*	*	*	**	*	*	*
Tuttle, 2017	*	*	*	*	**	*		
Oh, 2018	*		*	*	**	*	*	
Kwon, 2017	*		*	*	**	*	*	
Sugitani, 2010	*	*	*	*	*	*	*	
Sanabria, 2018	*	*	*	*	*	*	*	*
Oda, 2016	*		*	*	*	*	*	

Identify high quality choices with a "star". *. A maximum of one "star" for each item within the "Selection" and "Outcome Assessment" categories; maximum of two "stars" for "Comparability".

A total number of 4830 patients under AS were included in this review.

All studies assessed tumor growth during AS; a total of 451/4830 (9.4%) patients experienced an increase in diameter of up to 3 mm. Conversely, in five studies, a decrease in tumor size >3 mm was assessed in 172/1324 (12.9%) patients during AS.

DTS after AS was performed in 609/4830 (12.6%) patients, as reported by all authors. Ten authors reported involvement of cervical lymph nodes during AS in 88/4213 (2.1%) patients, while in six studies, 4/3589 (0.1%) patients were reported to have extra-nodal metastatic disease. No study reported mortality due to thyroid cancer during AS.

The results are summarized in Table 2.

Table 2. Characteristics of included studies.

First Author, Year	Patients, n	Age, Years	Female Sex, %	Tumor Growth, n	Delayed Surgery, n	Cervical Lymph Node Metastases, n	Localization of Metastasis	Distant Metastases, n	Death
Gorshtein, 2021	189	60.1 ± 13.1	89.2%	23	19	-	-	-	-
Rozenbaum, 2021	80	-	-	24	16	-	-	-	-
Hu, 2021	212	-	-	39	101	17	Central	2	-
Rosario, 2019	12	53 (median)	81.2%	1	2	1	-	-	-
Oh, 2019	273	51.1 (median)	75.8%	77	52	17	Central	-	-
Kim, 2018	126	51 ± 7	78.7%	25	18	1	-	-	-
Fukuoka, 2016	384	54 ± 11.9	86.1%	29	15	12	Central	-	-
Ito, 2014	1235	-	90%	58	191	19	-	-	-
Tuttle, 2017	291	51 ± 23	75.3%	11	5	-	-	-	-
Oh, 2018	370	51.1 ± 11.7	76.8%	86	58	5	-	-	-
Kwon, 2017	192	51.3 (median)	76 %	27	24	7	Central	2	-
Sugitani, 2010	230	56 (median)	50%	22	9	3	Central	-	-
Sanabria, 2018	57	51.9 (median)	84 %	2	5	-	-	-	-
Oda, 2016	1179	57 (median)	87 %	27	94	6	-	-	-

4. Discussion

DTC represents a heterogeneous pattern of different histological thyroid neoplasms [21]. With regard to histopathology, the most frequent variant is PTC, FTC represents 10–20% of cases, and medullary cancer is the rarest [22].

While the incidence of DTC continues to increase, mortality from thyroid cancer has declined over the last three decades. The prognosis for PMC is excellent, with a mortality rate of 0.3%; this includes patients with lymph node metastases and extra thyroidal extensions [23].

The mainstays of DTC therapy are surgical resection, radioiodine ablation, and thyroid-stimulating hormone (TSH) suppression; however, the benefits of active surveillance for selected cases have also been increasingly acknowledged in recent years [24,25]. Moreover, in 2016, encapsulated follicular variant papillary thyroid cancers (EFVPTC) were renamed non-invasive follicular thyroid neoplasms with papillary-like nuclear features (NIFTP) in an effort to avoid overtreatment arising from a diagnosis of cancer; the indolent nature of these neoplasms does not necessitate complete thyroidectomy or radioiodine ablation therapy [26].

The main risk factors for lymphatic recurrence are multifocality, infiltration of the thyroid capsule, positive margins, age, tumor size, and mutations of p53 or BRAF. The recurrence rate after surgery (thyroid lobectomy or total thyroidectomy) is 1–2% in all patients affected by unifocal PMC and less than 1% in patients without locoregional metastases. Conversely, sub-capsular location of the lesion, multifocal disease, and extrathyroidal microscopic extension are associated with a higher risk of recurrence and nodal metastases [27,28]. Many authors have shown that locoregional nodal metastases are also related to the male sex [29]. An age <45 years at diagnosis is considered as a risk factor for higher recurrence rate, as demonstrated in a recent meta-analysis [29,30].

Different prognostic scores have been proposed for DTC during the last ten years, taking into account the following elements:

- biomolecular features (BRAF status) [31,32]; while TERT-promoter mutations can be found in less than 10% of PMC, BRAF seems to be the most reliable as a predictor of natural behavior of the PMC [31]. BRAF mutations can be found in 30–57% of PMC patients and are related to nodal metastases, extrathyroidal extension, and higher risk of recurrence [33];
- histological features (fibrosis, distance between the lesion and the gland capsule, psammoma bodies) [23,32–34];
- tumor pathologic factors, such as cervical lymph node metastases, tumor size, multifocality, and extra-thyroid extension [32–34];
- patient factors such as male gender [34,35].

Based on these parameters, the scientific literature includes numerous studies in which patients with low-risk PTCM were safely and effectively managed with AS.

Furthermore, it has to be considered that thyroid surgery is not immune to complications; laryngeal nerve injury, hypoparathyroidism, and hypothyroidism are the most frequent adverse effects of total thyroidectomy, while post-surgical hematomas and surgical wound infections represent minor complications [36].

Currently, AS is not supported by ATA guidelines as the first-line treatment in patients with PMC, but is rather seen as an effective alternative, especially in high-risk surgical patients or in patients with more comorbid conditions. Molinaro and colleagues [37] confirmed the feasibility and safety of the AS approach for patients with very-low-risk tumors. High surgical risk, relatively short life expectancy, and cytologic biopsy with no aggressive disease were the characteristics for authors to identify patients eligible for AS.

In 2021, Lohia et al. [38] investigated patients >65 years with T1, N0, M0 PTC who received surgery and created a competing risk model to define patient groups with life expectancies of less than 10 and 15 years. They found, in their study of 3280 patients, that older patients with comorbidities have limited life expectancies but excellent Disease Specific Survival (DSS) from low-risk PTC and concluded that incorporating life expectancy into management criteria would likely promote less aggressive treatment such as AS.

A recent study by Tuttle et al. reported that AS was an appropriate strategy for patients with PTC less than 1.5 cm in diameter and isolated BRAF V600E mutations [39].

Oda et al. [15] compared surgically treated PMC patients with those who underwent simple surveillance. They showed an excellent outcome in both groups; however, logically, unfavourable events would be significantly higher in the surgical group.

The results of our review of 4830 patients confirm the safety and efficacy of AS. Only 9.4% of recorded patients experienced an increase of tumor diameter, and 12.6% of patients underwent delayed surgery after AS. Cervical lymph node metastasis was present in 2.1% patients, and only 0.1% had extra-nodal metastasis.

Recently, Jeon et al. [40] proposed an interesting prospective study for papillary thyroid microcarcinomas based on KoMPASS (Korean Multicenter Prospective cohort study of Active Surveillance or Surgery). This study enrolled patients with PTMCs from 6 to 10 mm in diameter, with a confirmed cytopathological diagnosis and no metastasis or extra thyroid involvement. From the results of this survey, we will able to establish a protocol for the clinical framework of patients eligible for AS.

As previously stated, it is of paramount importance to consider tumor characteristics, family history, age, and other risk factors for the appropriate selection of patients for AS; moreover, it is necessary to evaluate individual patient's attitudes, including anxiety and reliability, as an effective AS approach is based on patients' compliance with surveillance protocols and follow-up.

The possibility of disease progression must always be considered: tumor growth in a short time period or the onset of lymph node metastases must be diagnosed promptly in order to switch patients to surgery without delay.

In our opinion, in the future, we will be able to use a prognostic score in order to determine those patients who can be treated using AS for PTC; this will allow for a concrete therapeutic option to minimize surgical intervention risk for non-aggressive tumors.

Hospitals and regional or national health organizations are increasingly interested in cost-effective patient management. In this systematic review, unfortunately, we are not able to provide a cost analysis of active surveillance versus standard therapy. In addition, we did not find any studies during our literature review that focused on this topic.

In our opinion, it would be interesting to perform a cost analysis of physician review and molecular testing compared with the standard therapy. This will be a focus of our research in the near future.

Finally, the challenges presented by the COVID-19 pandemic further highlight the benefits of AS in minimizing surgeries in a context undermined by the possibility of contagion [41–43].

The limitations of the present study include its design: because no statistical analysis was carried out on the extracted data, no definitive conclusions can be reached. Further research, with a meta-analytic design, is needed to evaluate the weighted incidence of tumor growth and local/distant metastasis during AS in the included studies, thus avoiding possible bias related to patient demographics and tumor characteristics.

5. Conclusions

Active surveillance should be proposed for low-risk PMC only after clinical trials proving the validity of this approach. For high-risk PMC, (lymph node or distant metastasis, extra thyroid extension, closeness to recurrent laryngeal nerve or trachea, high-grade cytology, or growth during observation), a surgical approach (lobectomy with or without paratracheal dissection) is necessary. Better knowledge of papillary cancer natural history and biological behavior might be useful in the design of multimodal management.

Author Contributions: Conceptualization, R.P., N.V., and G.C.; methodology, N.V. and R.P.; validation, S.M., G.C.; formal analysis, C.C. and A.C.; investigation, V.G., F.I., D.T.; data curation, N.V. and R.P.; writing—original draft preparation, N.V. and R.P.; writing—review and editing, S.M., L.F., M.F., S.A., A.S., A.P.; supervision, R.P. and G.C. All authors have read and agreed to the published version of the manuscript.

Funding: This research received no external funding.

Conflicts of Interest: The authors declare no conflict of interest.

References

1. Bethesda, M.D.; SEER Cancer Stat Facts. Thyroid Cancer. National Cancer Institute. Available online: https://seer.cancer.gov/statfacts/html/thyro.html (accessed on 10 May 2021).
2. Stewart, L.A.; Kuo, J.H. Advancements in the treatment of differentiated thyroid cancer. *Ther. Adv. Endocrinol. Metab.* **2021**, *12*, 20420188211000251. [CrossRef] [PubMed]
3. Davies, L.; Welche, H.G. Current thyroid cancer trends in the United States. *JAMA Otolaryngol. Head Neck Surg.* **2014**, *140*, 317–322. [CrossRef] [PubMed]
4. Davies, L.; Morris, L.G.; Haymart, M.; Chen, A.Y.; Goldenberg, D.; Morris, J.; Ogilvie, J.B.; Terris, D.J.; Netterville, J.; Wong, R.J.; et al. AACE Endocrine Surgery Scientific Committee. The increasing incidence of thyroid cancer. American association of clinical endocrinologists and American college of endocrinology disease state clinical review. *Endocr. Pract.* **2015**, *21*, 686–696. [CrossRef] [PubMed]
5. Harach, H.R.; Franssila, K.O.; Wasenius, V.M. Occult papillary carcinoma of the thyroid. A "normal" finding in Finland. A systematic autopsy study. *Cancer* **1985**, *56*, 531–538. [CrossRef]
6. Ito, Y.; Uruno, T.; Nakano, K.; Takamura, Y.; Miya, A.; Kobayashi, K.; Yokozawa, T.; Matsuzuka, F.; Kuma, S.; Kuma, K.; et al. An observation trial without surgical treatment in patients with papillary microcarcinoma of the thyroid. *Thyroid.* **2003**, *13*, 381–387. [CrossRef] [PubMed]

7. Kim, H.I.; Jang, H.W.; Ahn, H.S.; Ahn, S.; Park, S.Y.; Oh, Y.L.; Hahn, S.Y.; Shin, J.H.; Kim, J.H.; Kim, J.S.; et al. High serum TSH level is associated with progression of papillary thyroid microcarcinoma during active surveillance. *J. Clin. Endocrinol. Metab.* **2018**, *103*, 446–451. [CrossRef]
8. Fukuoka, O.; Sugitani, I.; Ebina, A.; Toda, K.; Kawabata, K.; Yamada, K. Natural history of asymptomatic papillary thyroid microcarcinoma: Time-dependent changes in calcification and vascularity during active surveillance. *World J. Surg.* **2016**, *40*, 529–537. [CrossRef]
9. Ito, Y.; Miyauchi, A.; Kihara, M.; Higashiyama, T.; Kobayashi, K.; Miya, A. Patient age is significantly related to the progression of papillary microcarcinoma of the thyroid under observation. *Thyroid* **2014**, *24*, 27–34. [CrossRef]
10. Tuttle, R.M.; Fagin, J.A.; Minkowitz, G.; Wong, R.J.; Roman, B.; Patel, S.; Untch, B.; Ganly, I.; Shaha, A.R.; Shah, J.P.; et al. Natural history and tumor volume kinetics of papillary thyroid cancers during active surveillance. *JAMA Otolaryngol. Head Neck Surg.* **2017**, *143*, 1015–1020. [CrossRef] [PubMed]
11. Oh, H.-S.; Ha, J.; Kim, H.I.; Kim, T.H.; Kim, W.B.; Lim, D.-J.; Kim, S.W.; Shong, Y.K.; Chung, J.H.; Baek, J.H. Active surveillance of low-risk papillary thyroid microcarcinoma: A multi-center cohort study in Korea. *Thyroid* **2018**, *28*, 1587–1594. [CrossRef]
12. Kwon, H.; Oh, H.-S.; Kim, M.; Park, S.; Jeon, M.J.; Kim, W.B.; Shong, Y.K.; Song, D.E.; Baek, J.H.; Chung, K.-W.; et al. Active surveillance for patients with papillary thyroid microcarcinoma: A single center's experience in Korea. *J. Clin. Endocrinol. Metab.* **2017**, *102*, 1917–1925. [CrossRef] [PubMed]
13. Sugitani, I.; Toda, K.; Yamada, K.; Yamamoto, N.; Ikenaga, M.; Fujimoto, Y. Three distinctly different kinds of papillary thyroid microcarcinoma should be recognized: Our treatment strategies and outcomes. *World J. Surg.* **2010**, *34*, 1222–1231. [CrossRef] [PubMed]
14. Sanabria, A. Active surveillance in thyroid microcarcinoma in a Latin-American cohort. *JAMA Otolaryngol. Head Neck Surg.* **2018**, *144*, 947–948. [CrossRef] [PubMed]
15. Oda, H.; Miyauchi, A.; Ito, Y.; Yoshioka, K.; Nakayama, A.; Sasai, H.; Masuoka, H.; Yabuta, T.; Fukushima, M.; Higashiyama, T.; et al. Incidences of Unfavorable Events in the Management of Low-Risk Papillary Microcarcinoma of the Thyroid by Active Surveillance Versus Immediate Surgery. *Thyroid* **2016**, *26*, 150–155. [CrossRef]
16. Gorshtein, A.; Slutzky-Shraga, I.; Robenshtok, E.; Benbassat, C.; Hirsch, D. Adherence to Active Surveillance and Clinical Outcomes in Patients with Indeterminate Thyroid Nodules Not Referred for Thyroidectomy. *Eur. Thyroid J.* **2021**, *10*, 168–173. [CrossRef]
17. Rozenbaum, A.; Buffet, C.; Bigorgne, C.; Royer, B.; Rouxel, A.; Bienvenu, M.; Chereau, N.; Menegaux, F.; Leenhardt, L.; Russ, G. Outcomes of active surveillance of EU-TIRADS 5 thyroid nodules. *Eur. J. Endocrinol.* **2021**, *184*, 677–686. [CrossRef] [PubMed]
18. Hu, Y.L.; Cao, X.Y.; Zhou, Y.R.; Ye, X.H.; Wang, J.X.; Li, X.; Rong, R.; Shen, M.P.; Wu, X.H. Management of Sonographically Suspicious Thyroid Nodules 1 cm or Smaller and Candidacy for Active Surveillance: Experience of a Tertiary Center in China. *Endocr. Pract.* **2021**, *17*, S1530–S1891.
19. Rosario, P.W.; Mourão, G.F.; Calsolari, M.R. Active Surveillance in Adults with Low-Risk Papillary Thyroid microcarcinomas: A Prospective Study *Horm. Metab. Res.* **2019**, *51*, 703–708. [CrossRef]
20. Oh, H.S.; Kwon, H.; Song, E.; Jeon, M.J.; Kim, T.Y.; Lee, J.H.; Kim, W.B.; Shong, Y.K.; Chung, K.W.; Baek, J.H.; et al. Tumor Volume Doubling Time in Active Surveillance of Papillary Thyroid Carcinoma. *Thyroid* **2019**, *29*, 642–649. [CrossRef]
21. Davies, L.; Welch, H.G. Increasing incidence of thyroid cancer in the United States, 1973–2002. *JAMA* **2006**, *295*, 2164–2167. [CrossRef]
22. Mauriello, C.; Marte, G.; Canfora, A.; Napolitano, S.; Pezzolla, A.; Gambardella, C.; Tartaglia, E.; Lanza, M.; Candela, G. Bilateral Benign Multinodular Goiter: What Is the Adequate Surgical Therapy? A Review of Literature. *Int. J. Surg.* **2016**, *28*, S7–S12. [CrossRef]
23. Leboulleux, S.; Tuttle, R.M.; Pacini, F.; Schlumberger, M. Papillary thyroid microcarcinoma and active surveillance—Authors' reply. *Lancet. Diabetes Endocrinol.* **2016**, *4*, 976–977. [CrossRef]
24. Lechner, M.G.; Praw, S.S.; Angell, T.E. Treatment of differentiated thyroid carcinomas. *Surg. Pathol. Clin.* **2019**, *12*, 931–942. [CrossRef]
25. National Cancer Institute. Surveillance, Epidemiology, and End Results (SEER) Program. SEER Stat Fact Sheets: Thyroid Cancer. Available online: http://seer.cancer.gov/statfacts/html/thyro.html (accessed on 1 January 2016).
26. Bibbins-Domingo, K.; Grossman, D.C.; Curry, S.J.; Barry, M.J.; Davidson, K.W.; Doubeni, C.A.; Epling, J.W.; Jr Kemper, A.R.; Krist, A.H.; et al.; US Preventive Services Task Force. Screening for thyroid cancer: US preventive services task force recommendation statement. *JAMA* **2017**, *317*, 1882–1887. [PubMed]
27. Baudin, E.; Travagli, J.P.; Ropers, J.; Mancusi, F.; Bruno-Bossio, G.; Caillou, B.; Cailleux, A.F.; Lumbroso, J.D.; Parmentier, C.; Schlumberger, M. Microcarcinoma of the thyroid gland: The Gustave-Roussy Institute experience. *Cancer* **1998**, *83*, 553–559. [CrossRef]
28. Mehanna, H.; Al-Maqbili, T.; Carter, B.; Martin, E.; Campain, N.; Watkinson, J.; McCabe, C.; Boelaert, K.; Franklyn, J.A. Differences in the recurrence and mortality outcomes rates of incidental and nonincidental papillary thyroid microcarcinoma: A systematic review and meta-analysis of 21 329 person-years of follow-up. *J. Clin. Endocrinol. Metab.* **2014**, *99*, 2834–2843. [CrossRef] [PubMed]
29. Roti, E.; Degli Uberti, E.C.; Bondanelli, M.; Braverman, L.E. Thyroidpapillarymicrocarcinoma: A descriptive and meta-analysisstudy. *Eur. J. Endocrinol.* **2008**, *159*, 659–673. [CrossRef]

30. Ito, Y.; Miyauchi, A.; Oda, H.; Kobayashi, K.; Kihara, M.; Miya, A. Revisiting Low-Risk Thyroid Papillary Microcarcinomas Resected Without Observation: Was Immediate Surgery Necessary? *World J. Surg.* **2016**, *40*, 523–528. [CrossRef]
31. De Biase, D.; Gandolfi, G.; Ragazzi, M.; Eszlinger, M.; Sancisi, V.; Gugnoni, M.; Visani, M.; Pession, A.; Casadei, G.; Durante, C.; et al. TERT Promoter Mutations in Papillary Thyroid Microcarcinomas. *Thyroid* **2015**, *25*, 1013–1019. [CrossRef] [PubMed]
32. Somboonporn, C. Prognostic Scores for Predicting Recurrence in Patients with Differentiated Thyroid Cancer. *Asian Pac. J. Cancer Prev.* **2016**, *17*, 2369–2374.
33. Kimura, E.T.; Nikiforova, M.N.; Zhu, Z.; Knauf, J.A.; Nikiforov, Y.E.; Fagin, J.A. High prevalence of BRAF mutations in thyroid cancer: Genetic evidence for constitutive activation of the RET/PTC-RAS-BRAF signaling pathway in papillary thyroid carcinoma. *Cancer Res.* **2003**, *63*, 1454–1457.
34. Welsch, M.; Abeln, M.; Zaplatnikov, K.; Menzel, C.; Ackermann, H.; Döbert, N.; Grünwald, F. Multiparameter scoring system for the prognosis of differentiated thyroid cancer. *Nuklearmedizin* **2007**, *46*, 257–262. [CrossRef] [PubMed]
35. Onitilo, A.A.; Engel, J.M.; Lundgren, C.I.; Hall, P.; Thalib, L.; Doi, S.A. Simplifying the TNM system for clinical use in differentiated thyroid cancer. *J. Clin. Oncol.* **2009**, *27*, 1872–1878. [CrossRef]
36. Gambardella, C.; Polistena, A.; Sanguinetti, A.; Patrone, R.; Napolitano, S.; Esposito, D.; Testa, D.; Marotta, V.; Faggiano, A.; Calò, P.G.; et al. Unintentional recurrent laryngeal nerve injuries following thyroidectomy: Is it the surgeon who pays the bill? *Int. J. Surg.* **2017**, *1*, S55–S59. [CrossRef]
37. Molinaro, E.; Campopiano, M.C.; Elisei, R. Management of endocrine disease: Papillary thyroid microcarcinoma: Towards an active surveillance strategy. *Eur. J. Endocrinol.* **2021**, *1*, R23–R34.
38. Lohia, S.; Gupta, P.; Curry, M.; Morris, L.G.T.; Roman, B.R. Life Expectancy and Treatment Patterns in Elderly Patients With Low-Risk Papillary Thyroid Cancer: A Population-Based Analysis. *Endocr. Pract.* **2021**, *27*, 228–235. [CrossRef]
39. Tuttle, R.M.; Zhang, L.; Shaha, A. A clinical framework to facilitateselection of patients with differentiated thyroidcancer for activesurveillance or less aggressive initial surgical management. *Expert. Rev. Endocrinol. Metab.* **2018**, *13*, 77–85. [CrossRef] [PubMed]
40. Jeon, M.J.; Kang, Y.E.; Moon, J.H.; Lim, D.J.; Lee, C.Y.; Lee, Y.S.; Kim, S.W.; Kim, M.H.; Kim, B.H.; Kang, H.C.; et al. Protocol for a Korean Multicenter Prospective Cohort Study of Active Surveillance or Surgery (KoMPASS) in Papillary Thyroid Microcarcinoma. *Endocrinol. Metab.* **2021**, *36*, 359–364. [CrossRef]
41. Sawka, A.M.; Ghai, S.; Ihekire, O.; Jones, J.M.; Gafni, A.; Baxter, N.N.; Goldstein, D.P.; On Behalf Of The Canadian Thyroid Cancer Active Surveillance Study Group. Decision-making in Surgery or Active Surveillance for Low Risk Papillary Thyroid Cancer During the COVID-19 Pandemic. *Cancers* **2021**, *13*, 371. [CrossRef]
42. Medas, F.; Ansaldo, G.L.; Avenia, N.; Basili, G.; Boniardi, M.; Bononi, M.; Bove, A.; Carcoforo, P.; Casaril, A.; Cavallaro, G.; et al. The THYCOVIT (Thyroid Surgery during COVID-19 pandemic in Italy) study: Results from a nationwide, multicentric, case-controlled study. *Updat. Surg.* **2021**, *16*, 1–9.
43. Medas, F.; Ansaldo, G.L.; Avenia, N.; Basili, G.; Boniardi, M.; Bononi, M.; Bove, A.; Carcoforo, P.; Casaril, A.; Cavallaro, G.; et al. Italian Society of Endocrine Surgery (SIUEC) Collaborative Group. Impact of the COVID-19 pandemic on surgery for thyroid cancer in Italy: Nationwide retrospective study. *Br. J. Surg.* **2021**, *108*, e166–e167. [CrossRef] [PubMed]

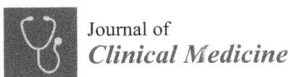 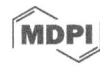

Article

The Role of IONM in Reducing the Occurrence of Shoulder Syndrome Following Lateral Neck Dissection for Thyroid Cancer

Andrea Polistena [1,2,*], Monia Ranalli [3], Stefano Avenia [4], Roberta Lucchini [1], Alessandro Sanguinetti [1], Sergio Galasse [1], Fabio Rondelli [1], Jacopo Vannucci [5], Renato Patrone [6], Nunzio Velotti [7], Giovanni Conzo [8] and Nicola Avenia [1]

1. Endocrine Surgery, Santa Maria University Hospital, Perugia University, 05100 Terni, Italy; r.lucchini@aospterni.it (R.L.); a.sanguinetti@aospterni.it (A.S.); s.galasse@aospterni.it (S.G.); fabio.rondelli@unipg.it (F.R.); nicola.avenia@unipg.it (N.A.)
2. Department of Surgery Pietro Valdoni, Oncologic and Laparoscopic Surgery, Sapienza University of Rome, University Hospital Policlinico Umberto I, 00161 Rome, Italy
3. Department of Statistical Sciences, Sapienza University of Rome, 00185 Rome, Italy; monia.ranalli@uniroma1.it
4. Residency Programme in General Surgery, Faculty of Medicine and Surgery, University of Perugia, 06123 Perugia, Italy; stefano_avenia@libero.it
5. Department of Surgery Paride Stefanini, Thoracic Surgery, Sapienza University of Rome, University Hospital Policlinico Umberto I, 00161 Rome, Italy; jacopo.vannucci@uniroma1.it
6. PhD ICHT, University of Naples Federico II, 80131 Napoli, Italy; dott.patrone@gmail.com
7. Department of Advanced Biomedical Science, University of Naples Federico II, 80131 Naples, Italy; nunzio.velotti@gmail.com
8. Department of Traslational Medical Sciences, Division of General and Oncologic Surgery, University of Campania "Luigi Vanvitelli", 80131 Naples, Italy; giovanni.conzo@un.campania.it
* Correspondence: andrea.polistena@uniroma1.it

Abstract: Lateral neck dissection (LND) leads to a significant morbidity involving accessory nerve injury. Modified radical neck dissection (MRND) aims at preservation of the accessory nerve, but patients often present with negative functional outcomes after surgery. The role of neuromonitoring (IONM) in the prevention of shoulder syndrome has not yet been defined in comparison to nerve visualization only. We retrospectively analyzed 56 thyroid cancer patients who underwent MRND over a period of six years (2015–2020) in a high-volume institution. Demographic variables, type of surgical procedure, removed lymph nodes and the metastatic node ratio, pathology, adoption of IONM and shoulder functional outcome were investigated. The mean number of lymph nodes removed was 15.61, with a metastatic node ratio of 0.2745. IONM was used in 41.07% of patients, with a prevalence of 68% in the period 2017–2020. IONM adoption showed an effect on post-operative shoulder function. There were no effects in 89.29% of cases, and temporary and permanent effects in 8.93% and 1.79%, respectively. Confidence intervals and two-sample tests for equality of proportions were used when applicable. Expertise in high-volume centres and IONM during MRND seem to be correlated with a reduced prevalence of accessory nerve lesions and limited functional impairments. These results need to be confirmed by larger prospective randomized controlled trials.

Keywords: IONM; accessory nerve; shoulder syndrome; thyroid cancer; neck dissection

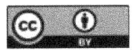

1. Introduction

Despite a general good prognosis, with a 10-year overall survival rate greater than 90%, regional lymph node metastases are frequently present at the time of diagnosis in patients with papillary carcinomas (PTC) and in a lower proportion of patients with follicular carcinomas (FTC) [1].

The N stage in differentiated thyroid carcinomas (DTC) is an important prognostic factor [2], and lateral neck lymph node dissection (LND) of compartments II–V provides a complete disease staging and may reduce the risk of recurrence and, possibly, mortality rates [1]. Consequently, LND has a pivotal role in the multidisciplinary management of DTC [3].

ATA guidelines provide clear indications for LND in DTC [1], and also for medullary (MTC) [4], anaplastic (ATC) or poorly differentiated thyroid carcinomas (PDTC) [5], which are also potentially characterized by metastases to cervical lymph nodes and are both associated with worse prognosis compared to DTC [6–9].

Although a specific oncologic role is proven, LND may lead to a significant morbidity characterized by potential severe complications [3]. Among nervous complications following LND, the lesion of the accessory nerve is one of the most severe affecting post-operative quality of life—being responsible for shoulder syndrome, characterized by decreased neck and shoulder mobility with reduced elevation, flexion and abduction of the shoulder joint, anesthesia, numbness, neuropathic pain and dysmorphy or hypotrophy of the upper trapezius and sternocleidomastoid muscles [10–13].

Despite the introduction of modified radical neck dissection (MRND) and selective neck dissection (SND)—aiming at the preservation of the anatomical integrity of the accessory nerve—as gold standards of treatment compared to radical neck dissection (RND) and extended radical neck dissection (ERND), a considerable number of patients present with impaired functional outcomes after surgery [14,15].

According to a recent systematic review, the estimated prevalence of shoulder syndrome following different types of LND is variably reported in the literature, ranging between 94.8% and 27.9%. MRND and SND are associated with a lower rate of accessory nerve lesions and shoulder syndrome compared to RND [16].

Intraoperative monitoring (IONM) of the accessory nerve during MRND is largely adopted [17–20].

The IONM records accessory nerve electrical transmission before, during and after dissection using subdermal needle electrodes inserted into the sternocleidomastoid and trapezius muscles that are innervated by the monitored nerve. As previously shown, usually patients without an electrophysiological threshold increase do not develop a postoperative clinical impairment [17–20]. IONM contributes to accessory nerve identification and theoretically supports the preservation of nerve integrity, providing an intra-operative feedback of nerve function during dissection [17].

However, evidence in the literature for the usefulness of IONM in potentially reducing injury to the accessory nerve and for predicting postoperative function in neck dissection patients is minimal and contradictory, as highlighted in a recent systematic review, with a need for randomized controlled trials to determine whether such monitoring is a valuable surgical adjunct [17].

Similarly, the role of IONM has not yet been defined for recurrent laryngeal nerve identification during thyroidectomy and central neck dissection (CND) [21,22].

The aim of the present research is the analysis of the use of IONM during MRND in a large institutional series, focusing on the potential benefits in terms of functional outcome and prevention of shoulder syndrome.

2. Patients and Methods

2.1. Study Design

In our institution, IONM has been regularly used for thyroid surgery since 2015 and progressively for MRND with standardization since 2017. We designed the present study to compare the outcomes, in terms of shoulder syndrome occurrence, of patients undergoing MRND with or without IONM, in addition to direct visualization. This retrospective observational cohort study was performed according to the Strengthening the Reporting of OBservational studies in Epidemiology (STROBE) guidelines [23]. The study was conducted in accordance with the Declaration of Helsinki, but the protocol was not submitted to the evaluation of the Ethics Committee of Umbria region or registered as a clinical trial due to the retrospective design of the research. All patients gave their informed consent to the use of their clinical data for research purposes at the time of surgery.

2.2. Setting and Participants

We retrospectively analyzed 56 patients undergoing MRND as a single procedure, or combined with total thyroidectomy (TT) and/or CND, in a population of 515 patients operated on for thyroid cancer by the same surgical team, with standard surgical techniques, over a period of 6 years (January 2015–December 2020) in the Unit of Endocrine Surgery, Santa Maria University Hospital, Terni, University of Perugia, Italy— which is the referral center for endocrine surgery in the Umbria Region, Italy. Patients were divided into two groups, respectively, according to the adoption of IONM during dissection or not. Direct visualization of the accessory nerve during dissection was carried out in all patients. The use of IONM during MRND, through the observation period, depended on the preliminary completion of the learning curve for recurrent laryngeal nerve monitoring, the availability of specific electrodes for the sternocleidomastoid and trapezius muscles and any technical problems with the monitoring system. Functional outcome was considered at post-operative (p.o.) day 3 and after 6 months by clinical evaluation and electromyography (EMG), when appropriate.

Inclusion criteria considered were: patients aged $\geq$ 18 years, undergoing MRND type III (with preservation of the spinal accessory nerve, internal jugular vein, and sternocleidomastoid muscle) with or without IONM, on biopsy-proven thyroid cancer with indication for lymphadenectomy according to ATA guidelines [1,4,24]. Patients who underwent more extended procedures (MRND type I and II or RND), or those with unavailable data regarding accessory nerve functional outcome, were excluded. Medical records in the observational period were collected from our database and analyzed anonymously.

2.3. Preoperative Work Out

Preoperative work-out included blood tests, ECG, chest X-ray and neck ultrasound with preoperative fine needle aspiration cytology (FNAC) when appropriate, and neck computed tomography scans in selected cases. According to ATA Guidelines [1], indications for MRND in DTC were evidence of lateral compartment pathologic-like lymph nodes at the preoperative ultrasound (US) with cytological confirmation, or thyroglobulin presence in the washout fluid of fine-needle aspiration (FNA). Only 3 patients with confirmed diagnoses of thyroid cancer, due to a large palpable mass in the lateral compartment and US-evident features of pathologic-like lymph nodes including enlargement, loss of the fatty hilum, a rounded shape, hyperechogenicity, calcifications, and peripheral vascularity underwent MRND without FNA. For MTC, MRND was carried out only if there was evidence of lateral compartment pathologic-like lymph nodes at ultrasound, calcitonin in the washout fluid of FNA or high serum calcitonin level. Bilateral MRND was considered if the basal serum calcitonin level was greater than 200 pg/mL [4]. In ATC/PDTC, MRND was selected for suitable patients, with consideration of the local invasiveness of the tumor [24].

2.4. Surgical Procedure

The surgical procedure for MRND and general clinical management were carried out as previously reported by our group [3,6,25]. Briefly, an MRND type III was adopted in all patients. It consisted of the removal of lymph nodes from levels II to V with preservation of the sternocleidomastoid muscle, accessory nerve and internal jugular vein. The incision was carried out along the anterior margin of the sternocleidomastoid muscle and a J-shaped prolongation was adopted in cases of combined thyroid surgery. After the skin incision, a flap in the subplatysmal plain above the superficial layer of the deep cervical fascia was elevated to the level of the inferior border of the mandible. The external jugular vein was identified and the dissection carried out, with careful maneuvers, superficially through the fascia of the sternocleidomastoid muscle, which was elevated around the edge and onto the medial surface where the accessory nerve entered the muscle. The small vessels close to the accessory nerve were divided and all branches of the nerve were preserved. The dissection continued posteriorly along the entire length of the muscle. The internal jugular vein, which lies immediately behind the proximal portion of the nerve, was exposed and the dissection was carried upward to the level of the posterior portion of the digastric muscle. The complete identification of the accessory nerve was obtained, completing the dissection in the upper part of the surgical field after the sternocleidomastoid muscle was retracted posteriorly and the digastric muscle was pulled superiorly. The lymph nodes at level 2B located between the spinal accessory nerve and internal jugular vein were dissected. In this phase, the nerve was exposed completely from the sternocleidomastoid muscle to the internal jugular vein, dividing the tissue overlying the nerve.

Once the accessory nerve was completely exposed, the tissue lying superior and posterior to the nerve was dissected from the splenius capitis and levator scapulae muscles. Then, the accessory nerve was identified at Erb's point, where it leaves the sternocleidomastoid muscle and courses through the posterior triangle of the neck to enter the anterior border of the trapezius muscle. The dissection proceeded while keeping the accessory nerve in view, with the removal of the fascia that still covered the posterior border of the sternocleidomastoid muscle and further from the anterior border of the trapezius muscle in a medial direction, including the lymphatic contents of the supraclavicular fossa.

During MRND the accessory nerve was always exposed and visually confirmed in both groups.

2.5. IONM System

In the study population, a NIM-Response 3.0 system (Medtronic, Minneapolis, MN, USA) set up for head and neck procedure/neck dissection was adopted to assess accessory nerve function during MRND. The IONM final reports were examined in order to verify the preserved or not-preserved transmission of the accessory nerve before, during and after dissection. Subdermal needle electrodes used as recording electrodes were inserted into the sternocleidomastoid and trapezius muscles. Additionally, a ground electrode and a stim return placed into the shoulder to complete the electrode setup and a monopolar stimulator probe (Medtronic, Minneapolis, MN, USA) were used during the procedure. When contemporary TT and CND were carried out, the NIM TriVantage tube (Medtronic, Minneapolis, MN, USA) was used for orotracheal intubation.

Muscle relaxant agents were avoided to keep the EMG responses of the examined muscle precisely assessable during general anesthesia. The accessory nerve was identified, usually proximal to its entrance into the sternocleidomastoid muscle, by application of a probe to deliver an electric stimulus that ranged from 1 to 2 mA, 100 ms, at 4 Hz. The correct identification of an intact nerve was confirmed through a series of audible acoustic signals that were generated by the system. Functional nerve integrity was once again confirmed during and at the end of the dissection by testing of the most proximal exposed portion of the nerve, and evaluating significant changes in M wave amplitude and waveform or an eventual threshold increase on electrophysiological monitoring after stimulation. The absence of a signal that was generated by the stimulator at any precise point along the nerve was accepted as evidence of loss of signal (LOS) and considered as a nerve injury. The troubleshooting protocol was always followed to check the IONM equipment for technical problems.

2.6. Variables

Demographic variables including sex and age, type of surgical procedure, side of MRND, number of removed lymph nodes and the metastatic node ratio, pathology on resected specimen and adoption of IONM during the observation period were investigated.

The primary functional outcome observed following MRND with and without IONM adoption, was evidence of any grade of shoulder syndrome which was defined at p.o. day 3 and after 6 months as regular accessory nerve function, or temporary or permanent nerve injuries by clinical examination and EMG when appropriate. Clinical evaluation of patients was performed after surgery using the Shoulder Pain and Disability Index (SPDI), for the evaluation of shoulder function, as previously reported [26]. The total SPDI score is the mean of the two subscales (Total pain score and Total disability score) and produces a total score ranging from 0 (best) to 100 (worst).

Patients with a negative clinical evaluation, presenting results not interfering with regular day life or working activity, were considered as negative for shoulder syndrome.

When clinical evaluation showed significant modifications in shoulder function, EMG confirmation was required. The degree of neurogenic involvement and the presence of spontaneous denervation potentials were investigated. Only partial axonal degeneration and total axonal degeneration were considered significant for persistent nerve lesions. All milder modifications observed at p.o. day 3 and recovered by a 6 months control period were considered to be transient nerve lesions. Between the two time points, all the involved patients received an intense rehabilitation program and corticosteroid treatment, when appropriate, as previously described [3].

2.7. Statistical Analysis

We analyzed the variables through descriptive statistics based on summary measures, plots and table distributions. We used Confidence Intervals (CI) and two sample tests for equality of proportions when applicable. A p-value < 0.05 or a confidence level equal to 0.95 was considered statistically significant. All of the data were analyzed using R statistical software (free open sources).

3. Results

3.1. Demographic and Surgical Results

The 56 cases included 30 females (53.57%) and 26 males (46.43%), with a mean age of 51.20 ± 17.59 years (Table 1). Median age was 51 years, and the corresponding interquartile range was 31 (range 22 and 88 years) (Figure 1).

Table 1. Patient demographic and clinical characteristics. Modified Radical Neck Dissection (MRND), Total Thyroidectomy (TT), Central Neck Dissection (CND), Papillary Thyroid Cancer (PTC), Follicular Thyroid Cancer (FTC), Medullary Thyroid Cancer (MTC), Poorly Differentiated Thyroid Cancer (PDTC).

	Years, Mean ± SD
Age	51.20 ± 17.59
	n (%)
Gender	
Female	30 (53.57)
Male	26 (46.43)
Surgical procedure	
MRND + TT	19 (33.93)
MRND + TT + CND	19 (33.93)
MRND + CND	3 (5.36)
MRND	15 (26.79)
Side of the procedure	
Right	28 (50)
Left	28 (50)
Thyroid cancer subtype	
PTC	40 (71.43)
FTC	7 (12.50)
MTC	6 (10.71)
PDTC	3 (5.36)

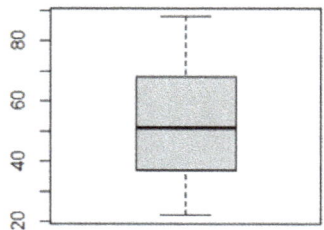

Figure 1. Boxplot of age distribution. Y-axis shows age in years.

Surgical procedures carried out were classified as: 19 (33.93%) MRND plus TT, 19 (33.93%) MRND plus TT and CND, 3 (5.36%) MRND plus CND and 15 (26.79%) MRND only (Table 1, Figure 2). Among patients, left and right lymphadenectomy were equally distributed. The corresponding CI was (0.37, 0.63). It follows that the proportion was not statistically different from 0.5.

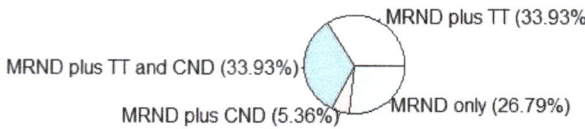

Figure 2. Pie chart showing the surgical procedures carried out in the series. Surgeries were classified as: 19 (33.93%) Modified Radical Neck Dissection (MRND) plus Total Thyroidectomy (TT), 19 (33.93%) MRND plus TT and Central Neck Dissection (CND), 3 (5.36%) MRND plus CND, 15 (26.79%) MRND only.

3.2. Lymph Node Retrieval

The mean of the number of removed lymph nodes was 15.61, while the median 14. Furthermore, the distribution seemed to be quite variable; its standard deviation was 7.85. The 95% CI was between 13.51 and 17.71. When we considered the ratio between the number of metastatic lymph nodes removed and the total number of lymph nodes, then its mean was 0.2745 with a standard deviation equal to 0.2358. The corresponding 95% CI was between 0.21 and 0.34.

3.3. Thyroid Cancer Subtypes

Different types of cancer were observed; the prevalence was 71.43% ($n = 40$), 12.50% ($n = 7$), 10.71% ($n = 6$) and 5.36% ($n = 3$) for PTC, FTC, MTC and PDTC respectively (Table 1, Figure 3).

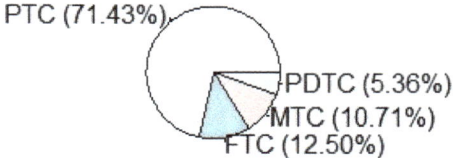

Figure 3. Pie Chart showing the different histotypes of cancer treated; the prevalence was 71.43% ($n = 40$) Papillary Thyroid Cancer (PTC), 12.50% ($n = 7$) Follicular Thyroid Cancer (FTC), 10.71% ($n = 6$) Medullary Thyroid Cancer (MTC) and 5.36% ($n = 3$) Poorly Differentiated Thyroid Cancer (PDTC).

3.4. IONM Use

In the observation cohort 41.07% of surgeries were supported by the use of IONM plus direct visualization of the accessory nerve. However, its use was different over the analyzed period; indeed, between 2015–2016 the prevalence was only 19.35%, while between 2017–2020 it increased to 68%. The different prevalence observed in the two periods was statistically significant ($p < 0.05$). We conducted a two-sample test for equality of proportions, where the alternative hypothesis was two-sided and the significance level was 0.05. The CI regarding the difference of proportions, $(-0.75, -0.22)$, showed only negative values since the increase in use of IONM was statistically significant.

3.5. Functional Outcome

Fifty patients out of 56 with MRND showed a post-operative SPDI at p.o. day 3 ranging between 0% and 10% and were considered negative for shoulder syndrome. All these patients maintained a low index around 0–5% at 6 months and EMG was not carried out. Six patients instead presented with significant increases on the SPDI following MRND at p.o. day 3 (Table 2) and were considered positive for a nervous lesion, with clinical evidence of shoulder syndrome. Two patients in the IONM plus visualization group who presented modification in the waveform and increases in the threshold of stimulation during surgery, and three patients in the visualization-only group, presented with significant improvement after 6 months, and the accessory nerve impairment was considered to be transient. Only one patient in the visualization-only group maintained a high SPDI at 6 months, attesting to a permanent nerve impairment with residual shoulder syndrome. EMG was carried out in the above six patients and showed at p.o. day 3, for those with transient impairment, denervation potentials referable to neuropraxia, which recovered at 6 months with normal EMG findings. The only patient with persistent nervous impairment presented EMG features of axonotmesis, almost stable at 6 months follow-up (Table 2).

Table 2. Shoulder Pain and Disability Index (SPDI) in patients with temporary and permanent lesion of the accessory nerve following MRND with or without IONM. The index is reported as total SPDI score. The total SPDI score is the mean of the two subscales (Total pain score and Total disability score) and produces a total score ranging from 0 (best) to 100 (worst).

SPDI p.o. day 3	SPDI 6 Months	Type of Nerve Lesion
IONM+ visualization ($n = 2$)		
57%	4%	transient
60%	5%	transient
Visualization only ($n = 4$)		
60%	10%	transient
38%	0%	transient
55%	5%	transient
75%	60%	permanent

The increase of IONM use during MRND seemed to have also had a mild effect on post-operative shoulder function. Overall, there were no effects in 89.29% (50) of cases, whereas transient and permanent effects were observed in 8.93% ($n = 5$) and 1.79% ($n = 1$) of patients, respectively. The distribution of the post-operative effects with IONM plus visualization or visualization only was summarized in Table 3.

According to Table 3, dependence was shown between the post-operative functional outcomes and the use of IONM; indeed, the conditional distributions were different. Furthermore, IONM decreased the incidence of shoulder syndrome, while direct visualization only, without IONM, increased both temporary and permanent nerve damage. However, statistical significance could not be analyzed since the number of observations was limited. To assess statistical significance, a larger sample size would have been needed. Indeed, considering three categories and fixing the significance level to 0.05, 108 and 141 units would have been needed to guarantee a power of 0.8 and 0.9, respectively, with a medium effect size (0.3)—and with a smaller difference, an even larger sample size. Unfortunately, since a relatively recent adoption of IONM during MRND in our institution, a proper number of cases was not available—thus attesting, for the present research, to the value of a pilot study for a larger future analysis.

Table 3. Post-operative effects distribution with IONM + visualization and visualization only and the unconditional distribution (overall).

Nerve Identification and Monitoring	No Lesion (*n*)	Temporary Lesion (*n*)	Permanent Lesion (*n*)
IONM+visualization	91.3% (21)	8.7% (2)	0% (0)
Visualization only	87.88% (29)	9.09% (3)	3.03% (1)
Overall	89.29% (50)	8.93% (5)	1.79% (1)

When considering the increased adoption of IONM in more recent years and its supposed value in supporting the identification and preservation of the accessory nerve during MRND, we expected a progressive reduction of the complications rate over the observation time. Despite the analysis of the accessory nerve lesion rates between the different years of observation, as similarly detected when comparing the rates in the two groups, statistical significance could not be assessed, since the number of observations was limited and the events were spread over the whole period.

4. Discussion

Our data showed that the use of IONM during MRND contributed to the containment of accessory nerve impairment, responsible for the clinical outcome of shoulder syndrome. In our experience, IONM adoption compared to direct visualization only, although not significantly, was associated to less temporary and permanent nerve lesions; indeed in recent years, it has become a standard procedure associated with MRND in the treatment of lateral neck lymph node metastases in our institution. However, statistical significance in our series could not be assessed, since the number of observations was limited—at least in the observation time. This is one of the main limits of the research. The prevalence of accessory nerve lesions observed was 10.7%, which could be considered quite low compared to data reported in the literature. A recent systematic review with metanalysis by Larsen et al. [16] studied the prevalence of nerve injuries following neck dissection and found a 33% prevalence of accessory nerve injuries after MRND.

The analysis reported a wide range of prevalence ranging from 1.3% to more than 80%. This spread distribution might be related to many factors; the included studies were published in different years (1981–2017), and this might reflect major changes in oncological treatments and the different adoption of new technologies such as neuromonitoring, which was not considered as a variable potentially affecting the results of the metanalysis. These factors could have a major impact on the number of nerve injuries reported and should be taken into consideration.

Furthermore, the series analyzed were significantly different with regards to the sample size of the studies. The main factor which might have affected a so large distribution of prevalence, relates to the modality of diagnosis of the nerve lesion. Some authors adopted standard EMG evaluation, others only clinical examination, or both. In our analysis, the low prevalence of accessory nerve lesions reported might be attributed to many factors. First of all, the size of the examined population, which was quite limited. Secondly, the modality of accessory nerve impairment was based on clinical evaluation in all patients and EMG was used only in those presenting a modification in the post-operative clinical score; this might imply that some minor nerve injuries which remained almost asymptomatic, and not evident with only clinical examination, were lost. According to this consideration, a systematic neuro-physio-pathologic evaluation by EMG would always be beneficial in determining a more realistic prevalence of accessory nerve dysfunction following MRND in future studies. Another criticism of the present series is that we reported, despite a large distribution, a not considerably high mean of lymph nodes removed compared to other studies [27–29].

This might reflect that some of the procedures considered and retrospectively classified, based on the surgical procedure code attributed in the clinical records, as MRND, should have been more properly considered as SND, with less lymph nodes excised, and most probably not including level II and V, which are at higher risk of accessory nerve iatrogenic injury [14,30].

Nevertheless, this bias was systematically spread over all the patients in the series, including both approaches, IONM and visualization only during MRND, thus not affecting the evidence that IONM seemed to decrease the eventuality of shoulder syndrome, while direct visualization only, without IONM, was associated, in our experience, with both temporary and permanent nerve injuries. On the other hand, the low prevalence of accessory nerve injuries observed in our series was certainly related to the large number of patients with thyroid cancer and neck metastases treated in our institution, which is a referral center for endocrine surgery [3].

Indeed, it has been proven that, in thyroid surgery, as in all surgical fields, morbidity is inversely related to the volume of patients treated, due to the increased expertise and the adequate technologies adopted [31–33].

The use of IONM requires an appropriate learning curve, which may optimize the clinical benefit of this device—mostly due to a more effective interpretation of the electrophysiological response during dissection—to prevent and eventually correct inappropriate maneuvers, as often experienced in recurrent laryngeal nerve dissection with IONM during thyroidectomy [34].

Another review by Gane et al. [15] examined the prevalence and incidence of shoulder and neck dysfunction after neck dissection and identified the risk factors for postoperative complications.

The authors showed an incidence of reduced shoulder active range of motion varying from 5% to 20%, but also observed a prevalence of reduced neck active range of motion, and prevalence rates for shoulder pain, following MRND of 1–13% and of (−100%, respectively. Again, clinical outcomes depended on the surgery carried out and on the modality of dysfunction measure used.

It is widely accepted that MRND, also known as functional neck dissection, is generally associated with considerably less morbidity, and for this reason, considering similar oncologic results, it also largely replaced RND and ERND in advanced disease [18–36].

Although the anatomical integrity of the accessory nerve is always supposed to be preserved following MRND, functional impairments are frequently reported, with a relevant number of patients complaining of at least chronic shoulder pain [16,37]. For this reason, during MRND, the accessory nerve should be preserved with careful dissection, avoiding even traction, potential thermal injury, extensive skeletonization and devascularization [3]. As previously shown, patients without an electrophysiological threshold increase usually do not develop a post-operative clinical impairment [19].

Evidence on the effective role of IONM in MRND are limited in the literature [17], with few prospective studies [19,20] and only one randomized trial [18] with a limited number of patients supporting the predictive value of IONM for determining shoulder function deterioration and activity restriction scores.

A fundamental point in shoulder impairment evaluation is the timing of the follow-up. Indeed, it is important to consider that shoulder function may improve 6 to 12 months after nerve-sparing operations [18]; thus, even prolonged clinical manifestations might recover with a longer follow-up period. In later controls—whereas in the literature the follow-up period is usually not standardized [16], and in our study a longer follow-up would also have been beneficial.

Another important issue is to quantify the real clinical impact of electrophysiological impairment observed post-operatively. Actually, some patients with insignificant IONM changes have a good functional prognosis and they may not present with a significant clinical counterpart due to a minor deterioration in shoulder function, and their activity restriction scores begin to improve earlier compared to those with poor prognostic findings on IONM [18].

Among different types of nerve injuries, neurotmesis and axonotmesis present with a worse prognosis, while neurapraxia, attributed to nerve motor fibers demyelination, results in short-term dysfunction, and usually recovers by remyelination within 6 to 8 weeks [11].

Furthermore, the function of trapezius muscle is often supported by an active motor branch from the cervical plexus, which may provide adequate vicarious innervation following accessory nerve injury without evident clinical effects on shoulder function [38]. Thus, as we experienced, clinically the majority of patients with neck dissection do not show shoulder movement deficits prior to discharge from the hospital because of the latent effects on trapezius muscle innervation that follow axonotmesis [11].

This can induce a delay in prompt rehabilitation programs and might affect the real estimate of shoulder function impairment, as probably occurred in our observation.

Again, EMG can help in detecting different degrees of nerve dysfunction, and it is recommended in the follow-up evaluation. An intensive program of rehabilitation with specific physiotherapy and physical therapy can improve shoulder function [11,18,39–42], as we also experienced in our current analysis and in a previous series [3], and should always be recommended [40].

Furthermore, the clinical impact of nerve injuries is also associated with a significant economic burden [43,44], with a necessity for future investigations on health-technology-assessment (HTA) and cost-effectiveness analysis, as already carried out for thyroid surgery [34]. Finally, a medico-legal issue has to be considered when dealing with technologies which might improve surgical outcomes. IONM at least provides a clinical, objective evaluation of nerve function during the surgical procedure and it certifies, despite possible functional outcomes, the correct identification and dissection of the accessory nerve, when a threshold increase in the final report is not shown [45].

5. Conclusions

Adoption of MRND as a standard of treatment for lateral lymph node metastases, appropriate surgical technique, expertise in high volume centres and IONM seem to be correlated with a reduced prevalence of accessory nerve lesions and consequent contained functional impairment [2,19,46–48].

Definitive evidence for the usefulness of IONM in reducing the prevalence of accessory nerve injury or as a method of predicting post-operative shoulder impairment outcomes following neck dissection is inconclusive at the moment. Although large prospective randomized controlled trials are required to determine the real impact of IONM in MRND, several experiences, including the results of the present research, support a potential benefit during dissection and show a correlation with improved functional outcomes.

Author Contributions: Conceptualization, All authors; Methodology, A.P. and M.R.; Software, M.R.; Validation, R.P., N.V. and G.C.; Formal Analysis, A.P. and M.R.; Investigation, S.A., R.L., S.G. and F.R.; Data Curation, S.A., R.L., A.S., S.G., F.R. and J.V.; Writing—Original Draft Preparation, A.P. and M.R.; Writing—Review & Editing, All authors; Visualization, All authors; Supervision, N.A. and A.S.; Project Administration, N.A. and G.C.; All authors have read and agreed to the published version of the manuscript.

Funding: This research received no external funding.

Institutional Review Board Statement: This study was conducted in accordance with the Declaration of Helsinki; the protocol was not submitted to the evaluation of the Ethics Committee of Umbria region and not registered as a clinical trial due to the retrospective design of the research.

Informed Consent Statement: All patients gave their written informed consent for the use of their clinical data for research purposes at the time of surgery.

Data Availability Statement: Data are available from the corresponding author upon request.

Acknowledgments: To Daniela Angelucci, Claudio Marcacci, Francesca Pennetti Pennella and Clara Salvador for data collection.

Conflicts of Interest: The authors declare no conflict of interest.

References

1. Haugen, B.R.; Alexander, E.K.; Bible, K.C.; Doherty, G.M.; Mandel, S.J.; Nikiforov, Y.E.; Pacini, F. Randolph, G.W.; Sawka, A.M.; Schlumberger, M.; et al. 2015 American Thyroid Association Management Guidelines for Adult Patients with Thyroid Nodules and Differentiated Thyroid Cancer: The American Thyroid Association Guidelines Task Force on Thyroid Nodules and Differentiated Thyroid Cancer. *Thyroid* 2016, 26, 1–133. [CrossRef]
2. Lindfors, H.; Ihre Lundgren, C.; Zedenius, J.; Juhlin, C.C.; Shabo, I. The Clinical Significance of Lymph Node Ratio and Ki-67 Expression in Papillary Thyroid Cancer. *World J. Surg.* 2021, 45, 2155–2164. [CrossRef] [PubMed]
3. Polistena, A.; Monacelli, M.; Lucchini, R.; Triola, R.; Conti, C.; Avenia, S.; Barillaro, I.; Sanguinetti, A.; Avenia, N. Surgical morbidity of cervical lymphadenectomy for thyroid cancer: A retrospective cohort study over 25 years. *Int. J. Surg.* 2015, 21, 128–134. [CrossRef] [PubMed]
4. Wells, S.A., Jr.; Asa, S.L.; Dralle, H.; Elisei, R.; Evans, D.B.; Gagel, R.F.; Lee, N.; Machens, A.; Moley J.F.; Pacini, F.; et al. American Thyroid Association Guidelines Task Force on Medullary Thyroid Carcinoma. Revised American Thyroid Association guidelines for the management of medullary thyroid carcinoma. *Thyroid* 2015, 25, 567–610. [CrossRef] [PubMed]
5. Bible, K.C.; Kebebew, E.; Brierley, J.; Brito, J.P.; Cabanillas, M.E.; Clark, T.J., Jr.; Di Cristofano, A.; Foote, R.; Giordano, T.; Kasperbauer, J.; et al. 2021 American Thyroid Association Guidelines for Management of Patients with Anaplastic Thyroid Cancer. *Thyroid* 2021, 31, 337–386. [CrossRef]
6. Polistena, A.; Sanguinetti, A.; Lucchini, R. Galasse, S.; Monacelli, M.; Avenia, S.; Boccolini, A.; Johnson, L.B.; Avenia, N. Timing and extension of lymphadenectomy in medullary thyroid carcinoma: A case series from a single institution. *Int. J. Surg.* 2017, 41 (Suppl. 1), S70–S74. [CrossRef] [PubMed]
7. Polistena, A.; Monacelli, M.; Lucchini, R.; Triola, R.; Conti, C.; Avenia, S.; Barillaro, I.; Sanguinetti, A.; Avenia, N. Approach to lymph node metastases in sporadic medullary thyroid carcinoma An istitutional experience. *Ann. Ital. Chir.* 2015, 86, 390–395.
8. Polistena, A.; Monacelli, M.; Lucchini, R.; Triola, R.; Conti, C.; Avenia, S.; Rondelli, F.; Bugiantella, W.; Barillaro, I.; Sanguinetti, A.; et al. The role of surgery in the treatment of thyroid anaplastic carcinoma in the elderly. *Int. J. Surg.* 2014, 12, S170–S176. [CrossRef]
9. Conzo, G.; Polistena, A.; Calò, P.G.; Bononi, P.; Gambardella, C.; Mauriello, C.; Tartaglia, E.; Avenia, S.; Sanguinetti, A.; Medas, F.; et al. Efficacy of combined treatment for anaplastic thyroid carcinoma: Results of a multinstitutional retrospective analysis. *Int. J. Surg.* 2014, 12 (Suppl. 1), S178–S182. [CrossRef] [PubMed]
10. Gane, E.M.; McPhail, S.M.; Hatton, A.L.; Panizza, B.J.; O'Leary, S.P. Neck and Shoulder Motor Function following Neck Dissection: A Comparison with Healthy Control Subjects. *Otolaryngol. Head Neck Surg.* 2019, 160, 1009–1018. [CrossRef]
11. McGarvey, A.C.; Chiarelli, P.E.; Osmotherly, P.G.; Hoffman, G.R. Physiotherapy for accessory nerve shoulder dysfunction following neck dissection surgery: A literature review. *Head Neck* 2011, 33, 274–280. [CrossRef]
12. Eickmeyer, S.M.; Walczak, C.K.; Myers, K.B.; Lindstrom, D.R.; Layde, P.; Campbell, B.H. Quality of life, shoulder range of motion, and spinal accessory nerve status in 5-year survivors of head and neck cancer. *PM R* 2014, 12, 1073–1080. [CrossRef]
13. Bradley, P.J.; Ferlito, A.; Silver, C.E.; Takes, R.P.; Woolgar, J.A.; Strojan, P.; Suárez, C.; Coskun, H.; Zbären, P.; Rinaldo, A. Neck treatment and shoulder morbidity: Still a challenge. *Head Neck* 2011, 33, 1060–1067. [CrossRef] [PubMed]
14. Lanisnik, B.; Zargi, M.; Rodi, Z. Electrophysiologic analysis of injury to cranial nerve XI during neck dissection. *Head Neck* 2016, 38 (Suppl. 1), E372–E376. [CrossRef] [PubMed]
15. Gane, E.M.; Michaleff, Z.A.; Cottrell, M.A.; McPhail, S.M.; Hatton, A.L.; Panizza, B.J.; O'Leary, S.P. Prevalence, incidence, and risk factors for shoulder and neck dysfunction after neck dissection: A systematic review. *Eur. J. Surg. Oncol.* 2017, 43, 1199–1218. [CrossRef] [PubMed]
16. Larsen, M.H.; Lorenzen, M.M.; Bakholdt, V.; Sørensen, J.A. The prevalence of nerve injuries following neck dissections—A systematic review and meta-analysis. *Dan. Med. J.* 2020, 67, A08190464.
17. McGarvey, A.C.; Hoffman, G.R.; Osmotherly, P.G.; Chiarelli, P.E. Intra-operative monitoring of the spinal accessory nerve: A systematic review. *J. Laryngol. Otol.* 2014, 128, 746–751. [CrossRef]
18. Birinci, Y.; Genc, A.; Ecevit, M.C.; Erdag, T.K.; Guneri, E.A.; Oztura, I.; Evlice, A.; Ikiz, A.O. Spinal Accessory Nerve Monitoring and Clinical Outcome Results of Nerve-Sparing Neck Dissections. *Otolaryngol. Head Neck Surg.* 2014, 151, 253–259. [CrossRef] [PubMed]
19. Witt, R.L.; Rejto, L. Spinal accessory nerve monitoring in selective and modified neck dissection. *Laryngoscope* 2007, 117, 776–780. [CrossRef] [PubMed]
20. Witt, R.L.; Gillis, T.; Pratt, R., Jr. Spinal accessory nerve monitoring with clinical outcome measures. *Ear Nose Throat J.* 2006, 85, 540–544. [CrossRef] [PubMed]

21. Cirocchi, R.; Arezzo, A.; D'Andrea, V.; Abraha, I.; Popivanov, G.I.; Avenia, N.; Gerardi, C.; Henry, B.M.; Randolph, J.; Barczyński, M. Intraoperative neuromonitoring versus visual nerve identification for prevention of recurrent laryngeal nerve injury in adults undergoing thyroid surgery. *Cochrane Database Syst. Rev.* **2019**, *1*, CD012483. [CrossRef] [PubMed]
22. Henry, B.M.; Graves, M.J.; Vikse, J.; Sanna, B.; Pękala, P.A.; Walocha, J.A.; Barczyński, M.; Tomaszewski, K.A. The current state of intermittent intraoperative neural monitoring for prevention of recurrent laryngeal nerve injury during thyroidectomy: A PRISMA-compliant systematic review of overlapping meta-analyses. *Langenbecks Arch. Surg.* **2017**, *402*, 663–673. [CrossRef] [PubMed]
23. Von Elm, E.; Altman, D.G.; Egger, M.; Pocock, S.J.; Gøtzsche, P.C.; Vandenbroucke, J.P. STROBE initiative. The strengthening the reporting of observational studies in epidemiology (STROBE) statement: Guidelines for reporting observational studies. *Int. J. Surg.* **2014**, *12*, 1495–1499. [CrossRef] [PubMed]
24. Smallridge, R.C.; Ain, K.B.; Asa, S.L.; Bible, K.C.; Brierley, J.D.; Burman, K.D.; Kebebew, E.; Lee, N.Y.; Nikiforov, Y.E.; Rosenthal, M.S.; et al. American Thyroid Association Anaplastic Thyroid Cancer Guidelines Taskforce. American Thyroid Association guidelines for management of patients with anaplastic thyroid cancer. *Thyroid* **2012**, *22*, 1104–1139. [CrossRef] [PubMed]
25. Rosato, L.; De Crea, C.; Bellantone, R.; Brandi, M.L.; De Toma, G.; Filetti, S.; Miccoli, P.; Pacini, F.; Pelizzo, M.R.; Pontecorvi, A.; et al. Diagnostic, therapeutic and health-care management protocol in thyroid surgery: A position statement of the Italian Association of Endocrine Surgery Units (U.E.C. CLUB). *J. Endocrinol. Investig.* **2016**, *39*, 939–953. [CrossRef] [PubMed]
26. Breckenridge, J.D.; McAuley, J.H. Shoulder Pain and Disability Index (SPADI). *J. Physiother.* **2011**, *57*, 197. [CrossRef]
27. Kang, S.W.; Lee, S.H.; Park, J.H.; Jeong, J.S.; Park, S.; Lee, C.R.; Jeong, J.J.; Nam, K.H.; Chung, W.Y.; Park, C.S. A comparative study of the surgical outcomes of robotic and conventional open modified radical neck dissection for papillary thyroid carcinoma with lateral neck node metastasis. *Surg. Endosc.* **2012**, *26*, 3251–3257. [CrossRef]
28. Ngo, D.Q.; Tran, T.D.; Le, D.T.; Ngo, Q.X.; Van Le, Q. Transoral Endoscopic Modified Radical Neck Dissection for Papillary Thyroid Carcinoma. *Ann. Surg. Oncol.* **2021**, *28*, 2766. [CrossRef]
29. Paek, S.H.; Lee, H.A.; Kwon, H.; Kang, K.H.; Park, S.J. Comparison of robot-assisted modified radical neck dissection using a bilateral axillary breast approach with a conventional open procedure after propensity score matching. *Surg. Endosc.* **2020**, *34*, 622–627. [CrossRef]
30. Dziegielewski, P.T.; McNeely, M.L.; Ashworth, N.; O'Connell, D.A.; Barber, B.; Courneya, K.S.; Debenham, B.J.; Seikaly, H. 2b or not 2b? Shoulder function after level 2b neck dissection: A double-blind randomized controlled clinical trial. *Cancer* **2020**, *126*, 1492–1501. [CrossRef]
31. Sharma, R.K.; Lee, J.; Liou, R.; McManus, C.; Lee, J.A.; Kuo, J.H. Optimal surgeon-volume threshold for neck dissections in the setting of primary thyroid malignancies. *Surgery* **2021**, *12*. [CrossRef]
32. Godballe, C.; Madsen, A.R.; Sørensen, C.H.; Schytte, S.; Trolle, W.; Helweg-Larsen, J.; Barfoed, L.; Kristiansen, L.; Sørensen, V.Z.; Samuelsen, G.; et al. Risk factors for recurrent nerve palsy after thyroid surgery: A national study of patients treated at Danish departments of ENT Head and Neck Surgery. *Eur. Arch. Otorhinolaryngol.* **2014**, *271*, 2267–2276. [CrossRef]
33. Loyo, M.; Tufano, R.P.; Gourin, C.G. National trends in thyroid surgery and the effect of volume on short-term outcomes. *Laryngoscope* **2013**, *123*, 2056–2063. [CrossRef] [PubMed]
34. Prete, F.P.; Sgaramella, L.I.; Di Meo, G.; Pasculli, A.; Calculli, G.; Protopapa, G.; Gurrado, A.; Testini, M. Introducing routine intraoperative nerve monitoring in a high-volume endocrine surgery centre: A health technology assessment. *Updates Surg.* **2021**, 1–11, Epub ahead of print. [CrossRef]
35. Ferlito, A.; Robbins, K.T.; Silver, C.E.; Hasegawa, Y.; Rinaldo, A. Classification of neck dissections: An evolving system. *Auris Nasus Larynx* **2009**, *36*, 127–134. [CrossRef] [PubMed]
36. Ferlito, A.; Robbins, K.T.; Shah, J.P.; Medina, J.E.; Silver, C.E.; Al-Tamimi, S.; Fagan, J.J.; Paleri, V.; Takes, R.P.; Bradford, C.R.; et al. Proposal for a rational classification of neck dissections. *Head Neck* **2011**, *33*, 445–450. [CrossRef] [PubMed]
37. Popovski, V.; Benedetti, A.; Popovic-Monevska, D.; Grcev, A.; Stamatoski, A.; Zhivadinovik, J. Spinal accessory nerve preservation in modified neck dissections: Surgical and functional outcomes. *Acta Otorhinolaryngol. Ital.* **2017**, *37*, 368–374. [CrossRef] [PubMed]
38. Svenberg Lind, C.; Lundberg, B.; Hammarstedt Nordenvall, L.; Heiwe, S.; Persson, J.K.; Hydman, J. Quantification of Trapezius Muscle Innervation During Neck Dissections: Cervical Plexus Versus the Spinal Accessory Nerve. *Ann. Otol. Rhinol. Laryngol.* **2015**, *124*, 881–885. [CrossRef]
39. McGarvey, A.C.; Hoffman, G.R.; Osmotherly, P.G.; Chiarelli, P.E. Maximizing shoulder function after accessory nerve injury and neck dissection surgery: A multicenter randomized controlled trial. *Head Neck* **2015**, *37*, 1022–1031. [CrossRef] [PubMed]
40. Harris, A.S. Do patients benefit from physiotherapy for shoulder dysfunction following neck dissection? A systematic review. *J. Laryngol. Otol.* **2020**, *134*, 104–108. [CrossRef] [PubMed]
41. Do, J.H.; Yoon, I.J.; Cho, Y.K.; Ahn, J.S.; Kim, J.K.; Jeon, J. Comparison of hospital based and home based exercise on quality of life, and neck and shoulder function in patients with spinal accessary nerve injury after head and neck cancer surgery. *Oral Oncol.* **2018**, *86*, 100–104. [CrossRef]
42. Barber, B.; McNeely, M.; Chan, K.M.; Beaudry, R.; Olson, J.; Harris, J.; Seikaly, H.; O'Connell, D. Intraoperative brief electrical stimulation (BES) for prevention of shoulder dysfunction after oncologic neck dissection: Study protocol for a randomized controlled trial. *Trials* **2015**, *16*, 240. [CrossRef]

43. Al-Qurayshi, Z.; Sullivan, C.B.; Pagedar, N.; Randolph, G.; Kandil, E. Prevalence of major structures injury in thyroid and neck surgeries: A national perspective. *Gland Surg.* **2020**, *9*, 1924–1932. [CrossRef]
44. Sahli, Z.T.; Zhou, S.; Sharma, A.K.; Segev, D.L.; Massie, A.; Zeiger, M.A.; Mathur, A. Rising Cost of Thyroid Surgery in Adult Patients. *J. Surg. Res.* **2021**, *260*, 28–37. [CrossRef]
45. Polistena, A.; Di Lorenzo, P.; Sanguinetti, A.; Buccelli, C.; Conzo, G.; Conti, A.; Niola, M.; Avenia, N. Medicolegal implications of surgical errors and complications in neck surgery: A review based on the Italian current legislation. *Open Med.* **2016**, *11*, 298–306. [CrossRef] [PubMed]
46. Li, F.; Sun, H. The application of intraoperative neuromonitoring in lateral neck dissections for thyroid cancers. *Ann. Thyroid* **2019**, *4*, 15. [CrossRef]
47. Lee, C.H.; Huang, N.C.; Chen, H.C.; Chen, M.K. Minimizing shoulder syndrome with intra-operative spinal accessory nerve monitoring for neck dissection. *Acta Otorhinolaryngol. Ital.* **2013**, *33*, 93–96. [PubMed]
48. Parmeggiani, D.; Gambardella, C.; Patrone, R.; Polistena, A.; De Falco, M.; Ruggiero, R.; Cirocchi, R.; Sanguinetti, A.; Cuccurullo, V.; Accardo, M.; et al. Radioguided thyroidectomy for follicular tumors: Multicentric experience. *Int. J. Surg.* **2017**, *41*, S75–S81. [CrossRef] [PubMed]

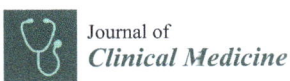

Article

Laser Ablation Treatment of Recurrent Lymph Node Metastases from Papillary Thyroid Carcinoma

Chiara Offi *, Claudia Misso, Giovanni Antonelli, Maria Grazia Esposito, Umberto Brancaccio and Stefano Spiezia

Department of Endocrine and Ultrasound-Guided Surgery, Ospedale del Mare, 80147 Naples, Italy; claudiamisso@hotmail.com (C.M.); giovanniantonelli81@libero.it (G.A.); mariagrazia.esposito@aslnapoli1centro.it (M.G.E.); umberto.brancaccio@aslnapoli1centro.it (U.B.); stefanospiezia@tiroide.org (S.S.)
* Correspondence: chiara.o@live.com; Tel.: +08-118-775-214

Abstract: (1) Background: The incidence of papillary thyroid cancers is increasing. Papillary neoplasm metastasizes to the central and lateral lymph nodes of the neck. The recurrence rate is less than 30%. The gold standard of treatment for lymph node recurrences is surgery, but surgery is burdened by a high rate of complications. Therefore, laser ablation of recurrent lymph nodes has been recognized as an alternative treatment with minimal invasiveness, a low complication rate and a curative effect. (2) Methods: We analyzed 10 patients who underwent a total thyroidectomy and metabolic radiotherapy and who developed a lymph node recurrence in the laterocervical compartment in the following 12–18 months. (3) Results: Patients developed lymph node recurrence at IV and Vb levels in 70% and 30% of cases, respectively. All patients were treated with a single laser ablative session. Hydrodissection was performed in all patients. The energy delivered was 1120 ± 159.3 Joules and 3–4 Watts in 362 ± 45.7 s. No complications were reported. All patients underwent a 6-month follow-up. A volumetric reduction of 40.12 ± 2.2%, 49.1 ± 2.13% and 59.8 ± 3.05%, respectively at 1-, 3- and 6-months of follow-up was reported. (4) Conclusions: At 6 months, a fine needle aspiration was performed, which was negative for malignant cells and negative for a dosage of Thyroglobulin in eluate. The laser ablation is an effective alternative to surgical treatment.

Keywords: thyroid carcinoma; laser ablation; papillary thyroid carcinoma; lymph nodes metastases; recurrence

Citation: Offi, C.; Misso, C.; Antonelli, G.; Esposito, M.G.; Brancaccio, U.; Spiezia, S. Laser Ablation Treatment of Recurrent Lymph Node Metastases from Papillary Thyroid Carcinoma. *J. Clin. Med.* **2021**, *10*, 5295. https://doi.org/10.3390/jcm10225295

Academic Editor:
Giuseppe Ingravallo

Received: 25 October 2021
Accepted: 12 November 2021
Published: 14 November 2021

Publisher's Note: MDPI stays neutral with regard to jurisdictional claims in published maps and institutional affiliations.

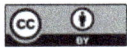

Copyright: © 2021 by the authors. Licensee MDPI, Basel, Switzerland. This article is an open access article distributed under the terms and conditions of the Creative Commons Attribution (CC BY) license (https://creativecommons.org/licenses/by/4.0/).

1. Introduction

In the last decade, we have seen an exponential increase in the incidence of microcarcinomas (PTMC) and papillary thyroid carcinoma (PTC) due to easier access to imaging methods. This is associated with an increase in the diagnosis of synchronous and metachronous lymph node metastases. This event has opened new clinical and therapeutic scenarios [1–3]. PTC spreads by the lymphatic route; in 30% of cases it can be associated with synchronous lymph node metastases and in 30% of cases with metachronous lymph node metastases [4]. The gold standard treatment of both synchronous and metachronous lymph node metastases is surgery, which involves an extensive lymphectomy of the laterocervical and/or central compartments or a lymphectomy of one or more compartments. Surgery is burdened by a higher rate of major complications in the case of reoperations and in patients treated with metabolic radiotherapy, greater than in the primary intervention [4,5]. In recent decades, due to complications, several minimally invasive techniques have been perfected such as percutaneous ethanol injection (PEI), percutaneous laser ablation (LA), microwave ablation and radiofrequency ablation (RFA) [6–9]. US-guided LA has played a prominent role due to the ability to perform ablations of small lesions safely [7].

In 1960 the first handcrafted laser with a ruby was made [10]. Since then, the laser technique has undergone considerable developments and it has been applied in various medical fields. In 1962 the ruby laser was used for the first time in medicine, retinal surgery and dentistry [11–13]. Today, there are various types of lasers. The LA is a type of minimally invasive procedure. The use of LA must always be supported by scientific evidence, due to the complications and the side effects deriving from incorrect use.

LA was first used in the treatment of thyroid disease in the 2000s. Today it is routinely used in the ablation of symptomatic benign thyroid nodules, recurrence, and lymph node metastases. LA is used in the treatment of metastatic lymph nodes lesions due to the possibility of inducing small volumes of well-defined and predictable tissues necrosis. This feature makes LA suitable for the ablative treatment of metachronous metastases, adjacent to delicate anatomical structures.

Our study analyzes retrospectively the first 10 cases that underwent LA of the metastatic lymph nodes after a total thyroidectomy and radiometabolic therapy for PTC. The treated lymph node metastases occurred in the 12–18 months following the radiometabolic treatment with I131. Recurrence was diagnosed by serum thyroglobulin (Tg) elevation, a positive ultrasound, a fine needle aspiration positive for malignant cells and positive Tg in the eluate.

2. Materials and Methods

We retrospectively collected data from 10 consecutive patients undergoing LA treatment of metachronous lymph node metastases at the Department of Endocrine and Ultrasound-Guided Surgery of the "Ospedale del Mare", Naples, Italy. The patients enrolled in the study were referred to our department in the period between December 2017 and June 2018 for the surgical treatment and in the period between June 2019 and December 2020 for the LA treatment. All included patients underwent a total thyroidectomy and subsequent metabolic radiotherapy (RAI) for the diagnosis of PTC, according to the American Thyroid Association (ATA) guidelines [4]. During oncological follow-up, all patients had an increase in serum Tg levels > 20 µg/L. Patients referred for LA treatment had a high surgical risk of comorbidities and/or had refused further surgery or were ineligible for a second RAI treatment. All cases were evaluated in the multidisciplinary oncological group prior to treatment.

The Campania Centro ethics committee approved the protocol and all patients signed a written informed consent. All procedures were performed in accordance with the Helsinki Declaration.

We included patients over 18 years with a histological diagnosis of PTC in the 12–18 months prior to ablative treatment. All patients were treated with a total thyroidectomy and RAI. During the follow-up, all patients showed an increase in serum Tg (values > 20 µg/L) and ultrasound evidence of pathological lymph nodes in the laterocervical compartment. All patients underwent a fine needle aspiration cytology (FNAC) of the lesion, which showed the presence of malignant cells and Tg values in the eluate >5000 µg/L. The volume of the lesion was calculated during the ultrasound examination. A complete history and preoperative hematological evaluation were collected in an electronic database. We evaluated patients' hematological tests: complete blood cells count, thyroid function and thyroid antibodies. The B-mode ultrasound examination was performed to evaluate the lymph node level, the lesion's volume and the presence of further metastases. Clinical and demographic data (age, sex, volume of nodal metastasis, level of metastasis) were collected in an electronic database.

Patients followed an ultrasound follow-up program after laser ablative treatment, with a timing of 1-, 3- and 6-months. During the follow-up, we calculated the treated lesion's volume in ml, the volumetric reduction in percentage compared to the pre-treatment volume and the serum Tg value. At the end of the 6-month follow-up, we performed a lesion's FNAC. In all treated cases we obtained a negative cytology for malignant cells and absence of Tg in the eluate.

The ultrasound examination was conducted with a 7.5–12 MHz linear probe (MyLab™ ClassC and MyLab™ 9 Platform, Esaote Biomedica, Genova, Italy). The basal volume of the lymph node lesion was calculated using the software. Vascularity was studied by Color Doppler (CD) examination and slow flow analysis.

We analyzed the number of laser fibers used, the Watts, the Joules and the time expressed in seconds. We used a continuous wave multi-source laser system with a length of 1064 nm (EchoLaser ModiLite^{TM}, Elesta SpA, Calenzano, Italy). The procedures were performed with ultrasound guidance and with a free hand technique. Currently, EchoLaser can now be used with a recently released new software (available with the ESI, EchoLaser Smart Interface) for a more precise and safer planning of the procedure. The laser generator, connected to the optical fiber, produces an illumination of the optical fiber which generates heat in tissues adjacent to the tip by. The temperature increase induces the denaturation of the proteins and irreversible cell damage. The energy produced decreases exponentially distancing from the tip of the optical fiber.

The patients underwent a single LA session. The procedure was performed by placing the patients in a supine position with a moderate hyperextension of the neck. We performed a pericapsular local anesthesia with 2% Lidocaine.

The applicators used were 21 Gauche (G) needles. The output power varied from 3 to 5 Watts (W) and in our population we used an output power of 3 W in nine cases and a power of 4 W in only one case, due to the lymph node's volume. The fibers used were quartz optical fibers with a flat tip and a diameter of 300 microns. The applicators were inserted into the target lesion through guides applied to the probe with different angles of incidence depending on the pre-treatment planning. The procedure began with the insertion of the 21G introducer into the target lesion along its major axis. The treatment was performed with a prefixed power, while the lighting time of the optical fiber varied according to the volume to be treated. The 21G applicators allow atraumatic, precise and multiple positioning of the fibers. More optical fibers can be used, as in one of the cases presented, with a distance of at least 0.8 cm. The tip of the fiber must have a minimum safety distance of 5–10 mm from the anatomical structures of the neck We performed a preliminary hydrodissection with a 5% glucose solution to ward off the lymph node metastases from the anatomical structures of the neck [14–16].

We performed the "pullback" technique in one case. The "pullback" technique can be used in the treatment of lesions with a major axis greater than 2 cm [7]. The technique allows the enlargement of the area to be ablated and the planning made at the beginning of the procedure to be respected. On the ultrasound, the ablated area appears hyperechoic due to the micro bubbles created by the evaporation of liquids. The hyperechoic area increases its size as the volume of the necrosis area increases. The treatment can be considered concluded when the volume of the hyperechoic area remains stable. The evaluation of the treatment's effectiveness is performed through the Color Doppler (CD) analysis [14–17]. The real volume of the area subjected to ablation can be determined 72 h after the end of the treatment, as the cell damage becomes permanent [14].

At the end of the procedure the functionality of the vocal cords was evaluated with an ecolaryngoscopy.

All patients were discharged two hours after the procedure in the absence of any type of symptoms. There were no cases of major or minor complications.

Statistical analysis was performed with SPSS version 23 (SPSS©, Chicago, IL, USA). Continuous variables were described as mean, standard deviation (SD) and range, while categorical variables were described as number of cases and the percentage.

3. Results

We retrospectively enrolled 10 patients (5 males and 5 females) treated with a single LA session for a single lymph node recurrence. All patients had a diagnosis of classic variant PTC that had been previously treated with a total thyroidectomy and RAI. The demographic characteristics are showed in Table 1. The mean age was 40.2 years (±17.98 SD). All patients were treated with suppressive therapy with L-thyroxine. During the oncological follow-up, all patients had an increase in the serum Tg value greater than 20 µg/L. The increase in serum Tg was followed by an ultrasound of the neck which revealed the presence of disease. There were seven metastatic lymph nodes at level IV and three at level Vb with a baseline volume of 1.82 mL (±3.45 SD). In all cases, a FNAC of the suspected lesion was performed with a Tg assay on the eluate. Data are reported in Tables 1 and 2.

Table 1. Demographic and clinical data of the study population (FNAC, fine needle aspiration cytology; Tg, thyroglobulin; mL, milliliter).

Data	Population
Gender	
Male	5 (50%)
Female	5 (50%)
Age	40.2 ± 17.98
FNAC	Positive for malignant cell
Eluate Tg	>5000 µg/L
Lymph node level	
IV	7 (70%)
Vb	3 (30%)
Side	
Right	4 (40%)
Left	6 (60%)
Lymph node volume	1.82 ± 3.45
Fiber optic	1.01 ± 0.31
Watt	3.1 ± 0.31
Time in second	531.86 ± 109.5
Joule	1256 ± 396
1-month volume in ml	1.12 ± 2.18
% reduction at 1 month	40.12 ± 2.2
3-months volume in ml	0.88 ± 1.65
% reduction at 3 months	49.1 ± 2.13
6-months volume in ml	0.706 ± 1.30
% reduction at 6 months	59.8 ± 3.05

Table 2. Demographic and clinical data of the included patients.

Patient	Gender	Age	FNAC	Eluate Tg (µg/L)	Lymph Node Level	Side	Lymph Node Volume (mL)	Fiber Optic	Watts	Time (Seconds)	Joules
1	Male	20	Positive	>5000	IV	Right	0.7	1	3	270	810
2	Male	19	Positive	>5000	IV	Right	0.35	1	3	365	1095
3	Male	19	Positive	>5000	IV	Right	0.25	1	3	365	1095
4	Female	59	Positive	>5000	Vb	Left	11.58	2	4	340	2720
5	Female	59	Positive	>5000	IV	Left	0.46	1	3	335	1005
6	Female	63	Positive	>5000	IV	Left	1.27	1	3	420	1260
7	Male	28	Positive	>5000	IV	Right	1.32	1	3	400	1200
8	Female	35	Positive	>5000	VB	Right	1.05	1	3	395	1185
9	Female	48	Positive	>5000	VB	Left	0.79	1	3	325	975
10	Female	52	Positive	>5000	IV	Left	0.98	1	3	405	1215

The size and margins of the metastases determined the number of laser fibers used. In metastases of less than 1 cm of maximum diameter (nine cases), only one fiber was used, while in metastases greater than 1 cm of maximum diameter (only one case), two laser fibers were used.

The treatment protocol, W and Joules, was planned before the start of the procedure by the expert operator (S.S.). An output power of 3 W was used in nine cases, while a power of 4 W was used in only one case for a mean of 531.86 s ($\pm$109.5 SD) and a mean of 1236 Joules ($\pm$396 SD). The data relating to individual cases analyzed are shown in Table 2.

After laser ablation treatment, the mean volume of the nodule was 1.12 ± 2.18 mL with a 40.12% reduction in volume 1 month after treatment. After 3 months the mean volume was 0.88 ± 1.65 mL with a 49.1% reduction in volume and after 6 months the mean volume was 0.706 ± 1.30 mL with a 59.8% reduction in volume (Table 3). The data showed a volume reduction of 60% after 6 months, but the most significant data were the absence of malignant cells at the FNAC performed after 6 months, the absence of Tg in the eluate and absent serum Tg values.

Table 3. Clinical data of volume reduction in the lymph nodes metastases treated with laser ablation.

Patients	1 Month Volume (mL)	% Reduction at 1 Month	3 Months Volume (mL)	% Reduction at 3 Months	6 Months Volume (mL)	% Reduction at 6-Months
1	0.1	42	0.08	50	0.07	60
2	0.22	37.2	0.19	45	0.16	55
3	0.15	40	0.13	48	0.11	56
4	7.3	37	5.56	52	4.4	62
5	0.22	43	0.2	47	0.26	57
6	0.74	42	0.62	51	0.48	62
7	0.76	42	0.64	51	0.49	63
8	0.61	41	0.53	50	0.38	64
9	0.48	39	0.4	49	0.32	59
10	0.61	38	0.51	48	0.39	60

The ablative techniques were conducted by one skilled operator (S.S.) of a tertiary thyroid center. There were no major complications or minor complications.

4. Discussion

The treatment of PTC is a total thyroidectomy with or without central lymphadenectomy followed or not followed by RAI therapy depending on the histotype and the presence of mutations [4]. Lymph node recurrence can occur in about 1–2% of patients after surgical and RAI therapy [4]. Lymph node recurrences can be treated with surgery or with additional RAI therapy, even if reoperations are burdened by a very high rate of major complications (25% of cases of vocal cord palsy) and metabolic radiotherapy is burdened by a very high failure rate when repeated [4]. In fact, various studies have shown that neoplastic cells subjected to repeated RAI therapies lose the ability to pick up radioactive iodine [4]. Ultrasound-guided mini-interventional procedures are an effective and safe alternative [6–9]. The minimally invasive ultrasound-guided procedures have been developed and validated. They can be performed repeatedly without an increased complication rate, without hospitalization and general anesthesia; all characteristics well accepted by patients. PEI was the first treatment used but was soon abandoned due to the unpredictable spread of alcohol [18]. Subsequently, RFA took over due to its ability to generate a complete necrosis of the lesion, even if burdened by high complication rates [19]. LA appears to be the safest and the most effective technique.

The LA technique of body tissues was proposed in 1983 by Bown and has undergone numerous revisions, standardizations and experiments [20]. Numerous data have emerged from the literature in support of minimally invasive ablative techniques. Dupuy et al. [21] treated eight cases of lymph node metastases with RFA; all healed with a single application but two cases of major complications were reported. Kim et al. [22] reported a series of 73 patients with lymph node recurrence, 27 treated with RFA and 46 treated with surgery. The study did not show statistical differences between the two groups in relation to disease free survival at 1 and 3 years. Unlike other techniques, LA is preferred in the treatment of thyroid pathologies due to the size of the introducers, which are reduced, easily reaching the target tissue with a low risk of tissue injury and bleeding. The thermic energy used allows a precise ablation of small volumes, reducing heat dissipation and the subsequent necrosis of the surrounding tissues. In cases of large lesions, multiple needles can be used simultaneously to increase the volume of the necrosis area. Mauri et al. [3] presented a series of 24 patients treated with LA for PTC's lymph node recurrence. The study showed that 86.9% of patients had a complete ablation 30 months after treatment and in 79.1% of patients no disease was detected on imaging methods. In only five cases a second session was required and no increase in the complications rate was reported. Zhou et al. [23] published a study on 81 patients with PTMC, 36 treated with LA and 45 treated with a lobectomy with a unilateral sixth compartment lymphectomy. The study showed that, with a mean follow-up of 49.2 months and 48.5 months, respectively, no patients developed lymph node recurrences. Therefore, LA can be considered an alternative treatment for patients who are unsuitable for or who refuse surgery.

Our series of 10 patients showed that a normalization of serum thyroglobulin levels, the absence of neoplastic cells in the control FNC and the absence of Tg in the eluate were recorded 6 months after the ablative treatment. In only one case we used two laser fibers due to the large size of the lesion and neither major nor minor complications were reported. The risk of ablative treatment in relation to lymph node recurrences is thermic injury to the nerve structures; we reduced this risk by practicing a hydrodissection, with a 5% glucose solution, of the lesion and reducing the power and increasing the application time. Figure 1 shows one of the cases included in our case series. Image A shows the lymph node recurrence prior to the treatment. Image B shows the tip of the laser fiber in the center of the lesion before the ablative treatment was started. Image C shows the ultrasound at 6 months. The lymph node lesion appears as a hypoechoic area with a hyperechoic halo (image of scarring fibrosis).

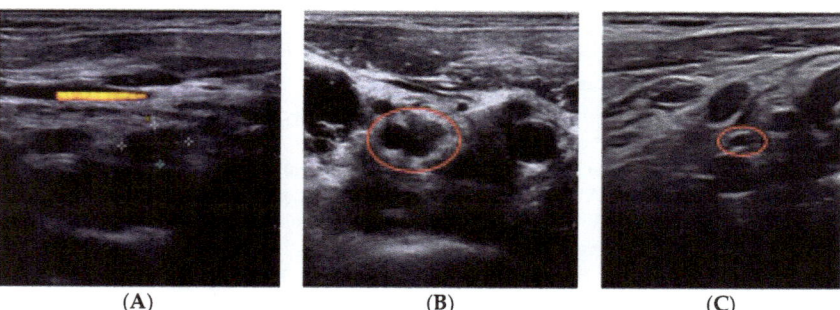

Figure 1. The images (**A**) show a lymph node recurrence to treat with laser ablation. Image (**B**) shows the tip of the laser fiber in the center of the lesion before the start of the ablative treatment. Image (**C**) shows the ultrasound follow-up at 6 months. The lymph node recurrence appears as a hypoechoic area with a hyperechoic halo (image of scarring fibrosis).

Our data demonstrate that LA of PTC's lymph node recurrence is a viable treatment. This technique allows a reduction in the surgical treatment of metachronous metastases from PTC with the reduction in morbidity associated with a reoperation.

It is useful in cases of multiple lymph node recurrences occurring during the follow-up, even after previous treatment. All these patients would be candidates for a lymphadenectomy with an exponential increase in complications.

However, our study had limitations: the sparse case history, the absence of randomization of the population, the impossibility of comparison with other techniques and the lack of follow-up at 5 and 10 years. This is a preliminary study; further analyses are needed.

5. Conclusions

LA represents a safe, effective and minimally invasive alternative to surgery in the treatment of lymph node recurrences from papillary thyroid carcinoma treated with surgical therapy and metabolic radiotherapy. This technique allows a total necrosis of the metastatic lesion associated with a reduced complications rate compared to surgical treatment.

Author Contributions: Conceptualization, C.O. and S.S.; Methodology, C.O. and S.S.; Software, C.C. and S.S.; Validation, C.O. and S.S.; Formal Analysis, C.O. and S.S.; Investigation, C.O. and S.S.; Resources, C.O. and S.S.; Data Curation, C.O. and S.S.; Writing—Original Draft Preparation, C.O. and S.S.; Writing—Review and Editing, C.O. and S.S.; Visualization, C.O., C M , G.A., M.G.E., U.B. and S.S.; Supervision, C.O. and S.S.; Project Administration, C.O. and S.S. All authors have read and agreed to the published version of the manuscript.

Funding: The APC was funded by Elesta SpA, Calenzano, Italy.

Institutional Review Board Statement: The study was conducted according to the guidelines of the Declaration of Helsinki and approved by the Ethics Committee "Campania Centro" (protocol code 0170338/E of 15 July 2021).

Informed Consent Statement: Informed consent was obtained from all subjects involved in the study.

Data Availability Statement: The data are deposited in an electronic database at the Department of Endocrine and Ultrasound-guided Surgery, "Ospedale del Mare", Naples, Italy.

Conflicts of Interest: The authors declare no conflict of interest.

References

1. Lim, H.; Devesa, S.S.; Sosa, J.A.; Check, D.; Kitahara, C.M. Trends in thyroid cancer incidence and mortality in the United States, 1974–2013. *JAMA* **2017**, *317*, 1338–1348. [CrossRef] [PubMed]
2. La Vecchia, C.; Malvezzi, M.; Bosetti, C.; Garavello, W.; Bertuccio, P.; Levi, F.; Negri, E. Thyroid cancer mortality and incidence: A global overview. *Int. J. Cancer.* **2015**, *136*, 2187–2195. [CrossRef] [PubMed]
3. Mauri, G.; Cova, L. Ierace, T.; Baroli, A.; Di Mauro, E.; Pacella, C.M.; Goldberg, S.N.; Solbiati, L. Treatment of Metastatic Lymph Nodes in the Neck from Papillary Thyroid Carcinoma with Percutaneous Laser Ablation. *Cardiovasc. Interv. Radiol.* **2016**, *39*, 1023–1030. [CrossRef] [PubMed]
4. Haugen, B.R. 2015 American Thyroid Association Management guidelines for adult patients with thyroid nodules and differentiated thyroid cancer: What is new and what has changed? *Cancer-Am. Cancer Soc.* **2017**, *123*, 372–381. [CrossRef] [PubMed]
5. Ito, Y.; Miyauchi, A. Lateral and mediastinal lymph node dissection in differentiated thyroid carcinoma: Indications, benefits, and risks. *World J. Surg.* **2007**, *31*, 905–915. [CrossRef]
6. Fontenot, T.E.; Denwar, A.; Bhatia, P.; Al-Qurayshi, Z.; Randolph, G.W.; Kandil, E. Percutaneous ethanol injection vs reoperation for locally recurrent papillary thyroid cancer: A systematic review and pooled analysis. *JAMA Otolaryngol. Head Neck Surg.* **2015**, *141*, 512–518. [CrossRef]
7. Papini, E.; Bizzarri, G.; Bianchini, A.; Valle, D.; Misischi, L.; Guglielmi, R.; Salvatori, M.; Solbiati, L.; Crescenzi, A.; Pacella, C.M.; et al. Percutaneous ultrasound-guided laser ablation is effective for treating selected nodal metastases in papillary thyroid cancer. *J. Clin. Endocrinol. Metab.* **2013**, *98*, E92–E97. [CrossRef]
8. Yue, W.; Chen, L.; Wang, S.; Yu, S. Locoregional control of recurrent papillary thyroid carcinoma by ultrasoundguided percutaneous microwave ablation: A prospective study. *Int. J. Hyperth.* **2015**, *31*, 403–408. [CrossRef]
9. Wang, L.; Ge, M.; Xu, D.; Chen, L.; Qian, C.; Shi, K.; Liu, J.; Chen, Y. Ultrasonography-guided percutaneous radiofrequency ablation for cervical lymph node metastasis from thyroid carcinoma. *J. Cancer. Res.* **2014**, *10*, C144–C149. [CrossRef]
10. Maiman, T.H. Optical and microwave-optical experiments in ruby. *Phys. Rev. Lett.* **1960**, *4*, 564–566. [CrossRef]
11. Zaret, M.M.; Breinin, G.M.; Schmidt, H.; Ripps, H.; Siegel, I.M.; Solon, L.R. Ocular lesions produced by an optical maser (laser). *Science* **1961**, *134*, 1525–1526. [CrossRef]
12. Goldman, L.; Hornby, P.; Meyer, R.; Goldman, B. Impact of the laser on dental caries. *Nature* **1964**, *25*, 203–417. [CrossRef] [PubMed]
13. Schena, E.; Saccomandi, P.; Fong, Y. Laser ablation for cancer: Past, present and future. *J. Funct. Biomater.* **2017**, *8*, 19. [CrossRef] [PubMed]
14. Ahmed, M.; Brace, C.L.; Lee, F.T., Jr.; Goldberg, S.N. Principles of and advances in percutaneous ablation. *Radiology* **2011**, *258*, 351–369. [CrossRef]
15. Thomsen, S. Pathologic analysis of photothermal and photomechanical effects of laser-tissue interactions. *Photochem. Photobiol.* **1991**, *53*, 825–835. [CrossRef] [PubMed]
16. Jacques, S.L. Laser-tissue interactions. Photochemical, photothermal and photomechanical. *Surg. Clin. North Am.* **1992**, *72*, 531–558. [CrossRef]
17. Stafford, R.J.; Fuentes, D.; Elliott, A.A.; Weinberg, J.S.; Ahrar, K. Laser-induced thermal therapy for tumor ablation. *Crit. Rev. Biomed. Eng.* **2010**, *38*, 79–100. [CrossRef] [PubMed]

18. Solbiati, L.; Giangrande, A.; De Pra, L.; Bellotti, E.; Cantù, P.; Ravetto, C. Percutaneous ethanol injection of parathyroid tumors under US guidance: Treatment for secondary hyperparathyroidism. *Radiology* **1985**, *155*, 607–610. [CrossRef] [PubMed]
19. Shin, J.E.; Baek, J.H.; Lee, J.H. Radiofrequency and ethanol ablation for the treatment of recurrent thyroid cancers: Current status and challenges. *Curr. Opin. Oncol.* **2013**, *25*, 14–19. [CrossRef]
20. Bown, S.G. Phototherapy in tumors. *World J. Surg.* **1983**, *7*, 700–709. [CrossRef] [PubMed]
21. Dupuy, D.E.; Monchik, J.M.; Decrea, C.; Pisharodi, L. Radiofrequency ablation of regional recurrence from well-differentiated thyroid malignancy. *Surgery* **2001**, *130*, 971–977. [CrossRef]
22. Kim, J.; Yoo, W.S.; Park, Y.J.; Park, D.J.; Yun, T.J.; Choi, S.H.; Sohn, C.H.; Lee, K.E.; Sung, M.W.; Youn, Y.K.; et al. Efficacy and safety of radiofrequency ablation for treatment of locally recurrent thyroid cancers smaller than 2 cm. *Radiology* **2015**, *276*, 909–918. [CrossRef]
23. Zhou, W.; Ni, X.; Xu, S.; Zhang, L.; Chen, L.; Zhan, W. Ultrasound-guided laser ablation versus surgery for solitary papillary thyroid microcarcinoma: A retrospective study. *Int. J. Hyperth.* **2019**, *36*, 897–904. [CrossRef]

Article

Preoperative Ultrasonography in the Evaluation of Suspected Familial Non-Medullary Thyroid Cancer: Are We Able to Predict Multifocality and Extrathyroidal Extension?

Giorgio Grani [1,†], Gianluca Cera [1,†], Giovanni Conzo [2], Valeria Del Gatto [1], Cira Rosaria Tiziana di Gioia [3], Marianna Maranghi [1], Piernatale Lucia [1], Vito Cantisani [3], Alessio Metere [4], Rossella Melcarne [4], Maria Carola Borcea [4], Chiara Scorziello [4], Rosa Menditto [4], Marco Summa [4], Marco Biffoni [4], Cosimo Durante [1,*] and Laura Giacomelli [4]

1. Department of Translational and Precision Medicine, Sapienza University of Rome, Viale del Policlinico, 155, I-00161 Rome, Italy; giorgio.grani@uniroma1.it (G.G.); Cera.1637917@studenti.uniroma1.it (G.C.); valeria.delgatto@uniroma1.it (V.D.G.); marianna.maranghi@uniroma1.it (M.M.); piernatale.lucia@uniroma1.it (P.L.)
2. Department of Cardiothoracic Sciences, University of Campania Luigi Vanvitelli, I-80131 Naples, Italy; giovanni.conzo@unicampania.it
3. Department of Radiological, Oncological and Pathological Sciences, Sapienza University of Rome, Viale del Policlinico, 155, I-00161 Rome, Italy; cira.digioia@uniroma1.it (C.R.T.d.G.); vito.cantisani@uniroma1.it (V.C.)
4. Department of Surgical Sciences, Sapienza University of Rome, Viale del Policlinico, 155, I-00161 Rome, Italy; alessio.metere@uniroma1.it (A.M.); rossella.melcarne@uniroma1.it (R.M.); mariacarola.borcea@uniroma1.it (M.C.B.); chiara.scorziello@uniroma1.it (C.S.); rosa.menditto@uniroma1.it (R.M.); marco.summa@uniroma1.it (M.S.); marco.biffoni@uniroma1.it (M.B.); laura.giacomelli@uniroma1.it (L.G.)
* Correspondence: cosimo.durante@uniroma1.it; Tel.: +39-0-649-975-130
† Equal contribution.

Abstract: Family history of thyroid cancer increases the risk of harboring thyroid malignancies that end up having extrathyroidal extension (ETE) and multifocality on histology; some authors suggest a more aggressive surgical approach. Their pre-operative identification could allow more conservative surgical procedures if none of these features are suspected. Our aim was to assess if neck ultrasonography could identify or exclude multifocality or ETE in these patients to tailor the extent of surgery. This retrospective study included patients with previous thyroid surgery, ≥1 first-grade relative with thyroid cancer, and who had undergone pre-surgical ultrasound. ETE was suspected in the case of thyroid border interruption or gross invasion of perithyroidal tissues. Multiple suspicious nodules were defined as suspicion of multifocal cancer. The cohort consisted of 45 patients (median age 49 years, 40 with thyroid cancer, 30 females). The positive predictive value of ultrasonography in predicting multifocality and ETE was 57.14% (25.25–84.03) and 41.67% (21.5–65.1%), respectively, while the negative predictive values were 63.2% (56.4–69.4%) and 72.7% (63.3–80.5%). Pre-operative ultrasound examination is unable to reliably identify or exclude multifocal disease or extrathyroidal extension. In patients scheduled for surgery and with a first-degree relative affected by DTC, a "negative" pre-operative US report does not exclude the potential finding of multifocality and ETE at final histopathology.

Keywords: TIRADS; thyroid cancer; thyroid nodules; multifocality

1. Introduction

Differentiated thyroid cancer (DTC) is commonly associated with a good prognosis and excellent survival rates [1]. Treatment strategies for DTC patients are increasingly tailored to individual patients' needs to guarantee that the benefits of more aggressive (or conservative) therapies outweigh the risks of adverse outcomes. This approach is advocated by international guidelines [2,3], with some issues still debated [4]. Given the low risk of death from DTC, treatment plans mostly rely on estimates of patients' risk of persistence or recurrence of disease, which guides decisions on surgery (e.g., lobectomy vs. total thyroidectomy vs. total thyroidectomy with prophylactic central neck dissection) and post-surgical treatment (e.g., radioiodine administration). Many tumor characteristics, including size, multifocality, extra-thyroidal extension (ETE), vascular invasion, incomplete surgical resection, lymph node involvement, and metastasis, have been associated with an increased risk of recurrence, warranting a more aggressive surgical approach and/or radioiodine treatment [2,3].

A family history of DTC is associated with some of these higher-risk features. Familial cases are characterized by younger age at presentation, increased risk of recurrence, and potentially more aggressive disease, with tumors showing multifocality and extra-thyroidal extension (ETE) more frequently than sporadic cases. However, the clinical implications of these findings on tumor screening, treatment, and prognosis remain controversial [5–7]. In total, 5–15% of DTC cases can be defined as familial in the context of multiple tumor syndromes (such as FAP, Gardner, Peutz–Jeghers syndromes, and Carney complex), or as familial non-medullary thyroid cancers (FNMTC) when at least two or three first-degree relatives are affected by DTC [6,8]. Having only one first-degree relative affected by DTC does not satisfy FNMTC criteria, but it has indeed been associated with some of its clinical features, including the histological presence of multifocality and ETE [5]. This may be partially explained by the fact that at least some of these cases are indeed familial forms that have not met diagnostic criteria yet [6].

Since familiarity increases the risk of both ETE and multifocality, more aggressive therapeutic approaches are advocated by default by some authors to prevent recurrences in patients with a family history of DTC. Nevertheless, a reliable preoperative assessment of ETE and multifocality may allow clinicians to propose a more conservative surgical approach (i.e., lobectomy) if none of these features are suspected. On the other hand, the identification of ETE and multifocality can favor total thyroidectomy and reduce the risk of having to perform a completion thyroidectomy [9]. Thyroid ultrasound (US) can be used to this scope, as it is the most informative imaging technique in evaluating number, size, location and characteristics of both thyroid nodules [10] and loco-regional lymph nodes [11]. US predictive power in identifying ETE when compared to post-surgical histopathological results is variable and suboptimal, and relevant interobserver variability has been reported; even so, neck US could be useful especially as a rule-out test given the higher negative predictive value reported in several studies [12,13].

In this study, we aimed to assess if preoperative neck US can identify or exclude multifocality and/or ETE in patients scheduled for surgery for a suspicious thyroid nodule and with family history of DTC, to clarify whether such history represents an "unpredictable" risk factor that warrants broader surgery, or if it is associated with detectable features allowing for tailored conservative treatment.

2. Materials and Methods

We carried out a retrospective observational study at the Thyroid Disease Clinic in Sapienza University of Rome. All patients met the following inclusion criteria: (a) previous thyroid surgery for sonographically and/or cytologically suspicious thyroid nodules; (b) complete histopathological report; (c) at least one first-grade relative affected by DTC (as known at the time of surgery); and (d) at least one pre-surgical neck ultrasound with available images and/or report, carried out to evaluate suspicious thyroid nodules, to perform FNA procedures, or as pre-surgical mapping. All patients were retained in the final analysis regardless of the final histological diagnosis. Ultrasound images and reports were examined by an experienced clinician (G.G.) to assess the suspicion of extra-thyroidal extension and/or multifocal disease between November 2015 and December 2020. While this specific analysis was retrospectively performed, the reporting and collection of sonographic features was part of a prospective, pre-specified study; sonographic examinations were performed at the Thyroid Disease Clinic following a standard ultrasound scanning protocol.

Specifically, extra-thyroidal extension was suspected in the presence of images suggestive of thyroid border interruption or of nodular invasion of perithyroidal tissues. Suspicion of multifocal disease was defined if multiple suspicious nodules were visible. American College of Radiology (ACR) Thyroid Imaging Reporting and Data System (TIRADS) scores were determined for each patient in order to estimate their malignancy risk.

Histopathological reports were examined to identify the description of microscopic or macroscopic extra-thyroidal extension and unilateral (including lesions in one lobe and isthmus) or bilateral multifocal disease.

US performance was assessed using the final histology report as the reference standard, using Fisher's exact test to determine the statistical significance of US findings, and estimating sensitivity, specificity, positive and negative LR, and accuracy, each with 95% CI. Statistical analysis was performed with Microsoft Excel and MedCalc Software.

The study was conducted according to the guidelines of the Declaration of Helsinki and approved by the Ethics Committee of Sapienza University of Rome (protocol code 4233, 12 December 2016). Informed consent was obtained from all subjects involved in the study.

3. Results

The final cohort consisted of 45 patients with a family history of thyroid cancer and complete sonographic data, aged 24 to 79 (median 49; IQR 3–63), mostly female (67%). Overall, 5 patients belonged to kindreds with 1 family member affected by DTC, 30 patients to kindreds with 2 DTCs, and 10 patients to kindreds with 3 or more DTCs. Relevant clinical features of this cohort are summarized in Table 1.

Table 1. Clinical, sonographic, and pathological features of the study cohort.

Clinical Features	n. or Median	% or IQR
Age (years)	49	39–63
Gender, female	30	67
Gender, male	15	33
Pre-Surgical Cytology [1]:		
Not available/nondiagnostic (category Tir 1)	8	18
Benign (category Tir 2) *	4	9
Indeterminate (categories Tir 3A and 3B)	15	33
Suspicious (category Tir 4)	9	20
Malignant (category Tir 5)	9	20
Sonographic Features	n.	%
Single nodule	9	20
Multiple nodules, unilateral	11	24
Multiple nodules, bilateral	25	56
Suspicion of:		
Multiple malignant foci, unilateral	0	0
Multiple malignant foci, bilateral	7	16
Extra-thyroidal extension	12	27
Histology Report	n. or median	% or IQR
Tumor size (mm) *	8	5–13.5
PTC, classic variant	23	51
PTC, follicular variant	10	22
PTC, solid variant	1	2
PTC, variant not specified	3	7
FTC, minimally invasive	2	4
Anaplastic thyroid cancer	1	2
Benign *	5	11

Table 1. Cont.

Clinical Features	n. or Median	% or IQR
Multiple malignant foci, unilateral	5	11
Multiple malignant foci, bilateral	13	29
ETE, microscopic	13	29
ETE, macroscopic	1	2
Total	45	100

[1] Results according to the Italian Thyroid Cytology Classification System. Abbreviations: ETE: extrathyroidal extension; FNAC: fine-needle aspiration cytology; FTC: follicular thyroid cancer; PTC: papillary thyroid cancer. * Small foci of thyroid cancer were reported in this study even when the nodule submitted to cytology was shown to be benign, given the specific aim of the study. Patients with final benign histology were retained in the analysis because the whole cohort was submitted to surgery for concerns of malignancy (cytological or sonographical suspicion, in the context of family history of thyroid cancer) and the pre-surgical sonographic evaluation was performed for suspected cancer.

Thirty-seven patients had undergone FNA of suspicious nodules, classified according to the Italian Thyroid Cytology Classification System [14] as TIR2 to TIR5 (with indeterminate TIR3 class divided in a lower-risk group, TIR3A, and a higher-risk group, TIR3B), which approximately correspond to Bethesda [15] classes II to VI. One other patient had a FNA result of TIR1 (non-diagnostic). Seven patients had no FNA reports (not performed or not available).

3.1. Ultrasound and Surgical Pathology Results

US neck images and reports review showed that 25 (56%) patients had bilateral nodules, and 11 (24%) had unilateral multinodular disease; 9 (20%) patients had a solitary nodule. Of the 25 patients with bilateral nodules, 7 (16%) had a suspicion of bilateral multifocal DTC because of the presence of at least two suspicious nodules in the two lobes. The remaining 18 patients with bilateral nodules and the 11 patients with unilateral nodules had only one suspicious lesion, therefore having no suspicion of multifocality. Disruption of the thyroid capsule or a clear invasion of perithyroidal tissue was observed in 12 patients (27%) (Table 1).

Histological examination revealed 5 cases of benign adenomas and 40 cases of thyroid cancer, mostly papillary thyroid cancer. The median diameter of malignant nodules was 8 mm (IQR 5–13.5). A total of 18 patients (40%) had bilateral ($n = 13$) or unilateral ($n = 5$) multifocal disease. Microscopic ETE was observed in 13 cases (29%), while macroscopic ETE was observed in just one case (Table 1).

3.2. Diagnostic Performance of US Examination

The crosstabulations of US and surgical pathology reports for multifocality and extrathyroidal extension are illustrated in Tables 2 and 3, respectively. Among the 7 patients with US suspicion of multifocality, 4 (57%) had multifocal disease according to pathology reports. 14 (37%) out of 38 patients without multiple suspicious nodules had multifocal disease anyway. ETE, on the other hand, was observed in 5 cases (42%) out of 12 suspicious US figures, and in 9 (27%) cases out of 33 without such appearances.

Table 2. Multifocality according to US and histopathological reports.

US Features	Histopathological Features		Total
	Multifocality	No multifocality	
Multifocality	4 (57%)	3 (43%)	7
No multifocality	14 (37%)	24 (63%)	38
Total	18	27	45

Table 3. Extrathyroidal extension according to US and histopathological reports.

US Features	Histopathological Features		Total
	ETE	No ETE	
ETE	5 (42%)	7 (58%)	12
No ETE	9 (27%)	24 (73%)	33
Total	14	31	45

Table 4 summarizes the diagnostic performance of US findings in predicting multifocality and ETE. Even though absolute frequencies of confirmed ETE and multifocality seem to be higher in patients with US suspicion of these characteristics, the performance is not statistically significant, nor clinically useful. This is reflected in the non-significant results of positive and negative likelihood ratios.

Table 4. Diagnostic performance of US findings in predicting multifocality and ETE.

	Multifocality		ETE	
	value	95% CI	value	95% CI
Sensitivity	22.2%	6.41% to 47.64%	35.71%	12.76% to 64.86%
Specificity	88.89%	70.84% to 97.65%	77.42%	58.90% to 90.41%
Positive LR	2.00	0.51 to 7.89	1.58	0.61 to 4.12
Negative LR	0.88	0.66 to 1.16	0.83	0.54 to 1.28
PPV	57.14%	25.25% to 84.03%	41.67%	21.50% to 65.07%
NPV	63.16%	56.42% to 69.42%	72.73%	63.33% to 80.46%
Accuracy	62.22%	46.54% to 76.23%	64.44%	48.78% to 78.13%

ETE: extra-thyroidal extension; LR: likelihood ratio; PPV: positive predictive value; NPV: negative predictive value.

We then evaluated whether more suspicious nodules, based on the ACR TIRADS classification, were more likely to have ETE or multifocal disease. Only nodules classified as TR5 have a higher rate of ETE at histology (Table 5).

Table 5. Extrathyroidal extension and multifocality according to ACR TIRADS classification.

		ETE		Multifocality		Total
		No	Yes	No	Yes	
ACR TIRADS	TR2	4 (100%)	0 (0%)	4 (100%)	0 (0%)	4
	TR3	2 (100%)	0 (0%)	2 (100%)	0 (0%)	2
	TR4	13 (81%)	3 (19%)	10 (63%)	6 (37%)	16
	TR5	12 (52%)	11 (48%)	11 (48%)	12 (52%)	23
p		0.077		0.141		
TR2 to TR4		19 (86%)	3 (14%)	16 (73%)	6 (27%)	22
TR5		12 (52%)	11 (48%)	11 (48%)	12 (52%)	23
p		0.023		0.130		
Total		31 (69%)	14 (31%)	27 (60%)	18 (40%)	45

ACR: American College of Radiology; ETE: extra-thyroidal extension; TIRADS: Thyroid Imaging Reporting and Data System.

4. Discussion

In recent years, the clinical guideline recommendations were revised in order to avoid over-diagnosis in patients with low-risk thyroid nodules, aiming to promptly identifying patients with advanced or high-risk tumors requiring aggressive treatment approaches [16]. This involved discouraging screening programs [17,18], biopsy of suspicious subcentimeter nodules [10], and favoring less extensive surgery [19,20] and radioiodine use [21], as well as reducing the burden of post-surgical follow-up examinations [22,23]. These efforts are consistent with the general trend in reducing low-value care [24]. Some of these recommendations do not apply to patients with one or more first-degree relatives with a history of thyroid cancer due to the potentially more aggressive nature of their neoplasms [6,25].

According to some reports, patients with first-degree relatives affected by DTC have an increased risk of multifocality and extrathyroidal extension: these findings, according to some authors, would justify a more extensive surgery [26]. Actually, when thyroid surgery is advocated for a suspected familial thyroid cancer, a number of consensus statements report data to favor total thyroidectomy (e.g., Japan Association of Endocrine Surgery [19], and the American Association of Endocrine Surgeons documents [27]). The debate on whether familiarity can be counted as a risk factor in DTC patients is still ongoing, with some studies reporting more aggressive behavior and a higher rate of recurrence [28–30], and other studies finding no differences [31]. Still, the impact of microscopic ETE on disease recurrence is not clear, as some studies reported no difference between patients with and without microscopic ETE [32], while a recent meta-analysis documented an increased risk (with no effect on survival) [33].

In this study, we evaluated whether pre-operative US examination of patients eligible for surgery for a suspicious thyroid nodule and a family history of thyroid cancer was able to identify features suggestive of multifocality and microscopic extrathyroidal extension in order to potentially restrict total thyroidectomy to individuals in which one of these situations was detected or suspected. We have found that ultrasonography was not able to reliably detect microscopic extrathyroidal involvement or multifocal disease, as reported by the surgical pathology report. These results are consistent with most of the studies conducted on not selected DTC cohorts [12,13,34]; in some cases, with sufficient NPV to rule out ETE [35]. Some authors reported better performance of neck US in detecting thyroid cancer minimal extrathyroidal extension (with a NPV of 76.2% and a PPV of 81.4%) [36]. The latter study, however, evaluated larger tumors (1.81 ± 0.61 cm in patients with ETE), and the matching of the nodule identified by sonography and histopathology was not guaranteed. Another possible explanation of this discrepancy is that in our cohort, we retained nodules that were confirmed to be benign, but were sonographically assessed as potentially malignant. This figure dilutes the number of nodules that may actually have an extrathyroid extension at final histology. Not surprisingly, we have only found that more suspicious nodules (classified as ACR TIRADS 5) are more likely to present with ETE: it was reported that irregular margins increase the risk of completion thyroidectomy [37].

The present study has some limitations. First of all, the sample size was quite small, and more insight may be derived by the study of larger cohorts; for the same reason, we were unable to stratify our cohort according to the number of affected relatives (FNMTC is usually defined as the occurrence of the disease in two or more first-degree relatives of the patient). Furthermore, in the case of multifocal cancer, the size of the non-dominant foci is not available in many cases, not allowing for a stratification of very small foci (<1 mm) and larger foci, potentially assessable by sonography.

It remains to be elucidated whether ETE or microscopic involvement of the same or contralateral lobe affects the short and long-term outcomes of DTC patients and justifies a more aggressive surgical approach: their impact in the context of a familial DTC occurrence is still uncertain [6,38].

5. Conclusions

In patients with one or more first-degree relatives with DTC scheduled for surgery for suspicion of thyroid malignancy, pre-operative ultrasound examination is unable to reliably identify or exclude multifocal disease or extrathyroidal extension. Thus, the extent of the surgical approach cannot be reduced by a "negative" US report if clinicians and patients are worried about the potential subsequent pathological findings of multifocality and ETE.

Author Contributions: Conceptualization, C.D.; data curation, G.C. (Gianluca Cera); formal analysis, G.G. and G.C. (Gianluca Cera); investigation, G.G., G.C. (Gianluca Cera), V.D.G., C.R.T.d.G., M.M., P.L., V.C., A.M., R.M. (Rossella Melcarne), M.C.B., C.S., R.M. (Rosa Menditto), M.S., M.B. and L.G.; methodology, G.G. and V.C.; supervision, G.C. (Giovanni Conzo), C.D. and L.G.; writing—original draft, G.G. and G.C. (Gianluca Cera); writing—review & editing, G.G., G.C. (Gianluca Cera), G.C. (Giovanni Conzo), V.D.G. and C.D. All authors have read and agreed to the published version of the manuscript.

Funding: This research received no external funding.

Institutional Review Board Statement: The study was conducted according to the guidelines of the Declaration of Helsinki and approved by the Institutional Review Board (or Ethics Committee) of Sapienza University of Rome (protocol code 4233, 12 December 2016).

Informed Consent Statement: Informed consent was obtained from all subjects involved in the study.

Data Availability Statement: The data presented in this study are available on request from the corresponding author. The data are not publicly available due to patients' data confidentiality.

Conflicts of Interest: The authors declare no conflict of interest.

References

1. Links, T.P. Life Expectancy in Differentiated Thyroid Cancer: A Novel Approach to Survival Analysis. *Endocr. Relat. Cancer* **2005**, *12*, 273–280. [CrossRef]
2. Haugen, B.R.; Alexander, E.K.; Bible, K.C.; Doherty, G.M.; Mandel, S.J.; Nikiforov, Y.E.; Pacini, F.; Randolph, G.W.; Sawka, A.M.; Schlumberger, M.; et al. 2015 American Thyroid Association Management Guidelines for Adult Patients with Thyroid Nodules and Differentiated Thyroid Cancer: The American Thyroid Association Guidelines Task Force on Thyroid Nodules and Differentiated Thyroid Cancer. *Thyroid* **2016**, *26*, 1–133. [CrossRef] [PubMed]
3. Filetti, S.; Durante, C.; Hartl, D.; Leboulleux, S.; Locati, L.D.; Newbold, K.; Papotti, M.G.; Berruti, A.; ESMO Guidelines Committee. Thyroid Cancer: ESMO Clinical Practice Guidelines for Diagnosis, Treatment and Follow-Up. *Ann. Oncol* **2019**, *30*, 1856–1883. [CrossRef]
4. Luster, M.; Aktolun, C.; Amendoeira, I.; Barczyński, M.; Bible, K.C.; Duntas, L.H.; Elisei, R.; Handkiewicz-Junak, D.; Hoffmann, M.; Jarzab, B.; et al. European Perspective on 2015 American Thyroid Association Management Guidelines for Adult Patients with Thyroid Nodules and Differentiated Thyroid Cancer: Proceedings of an Interactive International Symposium. *Thyroid* **2019**. [CrossRef] [PubMed]
5. Mazeh, H.; Benavidez, J.; Poehls, J.L.; Youngwirth, L.; Chen, H. Sippel, R.S. In Patients with Thyroid Cancer of Follicular Cell Origin, a Family History of Nonmedullary Thyroid Cancer in One First-Degree Relative Is Associated with More Aggressive Disease. *Thyroid* **2012**, *22*, 3–8. [CrossRef] [PubMed]
6. Capezzone, M.; Robenshtok, E.; Cantara, S.; Castagna, M.G. Familial Non-Medullary Thyroid Cancer: A Critical Review. *J. Endocrinol. Investig.* **2021**, *44*, 943–950. [CrossRef]
7. Nixon, I.J.; Suárez, C.; Simo, R.; Sanabria, A.; Angelos, P.; Rinaldo, A.; Rodrigo, J.P.; Kowalski, L.P.; Hartl, D.M.; Hinni, M.L.; et al. The Impact of Family History on Non-Medullary Thyroid Cancer. *Eur. J. Surg. Oncol.* **2016**, *42*, 1455–1463. [CrossRef]
8. Nosé, V. Familial Thyroid Cancer: A Review. *Mod. Pathol.* **2011**, *24*, S19–S33. [CrossRef]
9. Ito, Y.; Miyauchi, A.; Oda, H. Low-Risk Papillary Microcarcinoma of the Thyroid: A Review of Active Surveillance Trials. *Eur. J. Surg. Oncol.* **2018**, *44*, 307–315. [CrossRef]
10. Grani, G.; Sponziello, M.; Pecce, V.; Ramundo, V.; Durante, C. Contemporary Thyroid Nodule Evaluation and Management. *J. Clin. Endocrinol. Metab.* **2020**, *105*, 2869–2883. [CrossRef]
11. Lamartina, L.; Grani, G.; Biffoni, M.; Giacomelli, L.; Costante, G.; Lupo, S.; Maranghi, M.; Plasmati, K.; Sponziello, M.; Trulli, F.; et al. Risk Stratification of Neck Lesions Detected Sonographically During the Follow-Up of Differentiated Thyroid Cancer. *J. Clin. Endocrinol. Metab.* **2016**, *101*, 3036–3044. [CrossRef] [PubMed]
12. Ramundo, V.; Di Gioia, C.R.T.; Falcone, R.; Lamartina, L.; Biffoni, M.; Giacomelli, L.; Filetti, S.; Durante, C.; Grani, G. Diagnostic Performance of Neck Ultrasonography in the Preoperative Evaluation for Extrathyroidal Extension of Suspicious Thyroid Nodules. *World J. Surg.* **2020**, *44*, 2669–2674. [CrossRef] [PubMed]
13. Lamartina, L.; Bidault, S.; Hadoux, J.; Guerlain, J.; Girard, E.; Breuskin, I.; Attard, M.; Suciu, V.; Baudin, E.; Al Ghuzlan, A.; et al. Can Preoperative Ultrasound Predict Extrathyroidal Extension of Differentiated Thyroid Cancer? *Eur. J. Endocrinol.* **2021**, *185*, 13–22. [CrossRef]
14. Nardi, F.; Basolo, F.; Crescenzi, A.; Fadda, G.; Frasoldati, A.; Orlandi, F.; Palombini, L.; Papini, E.; Zini, M.; Pontecorvi, A.; et al. Italian Consensus for the Classification and Reporting of Thyroid Cytology. *J. Endocrinol. Investig.* **2014**, *37*, 593–599. [CrossRef] [PubMed]
15. Baloch, Z.; LiVolsi, V.A. The Bethesda System for Reporting Thyroid Cytology (TBSRTC): From Look-Backs to Look-Ahead. *Diagn. Cytopathol.* **2020**, *48*, 862–866. [CrossRef]

16. Lamartina, L.; Grani, G.; Durante, C.; Filetti, S. Recent Advances in Managing Differentiated Thyroid Cancer. *F1000Research* **2018**, *7*, 86. [CrossRef]
17. US Preventive Services Task Force; Bibbins-Domingo, K.; Grossman, D.C.; Curry, S.J.; Barry, M.J.; Davidson, K.W.; Doubeni, C.A.; Epling, J.W.; Kemper, A.R.; Krist, A.H.; et al. Screening for Thyroid Cancer: US Preventive Services Task Force Recommendation Statement. *JAMA* **2017**, *317*, 1882–1887. [CrossRef]
18. Lin, J.S.; Bowles, E.J.A.; Williams, S.B.; Morrison, C.C. Screening for Thyroid Cancer: Updated Evidence Report and Systematic Review for the US Preventive Services Task Force. *JAMA* **2017**, *317*, 1888. [CrossRef]
19. Sugitani, I.; Ito, Y.; Takeuchi, D.; Nakayama, H.; Masaki, C.; Shindo, H.; Teshima, M.; Horiguchi, K.; Yoshida, Y.; Kanai, T.; et al. Indications and Strategy for Active Surveillance of Adult Low-Risk Papillary Thyroid Microcarcinoma: Consensus Statements from the Japan Association of Endocrine Surgery Task Force on Management for Papillary Thyroid Microcarcinoma. *Thyroid* **2021**, *31*, 183–192. [CrossRef]
20. Hartl, D.M.; Guerlain, J.; Breuskin, I.; Hadoux, J.; Baudin, E.; Al Ghuzlan, A.; Terroir-Cassou-Mounat, M.; Lamartina, L.; Leboulleux, S. Thyroid Lobectomy for Low to Intermediate Risk Differentiated Thyroid Cancer. *Cancers* **2020**, *12*, 3282. [CrossRef]
21. Grani, G.; Lamartina, L.; Alfò, M.; Ramundo, V.; Falcone, R.; Giacomelli, L.; Biffoni, M.; Filetti, S.; Durante, C. Selective Use of Radioactive Iodine Therapy for Papillary Thyroid Cancers With Low or Lower-Intermediate Recurrence Risk. *J. Clin. Endocrinol. Metab.* **2021**, *106*, e1717–e1727. [CrossRef] [PubMed]
22. Peiling Yang, S.; Bach, A.M.; Tuttle, R.M.; Fish, S.A. Frequent Screening with Serial Neck Ultrasound Is More Likely to Identify False-Positive Abnormalities than Clinically Significant Disease in the Surveillance of Intermediate Risk Papillary Thyroid Cancer Patients without Suspicious Findings on Follow-up Ultrasound Evaluation. *J. Clin. Endocrinol. Metab.* **2015**, *100*, 1561–1567. [CrossRef] [PubMed]
23. Grani, G.; Ramundo, V.; Falcone, R.; Lamartina, L.; Montesano, T.; Biffoni, M.; Giacomelli, L.; Sponziello, M.; Verrienti, A.; Schlumberger, M.; et al. Thyroid Cancer Patients With No Evidence of Disease: The Need for Repeat Neck Ultrasound. *J. Clin. Endocrinol. Metab.* **2019**, *104*, 4981–4989. [CrossRef] [PubMed]
24. Ospina, N.S.; Salloum, R.G.; Maraka, S.; Brito, J.P. De-Implementing Low-Value Care in Endocrinology. *Endocrine* **2021**, *73*, 292–300. [CrossRef] [PubMed]
25. Lamartina, L.; Grani, G.; Durante, C.; Filetti, S.; Cooper, D.S. Screening for Differentiated Thyroid Cancer in Selected Populations. *Lancet Diabetes Endocrinol.* **2020**, *8*, 81–88. [CrossRef]
26. Kim, Y.S.; Seo, M.; Park, S.H.; Ju, S.Y.; Kim, E.S. Should Total Thyroidectomy Be Recommended for Patients with Familial Non-Medullary Thyroid Cancer? *World J. Surg.* **2020**, *44*, 3022–3027. [CrossRef]
27. Patel, K.N.; Yip, L.; Lubitz, C.C.; Grubbs, E.G.; Miller, B.S.; Shen, W.; Angelos, P.; Chen, H.; Doherty, G.M.; Fahey, T.J.; et al. The American Association of Endocrine Surgeons Guidelines for the Definitive Surgical Management of Thyroid Disease in Adults. *Ann. Surg.* **2020**, *271*, e21–e93. [CrossRef] [PubMed]
28. Cao, J.; Chen, C.; Chen, C.; Wang, Q.-L.; Ge, M.-H. Clinicopathological Features and Prognosis of Familial Papillary Thyroid Carcinoma—A Large-Scale, Matched, Case-Control Study. *Clin. Endocrinol.* **2016**, *84*, 598–606. [CrossRef]
29. Lee, Y.-M.; Yoon, J.H.; Yi, O.; Sung, T.-Y.; Chung, K.-W.; Kim, W.B.; Hong, S.J. Familial History of Non-Medullary Thyroid Cancer Is an Independent Prognostic Factor for Tumor Recurrence in Younger Patients with Conventional Papillary Thyroid Carcinoma: Familial History of Thyroid Cancer. *J. Surg. Oncol.* **2014**, *109*, 168–173. [CrossRef]
30. McDonald, T.J.; Driedger, A.A.; Garcia, B.M.; Van Uum, S.H.M.; Rachinsky, I.; Chevendra, V.; Breadner, D.; Feinn, R.; Walsh, S.J.; Malchoff, C.D. Familial Papillary Thyroid Carcinoma: A Retrospective Analysis. *J. Oncol.* **2011**, *2011*, 948786. [CrossRef]
31. Muallem Kalmovich, L.; Jabarin, B.; Koren, S.; Or, K.; Marcus, E.; Tkacheva, I.; Benbassat, C.; Steinschneider, M. Is Familial Nonmedullary Thyroid Cancer A More Aggressive Type of Thyroid Cancer? *Laryngoscope* **2021**, *131*. [CrossRef]
32. Liu, L.; Oh, C.; Heo, J.H.; Park, H.S.; Lee, K.; Chang, J.W.; Jung, S.-N.; Koo, B.S. Clinical Significance of Extrathyroidal Extension According to Primary Tumor Size in Papillary Thyroid Carcinoma. *Eur. J. Surg. Oncol.* **2018**, *44*, 1754–1759. [CrossRef]
33. Kim, H.; Kwon, H.; Moon, B.-I. Association of Multifocality with Prognosis of Papillary Thyroid Carcinoma: A Systematic Review and Meta-Analysis. *JAMA Otolaryngol. Head Neck Surg.* **2021**, *147*, 847–854. [CrossRef] [PubMed]
34. Chung, S.R.; Baek, J.H.; Choi, Y.J.; Sung, T.-Y.; Song, D.E.; Kim, T.Y.; Lee, J.H. Sonographic Assessment of the Extent of Extrathyroidal Extension in Thyroid Cancer. *Korean J. Radiol.* **2020**, *21*, 1187. [CrossRef] [PubMed]
35. Kuo, E.J.; Thi, W.J.; Zheng, F.; Zanocco, K.A.; Livhits, M.J.; Yeh, M.W. Individualizing Surgery in Papillary Thyroid Carcinoma Based on a Detailed Sonographic Assessment of Extrathyroidal Extension. *Thyroid* **2017**, *27*, 1544–1549. [CrossRef] [PubMed]
36. Hu, S.; Zhang, H.; Sun, Z.; Ge, Y.; Li, J.; Yu, C.; Deng, Z.; Dou, W.; Wang, X. Preoperative Assessment of Extrathyroidal Extension of Papillary Thyroid Carcinomas by Ultrasound and Magnetic Resonance Imaging: A Comparative Study. *Radiol. Med.* **2020**, *125*, 870–876. [CrossRef]
37. Leong, D.; Ng, K.; Nguyen, H.; Ryan, S. Preoperative Ultrasound Characteristics in Determining the Likelihood of Cytologically Confirmed (Bethesda VI), 1-4 Cm Papillary Thyroid Tumours Requiring Completion Thyroidectomy. *Asian J. Surg.* **2021**, in press. [CrossRef] [PubMed]
38. Bortz, M.D.; Kuchta, K.; Winchester, D.J.; Prinz, R.A.; Moo-Young, T.A. Extrathyroidal Extension Predicts Negative Clinical Outcomes in Papillary Thyroid Cancer. *Surgery* **2021**, *169*, 2–6. [CrossRef] [PubMed]

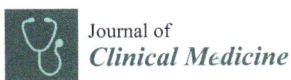

Article

Impact of Multifocality on the Recurrence of Papillary Thyroid Carcinoma

Joohyun Woo, Hyeonkyeong Kim and Hyungju Kwon *

Department of Surgery, Ewha Womans University Medical Center, 1071 Anyangcheon-ro, Yangcheon-Gu, Seoul 07985, Korea; jwoo@ewha.ac.kr (J.W.); cathy6280@naver.com (H.K.)
* Correspondence: hkwon@ewha.ac.kr; Tel.: +82-2-2650-5025

Abstract: The incidence of thyroid cancer has dramatically increased over the last few decades, and up to 60% of patients have multifocal tumors. However, the prognostic impact of multifocality in patients with papillary thyroid carcinoma (PTC) remains unestablished and controversial. We evaluate whether multifocality can predict the recurrence of PTC. A total of 1249 patients who underwent total thyroidectomy for PTC at the Ewha Medical Center between March 2012 and December 2019 were reviewed. In this study, multifocality was found in 487 patients (39.0%) and the mean follow-up period was 5.5 ± 2.7 years. Multifocality was associated with high-risk features for recurrence, including extrathyroidal extension, lymph node metastasis, and margin involvement. After adjustment of those clinicopathological features, 10-year disease-free survival was 93.3% in patients with multifocal tumors, whereas those with unifocal disease showed 97.6% ($p = 0.011$). Multivariate Cox regression analysis indicated that male sex (HR 2.185, 95% CI 1.047–4.559), tumor size (HR 1.806, 95% CI 1.337–2.441), N1b LN metastasis (HR 3.603, 95% CI 1.207–10.757), and multifocality (HR 1.986, 95% CI 1.015–3.888) were independent predictors of recurrence. In conclusion, multifocality increased the risk of recurrence in patients with PTC. Patients with multifocal PTCs may need judicious treatment and follow-up approaches.

Keywords: papillary thyroid carcinoma; multifocality; recurrence

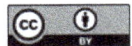

1. Introduction

Thyroid cancer is one of the more common cancers worldwide, and its incidence has rapidly increased over the last few decades [1]. In 2018, 567,233 patients were newly diagnosed with thyroid cancer, accounting for 3.1% of total cancer cases. Papillary thyroid carcinoma (PTC) represents more than 80% of all thyroid malignancies, which usually have a favorable prognosis [2]. Nevertheless, up to 50% of patients experience cancer relapse, including loco-regional recurrences or distant metastases [2,3]. Many studies have attempted to differentiate these patients at high risk from the population with excellent outcomes [4,5]. Several clinicopathological factors, including tumor size, extrathyroidal extension (ETE), and multifocality of tumor have been investigated to predict recurrence.

Multifocality has been considered as a prognostic marker for the recurrence of PTC [6,7]. The latest American Thyroid Association (ATA) and the European Thyroid Association (ETA) guidelines included multifocality as a risk factor for recurrence [8,9]. Although multifocality alone without other risk factors was classified as a low-risk category, these guidelines indicated that multifocality could assist in proper risk stratification for predicting recurrence. A consensus report of the European Society of Endocrine Surgeons suggested that multifocality might have a prognostic impact in overt PTC [6]. Other risk stratification systems also addressed the prognostic role of multifocality on cancer-specific survival [10]. However, recent studies raised questions about the impact of multifocality on the recurrence of PTC [11,12].

There is a controversy about the prognostic significance of multifocality in PTC. Several studies have suggested that multifocality is associated with a higher risk of recurrences and distant metastasis [13–15]. A few researchers further demonstrated that multifocal PTCs could decrease overall and cancer-specific survival [16]. On the contrary, other research has indicated that patients with multifocal disease showed a similar clinical course or comparable recurrence rates to those with unifocal disease [17,18]. A large multicenter study also suggested that multifocality of PTC had no independent impact on recurrences and mortality after adjustment of potential confounders [12]. Lim et al. further reported that patients with multifocal diseases might have lower risk of recurrences [19]. These conflicting data resulted from, at least in part, unadjusted clinicopathological characteristics or a limited number of patients.

In the present study, therefore, we investigated the effect of multifocality to the recurrence of PTC in a large cohort, using propensity score matching for adjustment of confounders.

2. Materials and Methods

Our institutional review board approved this retrospective cohort study (Approval No. 2021-07-015) and waived the requirement for written informed consent. This study included 1249 consecutive patients with thyroid cancer who underwent total thyroidectomy from March 2012 to December 2019. Neck ultrasonography and computed tomography was performed preoperatively in all patients to evaluate tumor location, multifocality, and cervical lymph node (LN) metastasis. Patients with suspicious LN enlargement underwent therapeutic LN dissection in addition to total thyroidectomy.

Demographic data, pathologic characteristics including tumor size, ETE, resection margin involvement, coexisting Hashimoto thyroiditis, LN metastasis, multifocality, and adjuvant radioiodine treatment were recorded. On the histopathological examination, entire thyroid glands were serially sectioned and examined. The World Health Organization criteria for PTC variants and the American Joint Committee on Cancer 7th edition were used for Tumor–Node–Metastasis (TNM) staging. Follow-up period and recurrence status were also collected and analyzed. The primary outcome measure was the recurrence-free survival (RFS).

To minimize selection bias and possible confounding effects, we performed 1:1 propensity score matching [20]. A propensity score measures the probability that a patient would have been treated using a covariates score. Thus, propensity score matching balances the covariates and increases the comparability between the patients with multifocal tumors and those with unifocal PTC. We selected 3 factors that could affect recurrences as follows: ETE, LN metastasis, and resection margin involvement. SPSS Statistics version 23.0 (IBM Corp., Armonk, NY, USA) was used for data analyses. Comparison of continuous data was performed using Student's t-tests. Dichotomous data were compared using chi-squared tests. RFS were assessed by using the log rank test and Kaplan–Meier plots. Cox proportional-hazards regression analysis was used to evaluate the relationship between prognostic factors and recurrence. A p-value less than 0.05 was considered statistically significant.

3. Results

3.1. Clinicopathological Characteristics of 1249 PTC Patients

The baseline characteristics of the included patients are summarized in Table 1. Mean age was 47.4 ± 11.4 years at the time of surgery and 1095 (87.7%) were women. The mean follow-up period was 5.5 ± 2.7 years (range, 1.0–11.1 years). Most patients (93.5%) had classical subtype of PTCs, while the remaining 81 patients with PTC variants included 53 patients with follicular variants including 7 encapsulated forms, 10 tall cell variants, 9 encapsulated variants, 4 oncocytic variants, 3 diffuse sclerosing variants, 1 columnar cell variant, and 1 hobnail variant.

Table 1. Comparison of clinicopathological characteristics between patients with multifocal PTCs and those with unifocal tumors.

Characteristics	Multifocal (n = 487)	Unifocal (n = 762)	p-Value
Age (years)	47.8 ± 11.5	47.1 ± 11.4	0.330
Female sex	425 (87.3%)	670 (87.9%)	0.730
Pathologic characteristics			
Subtype			0.244
Classical	460 (94.5%)	708 (92.9%)	
Follicular	20 (4.1%)	33 (4.3%)	
Tall cell	3 (0.6%)	7 (0.9%)	
Encapsulated	1 (0.2%)	8 (1.0%)	
Oncocytic	0 (0.0%)	4 (0.5%)	
Diffuse sclerosing	2 (0.4%)	1 (0.1%)	
Hobnail	1 (0.2%)	0 (0.0%)	
Columnar	0 (0.0%)	1 (0.1%)	
Tumor size (cm)	1.0 ± 0.7	1.0 ± 0.7	0.133
Microscopic ETE	327 (67.3%)	436 (57.3%)	<0.001
Lymphovascular invasion	10 (2.1%)	17 (2.2%)	0.833
Perineural invasion	1 (0.2%)	2 (0.3%)	0.841
LN metastasis			0.007
N0	258 (53.0%)	463 (60.8%)	
N1a	171 (35.1%)	240 (31.5%)	
N1b	58 (11.9%)	59 (7.7%)	
Margin involvement	22 (4.5%)	18 (2.4%)	0.035
Coexisting HT	130 (26.7%)	214 (28.1%)	0.592
Postoperative management			
^{131}I remnant ablation	227 (46.6%)	313 (41.1%)	0.054
^{131}I dose (mCi)	135.4 ± 38.2	134.6 ± 31.9	0.790
Follow-up period (years)	5.3 ± 2.8	5.6 ± 2.6	0.042
Recurrence	21 (4.3%)	15 (2.0%)	0.016

PTC, papillary thyroid carcinoma; ETE, extrathyroidal extension; LN, lymph node; HT, Hashimoto thyroiditis.

Of the 1249 patients enrolled, 487 patients (39.0%) had multifocal PTCs and 762 (61.0%) had unifocal tumor. Thyroid cancer in patients with multifocal PTCs showed a higher rate of ETE (67.3% vs. 57.3%; $p < 0.001$) and a microscopic resection margin involvement (4.5% vs. 2.4%; $p = 0.035$) than in patients with unifocal tumor (Table 1). LN metastasis was also more common in the multifocality group than in the unifocality group ($p = 0.007$). Distant metastasis was not observed in all patients. Other clinicopathological factors, including age, sex, and tumor size, showed no significant differences between the groups.

Recurrences were found in 21 patients (4.3%) in patients with multifocal PTCs, and 15 patients (2.0%) with unifocal tumor developed recurrence ($p = 0.013$). A log-rank test indicated that 10-year RFS was significantly lower in the multifocality group (93.3% vs. 97.1%; $p = 0.011$) than in the unifocality group (Figure 1a).

3.2. Comparison of Recurrence Rates in the Matched Cohorts

As LN metastasis or resection margin involvement could affect the risk of recurrence, we performed 1:1 propensity score matching and yielded 487 matched pairs. Table 2 shows the clinicopathological comparison between the multifocality group and the 1:1 matched unifocality group. The matched cohorts did not differ in terms of clinicopathological features including microscopic ETE, margin involvement, and LN metastasis.

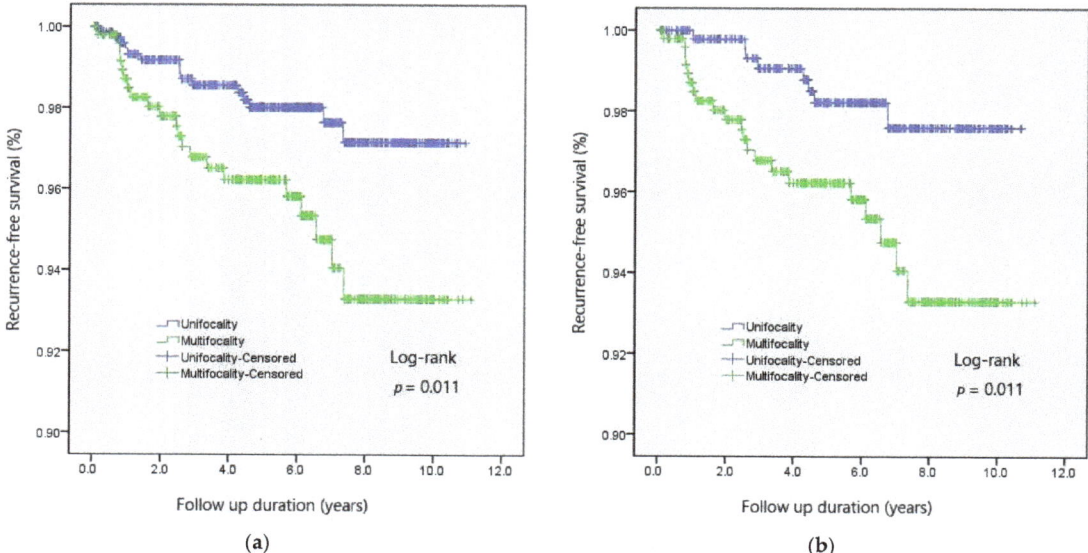

Figure 1. Recurrence-free survival according to the multifocality in patients with PTC, (**a**) before and (**b**) after propensity score matching.

Table 2. Comparison of clinicopathological characteristics between patients with multifocal PTCs and those with unifocal tumor after propensity score matching.

Characteristics	Multifocal (n = 487)	Unifocal (n = 487)	p-Value
Age (years)	47.8 ± 11.5	47.0 ± 12.0	0.279
Female sex	425 (87.3%)	426 (87.5%)	0.923
Pathologic characteristics			
Subtype			0.996
Classical	460 (94.5%)	460 (92.9%)	
Follicular	20 (4.1%)	21 (4.3%)	
Tall cell	3 (0.6%)	3 (0.9%)	
Encapsulated	1 (0.2%)	1 (1.0%)	
Oncocytic	0 (0.0%)	0 (0.5%)	
Diffuse sclerosing	2 (0.4%)	1 (0.1%)	
Hobnail	1 (0.2%)	0 (0.0%)	
Columnar	0 (0.0%)	0 (0.1%)	
Tumor size (cm)	1.0 ± 0.7	1.0 ± 0.7	0.864
Microscopic ETE	327 (67.3%)	319 (65.6%)	0.587
Lymphovascular invasion	10 (2.1%)	12 (2.5%)	0.666
Perineural invasion	1 (0.2%)	1 (0.2%)	1.000
LN metastasis			0.995
N0	258 (53.0%)	257 (52.8%)	
N1a	171 (35.1%)	171 (35.1%)	
N1b	58 (11.9%)	59 (12.1%)	
Margin involvement	22 (4.5%)	18 (3.7%)	0.518
Coexisting HT	130 (26.7%)	127 (26.1%)	0.827
Postoperative management			
^{131}I remnant ablation	227 (46.6%)	236 (48.6%)	0.543
^{131}I dose (mCi)	135.4 ± 38.2	136.3 ± 32.7	0.786
Follow-up period (years)	5.3 ± 2.8	5.6 ± 2.6	0.089
Recurrence	21 (4.3%)	8 (1.6%)	0.014

PTC, papillary thyroid carcinoma; ETE, extrathyroidal extension; LN, lymph node; HT, Hashimoto thyroiditis.

The overall recurrence rate was higher in the multifocality group than in the matched unifocality group (4.3% vs. 1.6%; p = 0.014), after adjustment of potential confounders. The 10-year RFS was also lower in the multifocality group (93.3% vs. 97.6%; p = 0.011) than in the matched group (Figure 1b).

3.3 Predictive Factors of Poor RFS in Patients with PTC

Univariate Cox proportional-hazards model indicated that male sex (HR 2.974, 95% CI 1.433–6.170), tumor size (HR 2.340, 95% CI 1.833–2.987), microscopic ETE (HR 2.708, 95% CI 1.186–6.182), LN metastasis (HR for N1a 3.858, 95% CI 1.587–9.380; HR for N1b 12.704, 95% CI 5.066–31.857), ^{131}I remnant ablation (HR 6.512, 95% CI 2.709–15.656), and multifocality (HR 2.294, 95% CI 1.183–4.451) were significantly associated with the recurrence (Table 3). Male sex (HR 2.185, 95% CI 1.047–4.559), tumor size (HR 1.806, 95% CI 1.337–2.441), N1b LN metastasis (HR 3.603, 95% CI 1.207–10.757), and multifocality (HR 1.986, 95% CI 1.015–3.888) retained statistical significance in multivariate analysis.

Table 3. Comparison of clinicopathological characteristics between patients with multifocal PTCs and those with unifocal tumor after propensity score matching.

Characteristics	Univariate Analysis		Multivariate Analysis	
	HR (95% CI)	p-Value	HR (95% CI)	p-Value
Age (years)	0.982 (0.952–1.012)	0.239		
Male sex	2.974 (1.433–6.170)	0.003	2.185 (1.047–4.559)	0.037
Tumor size (cm)	2.340 (1.833–2.987)	<0.001	1.806 (1.337–2.441)	<0.001
Microscopic ETE	2.708 (1.186–6.182)	0.018	1.311 (0.551–3.122)	0.541
LN metastasis				
N1a	3.858 (1.587–9.380)	0.003	1.859 (0.677–5.102)	0.229
N1b	12.704 (5.066–31.857)	<0.001	3.603 (1.207–10.757)	0.022
Margin involvement	2.071 (0.497–8.628)	0.317		
Hashimoto thyroiditis	0.643 (0.282–1.467)	0.294		
^{131}I remnant ablation	6.512 (2.709–15.656)	<0.001	2.345 (0.807–6.812)	0.117
Multifocality	2.294 (1.183–4.451)	0.014	1.986 (1.015–3.888)	0.045

HR, hazard ratio; CI, confidence interval; ETE, extrathyroidal extension; LN, lymph node.

4. Discussion

The present study demonstrates that multifocal PTCs are associated with a higher risk of recurrence. Multifocality is defined as the simultaneous presence of two or more anatomically separated foci within the thyroid gland [21]. Multifocal PTCs may result from intrathyroidal spread of original tumor or from multicentric independent PTCs [21]. The prevalence of multifocality in PTC ranges from 7.2 to 60.1% of the cases in the recent series [22,23]. The occurrence of multifocality varies according to the epidemiological and environmental factors [6]. Development of multifocal tumors can be associated with radiation, genetic disorders, or a family history of thyroid cancer [24,25]. A BRAF mutation also plays a role in inducing multifocality [26,27]. Furthermore, obese and overweight patients had a higher risk of multifocality [28].

Multifocality is associated with some high-risk features for the progression of PTC [7–9]. We demonstrated that multifocality was associated with higher ETE, LN metastasis, and microscopic resection margin involvement. Feng et al. showed that patients with multifocal PTCs had higher risk of large tumor size, ETE, vascular invasion, and LN metastasis [29]. Other researchers further indicated that multifocality was related with aggressive histologic subtype or higher ATA risk of recurrence [14,15]. A previous meta-analysis also suggested that multifocality was associated with an increased risk of tumor size >1 cm, ETE, and LN metastasis [13]. Hence, more radical treatments, including total thyroidectomy and radioactive iodine ablation, were commonly applied to patients with multifocal PTCs [6,7,30].

There is a controversy as to whether multifocality itself increases the risk of recurrence. Multifocality-associated high-risk features including ETE, LN metastasis, and margin involvement can affect the risk of recurrences. Previous studies further demonstrated that the impact of multifocality might be different according to the primary tumor size. In the present study, therefore, we performed propensity score matching to adjust potential confounders for minimizing biases. After propensity score matching, the overall recurrence rate was still higher in the multifocality group (4.3% vs. 1.6%; $p = 0.014$) than in the unifocality group. Survival analysis also indicated that patients with multifocal PTCs had a 1.986-fold higher risk of developing recurrences than those with unifocal tumors. Further validation studies may be helpful to confirm the impact of multifocality.

In the present study, male sex, tumor size, and N1b LN metastasis significantly increased the risk of recurrence, respectively. Data from the Canadian Collaborative Network for Cancer of the Thyroid indicated that men were at greater risk for recurrence than women (HR 2.31, 95% CI 1.48–3.60) [31]. Tumor size also has been widely accepted as a risk factor for recurrence in various risk stratification system, including AMES, AGES, and MACIS score [32]. N1b LN metastasis has been further recognized as a predictive factor for recurrence [33]. A meta-analysis suggested that a tumor size over 2 cm (OR 2.69, 95% CI 2.06–3.50) and LN metastasis (OR 3.24, 95% CI 2.61–4.02) were predictive factors for recurrence [34]. Wang et al. demonstrated that male sex, tumor size, and LN metastasis were associated with tumor recurrence of PTC in their large, multicenter study [12]. Our results are consistent with these previous reports.

This study has some limitations. First, our study was a retrospective cohort study, which was prone to a selection bias. Patient selection for receiving radioactive iodine ablation might be influenced by various factors and result in the difference of tumor recurrence. Second, we did not consider a family history or genetic mutation including BRAF mutation. Familial nonmedullary thyroid carcinoma can be more aggressive than the sporadic form [24,25]. However, because of the lack of data, we cannot evaluate the effect of family history or genetic mutation in the present study. Validation for the impact of multifocality is required in patients with family history or BRAF mutation. Third, we did not investigate the long-term prognosis including mortality. The mean follow-up period of 5.5 years was not sufficient for evaluating cancer-specific survival. Last, it is unclear whether patients with multifocal PTCs require aggressive treatment, although we demonstrated that multifocality increased the risk of recurrence. Further comparative studies are warranted to address these issues.

5. Conclusions

Multifocality increased the risk of recurrence in patients with PTC. Patients with multifocal PTCs may need judicious treatment and follow-up approaches.

Author Contributions: Conceptualization, J.W. and H.K. (Hyungju Kwon); methodology, H.K. (Hyeonkyeong Kim); validation, H.K. (Hyungju Kwon); formal analysis, J.W. and H.K. (Hyeonkyeong Kim); resources, H.K. (Hyeonkyeong Kim); data curation, H.K. (Hyeonkyeong Kim); writing—original draft preparation, H.K. (Hyeonkyeong Kim); writing—review and editing, J.W. and H.K. (Hyungju Kwon); project administration, H.K. (Hyungju Kwon). All authors have read and agreed to the published version of the manuscript.

Funding: This research received no external funding.

Institutional Review Board Statement: The study was conducted according to the guidelines of the Declaration of Helsinki and approved by the Institutional Review Board of the Ewha University Medical Center (Approval No. 15 July 2021).

Informed Consent Statement: Patient consent was waived by the institutional review board, because (1) this research involved no more than minimal risk to subjects, and (2) this research could be carried out practicably without the waiver.

Data Availability Statement: The data presented in this study are available on request from the corresponding author. The data are not publicly available due to institutional policy.

Conflicts of Interest: The authors declare no conflict of interest.

References

1. Bray, F.; Ferlay, J.; Soerjomataram, I.; Siegel, R.L.; Torre, L.A.; Jemal, A. Global cancer statistics 2018: GLOBOCAN estimates of incidence and mortality worldwide for 36 cancers in 185 countries. *CA Cancer J. Clin.* **2018**, *68*, 394–424. [CrossRef]
2. Cho, B.Y.; Choi, H.S.; Park, Y.J.; Lim, J.A.; Ahn, H.Y.; Lee, E.K.; Kim, K.W.; Yi, K.H.; Chung, J.-K.; Youn, Y.-K., et al. Changes in the Clinicopathological Characteristics and Outcomes of Thyroid Cancer in Korea over the Past Four Decades. *Thyroid* **2013**, *23*, 797–804. [CrossRef] [PubMed]
3. Tuttle, R.M.; Ball, D.W.; Byrd, D.; Dilawari, R.A.; Doherty, G.M.; Duh, Q.Y.; Ehya, H.; Farrar, W.B.; Haddad, R.I.; Kandeel, F.; et al. Thyroid carcinoma. *J. Natl. Compr. Cancer Netw.* **2010**, *8*, 1228–1274. [CrossRef]
4. Suh, Y.J.; Kwon, H.; Kim, S.J.; Choi, J.Y.; Lee, K.E.; Park, Y.J.; Park, D.J.; Youn, Y.K. Factors Affecting the Locoregional Recurrence of Conventional Papillary Thyroid Carcinoma After Surgery: A Retrospective Analysis of 3381 Patients. *Ann. Surg. Oncol.* **2015**, *22*, 3543–3549. [CrossRef] [PubMed]
5. Li, X.; Kwon, H. The Impact of BRAF Mutation on the Recurrence of Papillary Thyroid Carcinoma: A Meta-Analysis. *Cancers* **2020**, *12*, 2056. [CrossRef]
6. Iacobone, M.; Jansson, S.; Barczynski, M.; Goretzki, P. Multifocal papillary thyroid carcinoma—A consensus report of the European Society of Endocrine Surgeons (ESES). *Langenbecks Arch. Surg.* **2014**, *399*, 141–154. [CrossRef] [PubMed]
7. Filetti, S.; Durante, C.; Hartl, D.; Leboulleux, S.; Locati, L.; Newbold, K.; Papotti, M.; Berruti, A. Thyroid cancer: ESMO Clinical Practice Guidelines for diagnosis, treatment and follow-up. *Ann. Oncol.* **2019**, *30*, 1856–1883. [CrossRef] [PubMed]
8. Haugen, B.R.; Alexander, E.K.; Bible, K.C.; Doherty, G.M.; Mandel, S.J.; Nikiforov, Y.E.; Pacini, F.; Randolph, G.W.; Sawka, A.M.; Schlumberger, M.; et al. 2015 American Thyroid Association Management Guidelines for Adult Patients with Thyroid Nodules and Differentiated Thyroid Cancer: The American Thyroid Association Guidelines Task Force on Thyroid Nodules and Differentiated Thyroid Cancer. *Thyroid* **2016**, *26*, 1–133. [CrossRef]
9. Pacini, F.; Schlumberger, M.; Dralle, H.; Elisei, R.; Smit, J.W.; Wiersinga, W. European consensus for the management of patients with differentiated thyroid carcinoma of the follicular epithelium. *Eur. J. Endocrinol.* **2006**, *154*, 787–803. [CrossRef]
10. Momesso, D.P.; Tuttle, R.M. Update on Differentiated Thyroid Cancer Staging. *Endocrinol. Metab. Clin. N. Am.* **2014**, *43*, 401–421. [CrossRef]
11. Geron, Y.; Benbassat, C.; Shteinshneider, M.; Or, K.; Markus, E.; Hirsch, D.; Levy, S.; Ziv-Baran, T.; Muallem-Kalmovich, L. Multifocality Is not an Independent Prognostic Factor in Papillary Thyroid Cancer: A Propensity Score–Matching Analysis. *Thyroid* **2019**, *29*, 513–522. [CrossRef]
12. Wang, F.; Yu, X.; Shen, X.; Zhu, G.; Huang, Y.; Liu, R.; Viola, D.; Elisei, R.; Puxeddu, E.; Fugazzola, L.; et al. The Prognostic Value of Tumor Multifocality in Clinical Outcomes of Papillary Thyroid Cancer. *J. Clin. Endocrinol. Metab.* **2017**, *102*, 3241–3250. [CrossRef]
13. Joseph, K.R.; Edirimanne, S.; Eslick, G.D. Multifocality as a prognostic factor in thyroid cancer: A meta-analysis. *Int. J. Surg.* **2018**, *50*, 121–125. [CrossRef] [PubMed]
14. Vuong, H.G.; Duong, U.N.P.; Pham, T.Q.; Tran, H.M.; Oishi, N.; Mochizuki, K.; Nakazawa, T.; Hassell, L.; Katoh, R.; Kondo, T. Clinicopathological Risk Factors for Distant Metastasis in Differentiated Thyroid Carcinoma: A Meta-analysis. *World J. Surg.* **2018**, *42*, 1005–1017. [CrossRef] [PubMed]
15. Qu, N.; Zhang, L.; Lu, Z.W.; Ji, Q.H.; Yang, S.W.; Wei, W.J.; Zhang, Y. Predictive factors for recurrence of differentiated thyroid cancer in patients under 21 years of age and a meta-analysis of the current literature. *Tumor Biol.* **2016**, *37*, 7797–7808. [CrossRef] [PubMed]
16. Markovic, I.; Goran, M.; Besic, N.; Buta, M.; Djurisic, I.; Stojiljkovic, D.; Zegarac, M.; Pupic, G.; Inic, Z.; Dzodic, R. Multifocality as independent prognostic factor in papillary thyroid cancer—A multivariate analysis. *J. BUON* **2018**, *23*, 1049–1054.
17. Guo, K.; Wang, Z. Risk factors influencing the recurrence of papillary thyroid carcinoma: A systematic review and meta-analysis. *Int. J. Clin. Exp. Pathol.* **2014**, *7*, 5393–5403.
18. Kim, J.K.; Kim, M.J.; Choi, S.H.; Choi, S.M.; Choi, H.R.; Lee, C.R.; Kang, S.; Lee, J.; Jeong, J.J.; Nam, K.; et al. Cystic Lateral Lymph Node Metastases From Papillary Thyroid Cancer Patients. *Laryngoscope* **2020**, *130*. [CrossRef]
19. Lim, Y.C.; Liu, L.; Chang, J.W.; Koo, B.S. Lateral lymph node recurrence after total thyroidectomy and central neck dissection in patients with papillary thyroid cancer without clinical evidence of lateral neck metastasis. *Oral Oncol.* **2016**, *62*, 109–113. [CrossRef]
20. Lee, K.E.; Koo, D.H.; Im, H.J.; Park, S.K.; Choi, J.Y.; Paeng, J.C.; Chung, J.-K.; Oh, S.K.; Youn, Y.-K. Surgical completeness of bilateral axillo-breast approach robotic thyroidectomy: Comparison with conventional open thyroidectomy after propensity score matching. *Surgery* **2011**, *150*, 1266–1274. [CrossRef]
21. Kuhn, E.; Teller, L.; Piana, S.; Rosai, J.; Merino, M.J. Different Clonal Origin of Bilateral Papillary Thyroid Carcinoma, with a Review of the Literature. *Endocr. Pathol.* **2012**, *23*, 101–107. [CrossRef] [PubMed]
22. Wang, Z.; Xiang, J.; Gui, Z.; Qin, Y.; Sun, W.; Huang, J.; He, L.; Dong, W.; Zhang, D.; Zhang, T.; et al. Unilateral Tnm T1 and T2 thyroid papillary carcinoma with lateral Cervical lymph node metastasis: Total thyroidectomy or lobectomy? *Endocr. Pract.* **2020**, *26*, 1085–1092. [CrossRef] [PubMed]
23. Qu, N.; Zhang, L.; Ji, Q.-H.; Zhu, Y.-X.; Wang, Z.-Y.; Shen, Q.; Wang, Y.; Li, D.-S. Number of tumor foci predicts prognosis in papillary thyroid cancer. *BMC Cancer* **2014**, *14*, 914. [CrossRef] [PubMed]
24. Lupoli, G.; Vitale, G.; Caraglia, M.; Fittipaldi, M.R.; Abbruzzese, A.; Tagliaferri, P.; Bianco, A.R. Familial papillary thyroid microcarcinoma: A new clinical entity. *Lancet* **1999**, *353*, 637–639. [CrossRef]

25. Cirello, V. Familial non-medullary thyroid carcinoma: Clinico-pathological features, current knowledge and novelty regarding genetic risk factors. *Minerva Endocrinol.* **2020**, *46*, 5–20.
26. Wang, Z.; Chen, J.Q.; Liu, J.L.; Qin, X.G. Clinical impact of BRAF mutation on the diagnosis and prognosis of papillary thyroid carcinoma: A systematic review and meta-analysis. *Eur. J. Clin. Investig.* **2016**, *46*, 146–157. [CrossRef]
27. Zhang, Q.; Liu, S.Z.; Zhang, Q.; Guan, Y.X.; Chen, Q.J.; Zhu, Q.Y. Meta-Analyses of Association Between BRAF(V600E) Mutation and Clinicopathological Features of Papillary Thyroid Carcinoma. *Cell Physiol. Biochem.* **2016**, *38*, 763–776. [CrossRef]
28. Kaliszewski, K.; Diakowska, D.; Rzeszutko, M.; Rudnicki, J. Obesity and Overweight Are Associated with Minimal Extrathyroidal Extension, Multifocality and Bilaterality of Papillary Thyroid Cancer. *J. Clin. Med.* **2021**, *10*, 970. [CrossRef]
29. Feng, J.W.; Qu, Z.; Qin, A.C.; Pan, H.; Ye, J.; Jiang, Y. Significance of multifocality in papillary thyroid carcinoma. *Eur. J. Surg. Oncol.* **2020**, *46*, 1820–1828. [CrossRef]
30. Kim, K.J.; Kim, S.M.; Lee, Y.S.; Chung, W.Y.; Chang, H.S.; Park, C.S. Prognostic significance of tumor multifocality in papillary thyroid carcinoma and its relationship with primary tumor size: A retrospective study of 2309 consecutive patients. *Ann. Surg. Oncol.* **2015**, *22*, 125–131. [CrossRef]
31. Zahedi, A.; Bondaz, L.; Rajaraman, M.; Leslie, W.D.; Jefford, C.; Young, J.E.; Pathak, K.A.; Bureau, Y.; Rachinsky, I.; Badreddine, M.; et al. Risk for Thyroid Cancer Recurrence Is Higher in Men Than in Women Independent of Disease Stage at Presentation. *Thyroid* **2020**, *30*, 871–877. [CrossRef] [PubMed]
32. Dean, D.S.; Hay, I.D. Prognostic Indicators in Differentiated Thyroid Carcinoma. *Cancer Control.* **2000**, *7*, 229–239. [CrossRef] [PubMed]
33. Kwon, H.; Moon, B.-I. Prognosis of papillary thyroid cancer in patients with Graves' disease: A propensity score-matched analysis. *World J. Surg. Oncol.* **2020**, *18*, 266. [CrossRef] [PubMed]
34. Suh, S.; Goh, T.S.; Kim, Y.H.; Oh, S.-O.; Pak, K.; Seok, J.W.; Kim, I.J. Development and Validation of a Risk Scoring System Derived from Meta-Analyses of Papillary Thyroid Cancer. *Endocrinol. Metab.* **2020**, *35*, 435–442. [CrossRef]

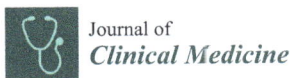

Article

Impact of Epithelial–Mesenchymal Immunophenotype on Local Aggressiveness in Papillary Thyroid Carcinoma Invading the Airway

Martina Mandarano [1,†], Marco Andolfi [2,†], Renato Colella [1], Massimo Monacelli [3], Andrea Polistena [4], Sonia Moretti [5], Guido Bellezza [1], Efisio Puxeddu [5], Alessandro Sanguinetti [6], Angelo Sidoni [1], Nicola Avenia [6], Francesco Puma [3] and Jacopo Vannucci [7,*]

1. Section of Anatomic Pathology and Histology, Department of Medicine and Surgery, University of Perugia, 06132 Perugia, Italy; martina.mandarano@unipg.it (M.M.); renato.colella75@gmail.com (R.C.); guido.bellezza@unipg.it (G.B.); angelo.sidoni@unipg.it (A.S.)
2. Thoracic Surgery Unit, AOU Ospedali Riuniti di Ancona, 60126 Ancona, Italy; marcoandolfi@hotmail.com
3. Thoracic Surgery Unit, University of Perugia Medical School, 06132 Perugia, Italy; massimo.monacelli@gmail.com (M.M.); francesco.puma@unipg.it (F.P.)
4. Department of Surgery "Pietro Valdoni", Policlinico Umberto I, University of Rome "Sapienza", 00161 Rome, Italy; andrea.polistena@uniroma1.it
5. Internal Medicine and Endocrine and Metabolic Sciences Unit, University of Perugia Medical School, 06132 Perugia, Italy; sonia.moretti@unipg.it (S.M.); efisio.puxeddu@unipg.it (E.P.)
6. General and Specialized Surgery, University of Perugia Medical School, Santa Maria Hospital, 05100 Terni, Italy; a.sanguinetti@aospterni.it (A.S.); nicola.avenia@unipg.it (N.A.)
7. Thoracic Surgery and Lung Transplantation Unit, Policlinico Umberto I, University of Rome "Sapienza", 00161 Rome, Italy
* Correspondence: jacopo.vannucci@uniroma1.it; Tel.: +39-06-49970220
† These Authors equally contributed to this study.

Abstract: Primary thyroid tumours show different levels of aggressiveness, from indolent to rapidly growing infiltrating malignancies. The most effective therapeutic option is surgery when radical resection is feasible. Biomarkers of aggressiveness may help in scheduling extended resections such as airway infiltration, avoiding a non-radical approach. The aim of the study is to evaluate the prognostic role of E-cadherin, N-cadherin, Aryl hydrocarbon receptor (AhR), and CD147 in different biological behaviours. Fifty-five samples from three groups of thyroid carcinomas were stained: papillary thyroid carcinomas (PTCs) infiltrating the airway (PTC-A), papillary intra-thyroid carcinomas (PTC-B) and poorly differentiated or anaplastic thyroid carcinomas (PDTC/ATC). High expressions of N-cadherin and AhR were associated with higher locoregional tumour aggressiveness ($p = 0.005$ and $p < 0.001$ respectively); PDTC/ATC more frequently showed a high expression of CD147 ($p = 0.011$), and a trend of lower expression of E-cadherin was registered in more aggressive neoplasms. Moreover, high levels of AhR were found with recurrent/persistent diseases ($p = 0.031$), particularly when tumours showed a concomitant high N-cadherin expression ($p = 0.043$). The study suggests that knowing in advance onco-biological factors with a potential role to discriminate between different subsets of patients could help the decision-making process, providing a more solid therapeutic indication and an increased expectation for radical surgery.

Keywords: thyroid cancer; papillary thyroid carcinoma; poorly differentiated thyroid carcinoma; airway; trachea; neck; endocrine tumours; biomarkers; immunohistochemistry

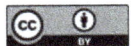

1. Introduction

Thyroid cancer is the most common endocrine malignancy. This disease varies from indolent tumour to highly aggressive disease [1]. Indeed, although early-stage well-differentiated thyroid cancer (DTC) has a good prognosis after surgery [2–4], those tumours invading surrounding tissues (extra-thyroid extension) show an increased persistence/recurrence of disease and decreased survival [5–7].

Airway invasion is found in approximately 6% of the total thyroid tumours and can determine different clinical conditions. These patients can show normal breathing or severe obstruction in the most advanced disease progression [5,6]. In such conditions, the ideal surgical treatment is still a matter of debate. Many approaches, single or combined multi-modality treatment, have been described with disputed results [8]. In particular, concerning the airway invasion, the shaving-off of the tumour from the airway or tracheal window resection is performed in the case of superficial invasion, while segmental resection is preferred when the airway invasion is deeper in the laryngo-tracheal wall [4]. However, some authors underline the weakness of the shaving and tracheal window [4,8], emphasising that segmental resection with end-to-end anastomosis should be preferred even in limited infiltration to reduce risk for recurrence and airway damage. Moreover, other conventional therapies, such as radioactive iodine, thyroid hormone therapy and chemotherapy, have been developed and performed with growing trends and promising perspectives [9–12].

Despite the progress obtained in the recent past in terms of diagnosis, staging and therapeutic options [13–15], and in view of the lack of markers to predict the oncological outcome, there is still a need for biological, genetic and immunohistochemical (IHC) indicators to develop a more effectively tailored approach. Based on the current knowledge regarding potential biomarkers of tumour aggressiveness, Aryl hydrocarbon receptor (AhR), N-cadherin, E-cadherin and CD147 were selected to be analysed in thyroid carcinomas for the following reasons. AhR has been widely analysed and seems to be associated with tumour genesis and different disease progression phases [16]. In a poorly differentiated thyroid carcinoma (PDTC) cell line, kynurenine-driven activation of AhR induced epithelial–mesenchymal transition (EMT) involving cadherins [17]. The transmembrane glycoprotein CD147 is known to facilitate tumour cell migration and invasion in several cancers [18]; matrix metalloproteinases (MMPs) seem to be activated [19], and CD147 possibly promotes the mesenchymal phenotype with cadherin expression variations [20,21]. A high expression of CD147 was described in DTC [22], with an emphasis on lymph node metastasis and tumour invasion [23].

The aim of the study is to compare the immunophenotypic characteristics of thyroid tumours invading the airway and complete intra-thyroid tumours in order to generate a hypothesis for possible new markers of local aggressiveness and to determine how the aggressive tumour attitude could be predicted.

2. Material and Methods

A comparative retrospective observational study on the expression of E-cadherin, N-cadherin, AhR and CD147 was performed on a series of patients undergoing surgery (2010–2017) for papillary thyroid cancer. The presence of accurate pathological reports, information regarding nodal status at the diagnosis and/or data regarding the recurrence and/or persistence of disease were used to select the patients eligible for the study. Subsequently, 3 groups of patients were considered: patients with papillary thyroid carcinoma (PTC) invading larynx and trachea undergoing total thyroidectomy with segmental resection of the airway (PTC-A group); patients with completely intrathyroidal PTC (PTC-B group); and patients with PDTC or anaplastic thyroid carcinomas (ATC) (PDTC/ATC group), which served as a control group for more locally aggressive neoplasms. The study was approved by the local ethics committee (N. 23665/10/AV of 26 January 2010).

2.1. Study Population

Patients were included the analysis if they were over 18 years of age; histologically diagnosed for PTC, PDTC or ATC; and followed up by the Internal Medicine and Endocrine and Metabolic Sciences Unit, University of Perugia. Patients with follicular and medullary tumours were excluded. Medical history, endoscopic findings, pathological reports, work for the assessment of possible resection with curative intent, indication to airway resection or other therapeutic options, histo-pathological aspects, immunophenotypic profile and adjuvant therapies were evaluated. At admission, all the patients underwent routinary tests for an appropriate preoperative assessment.

2.2. Surgical Procedures

Based on the different disease characteristics, two different procedures of surgical resection were carried out: total thyroidectomy with central compartment lymphectomy and latero-cervical lymphectomy (in the case of positive ultrasound (US) lymph node involvement) was performed for all cyto-histologically proven PTCs or early-stage PDTCs. In the cases of tumours infiltrating the airway, total thyroidectomy + lymphectomy was associated with resection and end-to-end anastomosis of the airway according to Grillo's technique [24]. Diagnosed ATCs were excluded from radical surgery due to stage and local conditions but were submitted to palliative procedures (endoscopy or tracheotomy) and alternative treatment.

2.3. Histopathological and Immunohistochemical Determinations

The surgical specimens were fixed in 4% buffered formalin and paraffin embedded (FFPE). Four-micrometer-thick sections were used to obtain both the haematoxylin and eosin (H&E) (Leica ST5020 Multistainer (Leica Biosystems, Nußloch, Germany)), using the ST Infinity H&E Staining System kit (Leica Biosystems, Richmond, IL USA), and the IHC stains (BOND-III fully automated immunohistochemistry stainer (LeicaBiosystems, Nußloch, Germany)) and peroxidase immunoenzymatic reaction with development in diaminobenzidine, including proper positive and negative controls.

The tumour areas and the tumour histotypes, according to the World Health Organization's classification of endocrine organ tumours, 2017, 4th Ed.—in force at the time of the study—were identified on H&E slides, allowing the identification of 3 groups of tumours: PTC, PDTC and ATC. Among these last two groups, tumours without a pure histotype were not considered for the analyses. Moreover, the presence of extra-thyroid infiltration was assessed on H&E slides.

The IHC stains were set up using antibodies against E-cadherin (Leica Biosystems, Newcastle Upon Tyne, United Kingdom, Cat# PA0387, RRID:AB_442084, ready-to-use), N-cadherin (ThermoFisher Scientific, Rockford, IL, USA, Cat# 33-3900, RRID:AB_2313779, dilution 1:150), AhR (ThermoFisher Scientific, Rockford, IL, USA, Cat# MA1-514, RRID: AB_2273723, dilution 1: 250) and CD147 (ThermoFisher Scientific, Rockford, IL, USA, Cat# MA1-19201, RRID: AB_1071293, dilution 1:100). Two trained pathologists (M.Ma. and R.C.) separately performed a semi-quantitative evaluation of the immunostains, using a H-Score—as previously reported for AhR [17]—which was the result of the intensity of the staining (0 = absent, 1 = mild, 2 = moderate, 3 = intense) multiplied by the percentage of labelled tumour cells. Two other expert pathologists (G.B. and A.Si.) convened to compare discordant cases in order to assign a definitive H-score. Afterwards, the low and the high classes of expression were obtained, depending on whether the H-score was lower or higher than the internally validated cut-offs—laboratory developed test (LDT)—for each protein investigated (Table 1). As regards E-cadherin, the tumour belonged to the normal expression group when the H-score was >200 and to the lost/low group when the H-score was ≤200.

Table 1. H-score cut-offs for N-cadherin, AhR and CD147 groups of expression.

Protein (IHC)	H-Scores for Expression Groups	
	Low	High
N-Cadherin	0–40	41–300
AhR	0–70	71–300
CD147	0–40	41–300

2.4. Statistical Analysis

Descriptive statistics were used for the analysis of immunomarker expressions. Linear correlations between the expressions of the immunomarkers were analysed using the Pearson correlation coefficient. Categorical variables were presented as frequencies with row and column percentages and compared between the groups using chi-square test or Fisher's exact test as appropriate. Values of $p < 0.05$ were assumed as significant.

3. Results

3.1. Histopathological Findings

The H&E slides examination identified 8 (15%) PTC-A out of 55 enrolled cases, 27 (49%) PTC-B and 20 (36%) PDTC/ATC. Moreover, H&E enabled the choice of the appropriate tumour areas for the following IHC analysis. Among the PDTC/ATC (13/7), 4/13 PDTC and 1/7 ATC showed more differentiated tumour areas and were therefore not considered for further analysis between immunomarker expressions and clinical–pathological characteristics of the tumours. The clinical characteristics of the PTC-A patients are summarised in Table 2.

Table 2. Clinical characteristics of patients with PTC invading the airway.

ID	Sex	Age	Pathological Diagnosis	Extrathyroidal Invasion	Multifocality	Tumour Size (cm)	pT	Lymph Node Metastasis	N Tot	N+	AJCC Stage at Diagnosis	Recurrence or Persistence
1	F	69	PTC	yes	yes	4.0	pT3	yes	5	5	II	-
2	F	75	PTC	yes	yes	2.4	pT4	no	10	0	III	Persistence
3	F	59	PTC	yes	yes	1.8	pT3	yes	1	1	II	Recurrence
4	F	45	PTC	yes	no	1.8	pT4	no	0	0	III	Recurrence
5	M	49	PTC	yes	no	2.4	pT3	no	3	0	II	Persistence
6	F	72	PTC	yes	no	2.0	pT4	yes	11	2	III	Persistence
7	F	55	PTC	yes	no	1.2	pT4	no	0	0	III	Persistence
8	M	43	PTC	yes	yes	2.2	pT4	yes	5	5	I	Recurrence

3.2. Immunohistochemical Analyses

The obtained H-score values showed a mean value of 62.49 ± 73.49 (range 0–210) for N-cadherin, 106.6 ± 78.19 (range 5–294) for AhR, 121.5 ± 80.34 (range 0–285) for CD147 and 75.80 ± 78.66 (range 0–270) for E-cadherin (Figure 1).

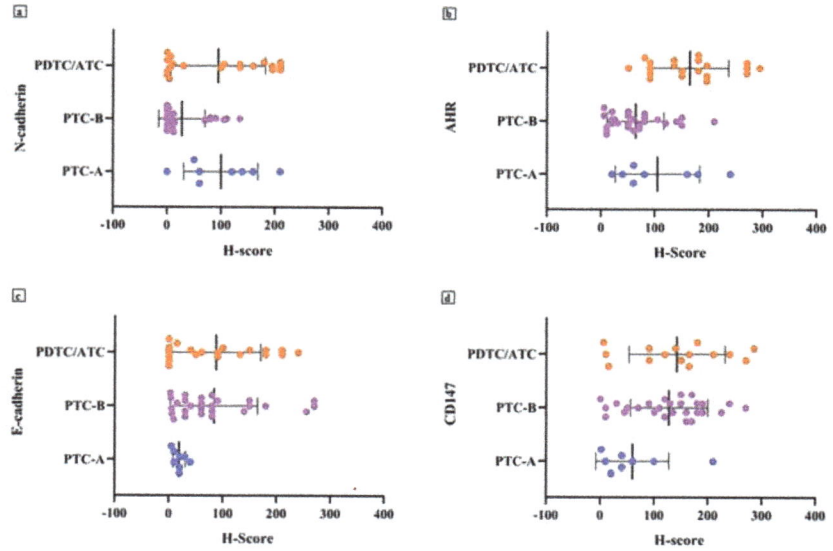

Figure 1. Scatter plots of H-score distribution for N-cadherin (**a**), AhR (**b**), E-cadherin (**c**) and CD147 (**d**) according to tumour groups analysed.

Regarding N-cadherin expression, 30 cases (55%) belonged to the low expression class for this protein; 7 (87%) PTC-A and 11 (55%) PDTC/ATC showed high N-cadherin expression. Therefore, the higher the tumour aggressiveness, the higher the N-cadherin expression (p = 0.005; Table 3, Figure 2).

Thirty-two tumours (58%) showed a high expression of AhR, and 19 of these (95%) belonged to the PDTC/ATC group (p < 0.001; Table 3). A higher expression of AhR was found in PTC infiltrating the airway compared to intrathyroid tumours (50% of PTC-A vs. 33% of PTC-B; Figure 2).

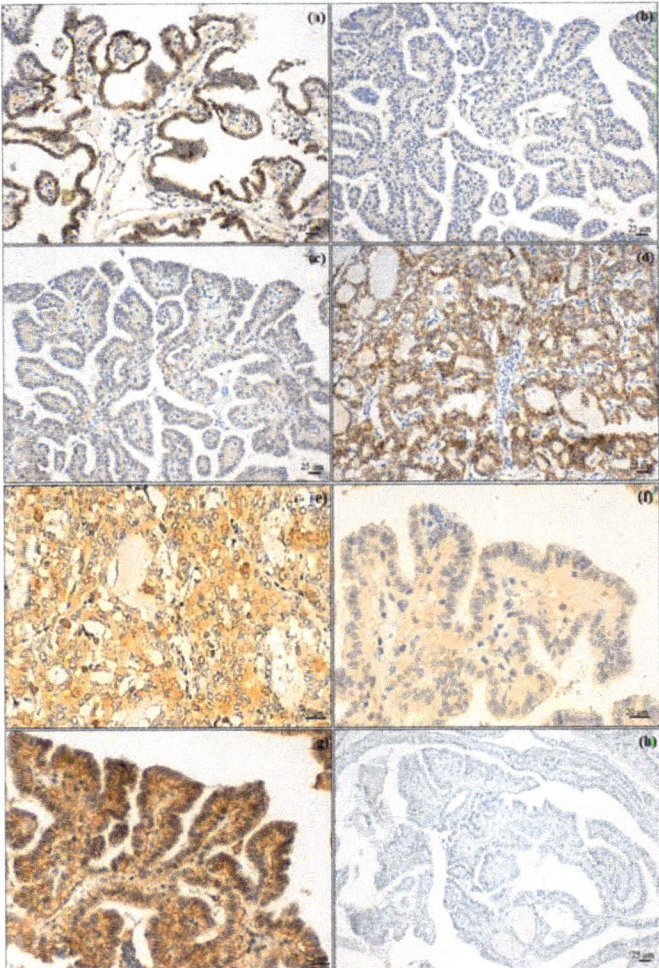

Figure 2. Biomarker immunohistochemical expression. (**a**) Membranous high expression of N-cadherin on tumour cells of PTC infiltrating the airway (PTC-A) compared with (**b**) an intrathyroid PTC (PTC-B); (**c**) PTC-A presented a low expression of E-cadherin and (**d**) PTC-B (follicular variant) with retained expression of this molecule; (**e**) PTC-A showing a high expression of AhR in contrast with (**f**), which shows low expression of the same immunomarker in a PTC-B; (**g**) CD147 high expression of PTC-B and (**h**) absent expression in PTC-A. Original magnification: (**a–d,h**) 200×; (**e–g**) 400×.

Table 3. N-cadherin, AhR and CD147 expression among tumour groups.

Histotype	N-Cadherin			AhR			CD147		
	Low n. (%)	High n. (%)	p	Low n. (%)	High n. (%)	p	Low n. (%)	High n. (%)	p
PTC-A [1]	1 (13)	7 (87)		4 (50)	4 (50)		5 (63)	3 (37)	
PTC-B [2]	20 (74)	7 (26)	0.005	18 (67)	9 (33)	<0.001	4 (15)	23 (85)	0.011
PDTC/ATC	9 (45)	11 (55)		1 (5)	19 (95)		3 (15)	17 (85)	

[1] PTC-A: PTC infiltrating the airway. [2] PTC-B: PTC without airway infiltration.

CD147 presented a high expression in 43 cases (78% of the total caseload), with 23 (85%) in the PTC-B group and 17 in the PDTC/ATC group (85%) ($p = 0.011$; Table 3, Figure 2).

Most tumours (49, 89%) presented a lost/low expression of the E-cadherin; all 8 PTC-A cases (100%) presented a lower expression of E-cadherin, while 3 out of 20 PDTC/ATC cases (15%) retained its expression (Table 4; Figure 2).

Table 4. E-cadherin distribution among tumour groups.

Histotype	E-Cadherin		
	Normal n. (%)	Lost/Low n. (%)	p
PTC-A [1]	0 (0)	8 (100)	
PTC-B [2]	3 (11)	24 (89)	0.516
PDTC/ATC	3 (15)	17 (85)	

[1] PTC-A: PTC infiltrating the airway. [2] PTC-B: PTC without airway infiltration.

3.3. Correlations between Immunomarkers

A moderate positive correlation between the expression of N-cadherin and AhR is reported if H-score values are considered as continuous variables; i.e., the increase in N-cadherin expression follows the increase in AhR and vice versa ($\rho = 0.540$; $p < 0.001$; Figure 3a).

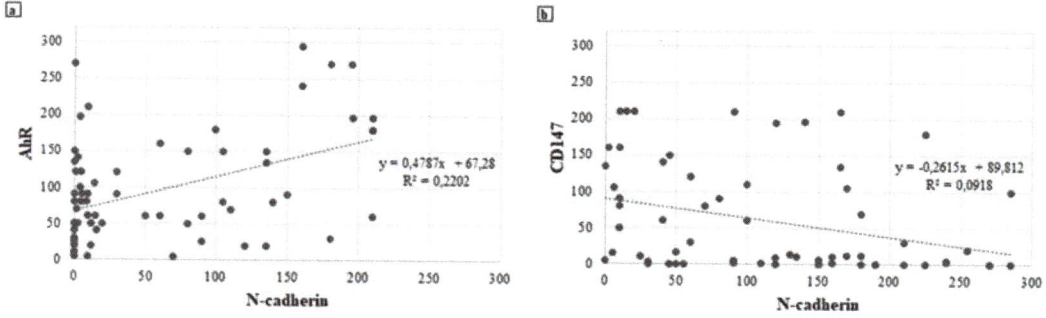

Figure 3. (a) Positive relationship between the expression of N-cadherin and AhR. (b) Negative relationship between the expression of N-cadherin and CD147.

Furthermore, the higher the expression of N-cadherin, the lower the expression of CD147 ($\rho = -0.426$; $p = 0.002$; Figure 3b). An inverse correlation trend was observed between the other tested immunomarkers. When the expression of CD147 increases, both E-cadherin ($\rho = -0.112$; $p = 0.438$) and AhR ($\rho = -0.256$; $p = 0.073$) decrease (Figure S1a,b, respectively). On the other hand, there was a positive correlation between the expressions of AhR and E-cadherin, but this was not statistically significant ($\rho = 0.124$; $p = 0.366$; Figure S2).

3.4. Immunomarker Expression and Clinical–Pathological Associations

The results regarding the analysis of the associations between the IHC expression of N-cadherin, AhR, CD147 or E-cadherin and histotype, multifocality of the disease, nodal status and tumour recurrence/persistence are shown in Table 5. Some data were not available when the series review was performed.

Table 5. Expression of N-cadherin, AhR, CD147 or E-cadherin associations with clinical–pathological characteristics.

Parameter	N-Cadherin			AhR			CD147			E-Cadherin			Total
	Low n. (%)	High n. (%)	p	Low n. (%)	High n. (%)	p	Low n. (%)	High n. (%)	p	N [1] n. (%)	L/L [2] n. (%)	p	n. (%)
Histotype													50 (91)
PTC	21 (60)	14 (40)	0.193	22 (63)	13 (37)	<0.001	9 (26)	26 (74)	0.910	3 (9)	32 (91)	0.607	35 (70)
PDTC/ATC	6 (40)	9 (60)		1 (7)	14 (93)		3 (20)	12 (80)		2 (13)	13 (87)		15 (30)
Multifocality													38 (69)
No	11 (55)	9 (45)	0.973	9 (45)	11 (55)	0.090	4 (20)	16 (80)	0.573	1 (5)	19 (95)	0.485	20 (53)
Yes	10 (56)	8 (44)		13 (72)	5 (28)		5 (28)	13 (72)		2 (11)	16 (89)		18 (47)
Nodal Status													36 (65)
N−	9 (60)	6 (40)	0.864	7 (47)	8 (53)	0.230	1 (7)	14 (93)	0.058	1 (7)	14 (93)	0.760	15 (42)
N+	12 (57)	9 (43)		14 (67)	7 (33)		7 (33)	14 (67)		2 (10)	19 (90)		21 (58)
Recurrence/Persistence													45 (82)
No	12 (60)	8 (40)	0.182	12 (60)	8 (40)	0.031	4 (20)	16 (80)	0.366	1 (5)	19 (95)	0.243	20 (44)
Yes	10 (40)	15 (60)		7 (28)	18 (72)		8 (32)	17 (68)		4 (16)	21 (84)		25 (56)

[1] N: normal expression. [2] L/L: lost/low expression.

In particular, high expression of AhR was statistically correlated with a more aggressive histotype of thyroid cancer: 14 PDTC/ATC (93%) showed a high AhR expression ($p < 0.001$, Table 5). Moreover, the cases with recurrence/persistence of disease more frequently expressed high levels of AhR (18 cases, 72%; $p = 0.031$, Table 5). N-cadherin was more frequently observed in PDTC/ATC histotype (9 cases, 60%, not significant, $p = 0.193$, Table 5) and in tumours presenting a recurrence/persistence of the disease (15 cases, 60%, not significant, $p = 0.182$, Table 5). CD147 and E-cadherin did not show a statistically significant association with the clinical–pathological parameters considered (Table 5).

Concomitant high levels of AhR and N-cadherin (9 PDTC/ATC cases, 90%) seemed to be associated with a more aggressive tumoural behaviour ($p = 0.002$; Table 6), as already shown in cases of the expression of both AhR (statistically significant, $p < 0.001$) and N-cadherin (showing just a trend, $p = 0.193$) when singularly analysed (Table 5). Moreover, 12 cases (75%) with high AhR and N-cadherin showed a recurrence/persistence of the disease ($p = 0.043$; Table 6).

Table 6. Associations between tumours examined according to the concurrent expression of AhR and N-cadherin and clinical–pathological parameters.

Parameter	AhR and N-Cadherin			Total
	Low n. (%)	High n. (%)	p	n. (%)
Histotype				30 (100)
PTC	14 (70)	6 (30)	0.002	20 (67)
PDTC/ATC	1 (10)	9 (90)		10 (33)
Multifocality				23 (100)
No	5 (50)	5 (50)	0.417	10 (43)
Yes	9 (31)	4 (69)		13 (57)
Nodal Status				22 (100)
N−	6 (55)	5 (45)	0.659	11 (50)
N+	8 (73)	3 (27)		11 (50)
Recurrence/Persistence				26 (100)
No	7 (70)	3 (30)	0.043	10 (38)
Yes	4 (25)	12 (75)		16 (62)

When immunomarker expressions were evaluated in PTC cases in view of the presence (PTC-A) or absence (PTC-B) of the infiltration of the airway, high N-cadherin was statistically associated with the tumours presenting airway infiltration ($p = 0.003$; Table 7). CD147 expression was lower in PTC-A (5 cases, 56%; $p = 0.015$, Table 7), supporting the finding of an inverse correlation between this protein and N-cadherin ($p = 0.002$; Figure 3b).

Table 7. PTC-A and PTC-B associations with immunomarkers.

Parameter	PTC			Total
	PTC-A [1] n. (%) 8 (23)	PTC-B [2] n. (%) 27 (77)	p	n. (%) 35 (100)
N-cadherin				
Low	1 (5)	20 (95)	0.003	21 (60)
High	7 (50)	7 (50)		14 (40)
AhR				
Low	4 (18)	18 (82)	0.433	22 (63)
High	4 (31)	9 (69)		13 (37)
CD147				
Low	5 (56)	4 (44)	0.015	9 (26)
High	3 (12)	23 (88)		26 (74)
E-cadherin				
N [3]	0 (0)	3 (100)	1.000	3 (9)
L/L [4]	8 (25)	24 (75)		32 (91)

[1] PTC-A: PTC infiltrating the airway. [2] PTC-B: PTC without airway infiltration. [3] N: normal expression. [4] L/L: lost/low expression.

4. Discussion

Thyroid carcinoma is a very heterogeneous disease with a different prognosis based mainly on histology [4]. Surgery is still the best therapeutic option with a generally good prognosis, especially in small-sized completely intra-thyroid DTC without lymph nodal or distant metastases [4,14]. Conversely, PDTC and ATC are more aggressive with a severe natural history. In these cases, there is usually no chance for curative surgery, only palliative procedures [25,26].

Between these two last extremes described, there are several intermediate conditions showing a locally advanced tumour that might benefit from a radical resection but need more complex procedures than total thyroidectomy. Indeed, considering the neck's anatomy, when thyroid tumours acquire the capacity to infiltrate the neighbourhood, a radical resection is a difficult goal. In this regard, infiltration of the airway represents the most challenging condition, but, in a consistent number of patients, radical surgery can be performed and increases the chances for cure [8]. The shaving-off of the tumour from the airway, tracheal window resection or segmental resection are performed in relation to the degree of airway invasion [4]. These procedures, already described and still disputed in some technical aspects and indications [8,24], are effective in expert hands but must be strictly planned [27]. The preoperative US evaluation of thyroid nodules allows the identification of some characteristics, such as the higher tumour size or the irregular tumour margins, typically associated with an already locally advanced disease and more aggressive histotype [15]. However, although the US examination aims at also assessing lymph node status, it might fail to adequately investigate the deep neck. Furthermore, the cytological information derived from FNAs cannot currently predict the biological aggressiveness of well-differentiated carcinomas.

In particular, this lack of knowledge prevents us from gaining specific information on the tumour trend to present local infiltration, early lymphatic spread or both. To fill this gap, we attempted to investigate the IHC expression of AhR, N-cadherin, E-cadherin and CD147, considering the correlation found in various cancer types between their expression and tumour aggressive behaviour [16–23].

Indeed, based on the study findings, we could advance the potential role of AhR/N-cadherin as a prognostic marker, being able to suggest a more aggressive phenotype in thyroid carcinoma as evidenced by the high levels of AhR/N-cadherin found in most patients of the PTC-A and PDTC/ATC groups.

These findings are consistent with previously reported data that showed how the increased expression of AhR may play an oncogenic enhancing function not only through the induction of an immune-tolerant microenvironment but also through the expression of proteins such as N-cadherin involved in the regulation and initiation of the EMT [17,28,29].

In our case series, AhR seems to be an important prognostic marker, highly expressed in patients with a persistence or recurrence of disease in addition to being a marker of aggression and histologic de-differentiation.

N-cadherin expression still remains a matter of debate in the context of thyroid oncogenesis [17,30]. This study could find that expression of this protein plays a significant role in promoting invasiveness, being expressed in both PTC-A and PDTC/ATC groups and displaying a low expression rate in the PTC-B group.

The role of E-cadherin and CD147 remains to be defined: despite the available data reported [31–36], they showed only marginal roles as markers of aggressive biological behaviour in this analysis. In particular, although E-cadherin expression is not significantly associated with all of the analysed variables, we could observe a trend of increased aggressiveness (PTC-A and PDTC/ATC) with absent or very low E-cadherin. CD147 was highly expressed both in PTC-B and PDTC/ATC groups and increased with a decrease in E-cadherin. Nevertheless, as CD147 levels increased, both AhR and N-cadherin expressions decreased; some authors hypothesised that the reason behind the biological aggressiveness related to the overexpression of CD147 could be the enhancement of the EMT process with cancer migration and invasion as also described in other tumours [37–39].

The current study has some limitations: this is a retrospective clinical study and poor a priori knowledge is available to formally attribute an effective correlation between AhR/N-cadherin expression and biologic aggressiveness. The study timeframe is almost two decades and does not guarantee homogeneous diagnostic–therapeutic management in all patients; moreover, the number of patients in group A is limited, despite it representing a good experience for a very rare condition, and, hence, it cannot fully show an independent impact of these findings. However, to have a more homogeneous caseload, the study was designed to only analyse PTCs among the most differentiated histotypes. In addition, considering that one of the goals of the study was to preoperatively identify non-infiltrating airway carcinomas and infiltrating ones, we considered only PTCs since the preoperative FNAs do not allow the cytological diagnosis of follicular thyroid carcinomas. Therefore, the assessment of the analysed biomarkers on such specimens would not change the surgical management of preoperative follicular lesions. Moreover, since BRAFV600E mutation was demonstrated to be associated with an increased expression of AhR, particularly at the infiltrative tumour edge, in thyroid cancer murine models [17], and the associations between the molecules here investigated and other mutations implied in thyroid cancer pathogenesis, progression and prognosis (e.g., RET/PTC, TP53, TERT, ATK1 and RAS) have not yet been described [40], additional studies at the molecular level of these aspects should be conducted.

This study suggests that knowing in advance the most important onco-biological factors might be helpful in the decision-making process, providing a more solid therapeutic indication and an increased expectation for radical surgery when markers of local aggressiveness are negative. Hence, there is the need for further studies to confirm these preliminary findings. When prognosticators and biomarkers for local aggressiveness can be translated into clinical practice, they may be supportive in better planning the most appropriate surgical procedure to be performed. A biological tumour profile could change the current paradigm to plan treatments based on "static" instrumental examination, giving a more "dynamic" assessment of tumour behaviour from the cytological immunophenotyping of the FNA-derived material.

In conclusion, thyroid cancer is a varied disease with a positive outcome after resection, if the tumour is intrathyroid. Our study suggests that several markers deserve to be further investigated in view of a potential role to discriminate, among the same histotype, between different subsets of a patient's risk. Knowing in advance tumour aggressiveness could be helpful in avoiding suboptimal surgery if the tumour has an inner trend to recur or to infiltrate the neighbouring anatomical structures.

Supplementary Materials: The following are available online at https://www.mdpi.com/article/10.3390/jcm10194351/s1. Figure S1: (a) Negative correlation between the expression of CD147, E-cadherin and (b) AhR. Figure S2: positive correlation between the expression of AhR and E-cadherin.

Author Contributions: Conceptualisation, J.V., M.A., M.M. (Martina Mandarano), R.C. and F.P.; methodology, J.V., N.A., and F.P.; formal analysis, M.A., M.M. (Martina Mandarano), R.C., S.M. and E.P; data curation, M.M. (Martina Mandarano), A.P., S.M., G.B., A.S. (Angelo Sidoni) and E.P.; writing—original draft preparation, J.V., M.A., M.M. (Martina Mandarano) and R.C.; writing—review and editing, M.M. (Massimo Monacelli), A.P and E.P.; visualisation, M.M. (Martina Mandarano); supervision, A.S. (Alessandro Sanguinetti), A.S. (Angelo Sidoni), N.A. and F.P.; funding acquisition, A.S. (Alessandro Sanguinetti), J.V. and F.P. All authors have read and agreed to the published version of the manuscript.

Funding: This research was funded by the Department of Surgical and Biomedical Sciences Research Fund 2017, University of Perugia Medical School.

Institutional Review Board Statement: This study was approved by the local ethics committee (N. 23665/10/AV of 26 January 2010).

Informed Consent Statement: Patient consent was obtained from all patients at admission for clinical research.

Acknowledgments: The authors thank Elisabetta Loreti for the invaluable technical support in the research laboratory.

Conflicts of Interest: The authors declare no conflict of interest.

References

1. Siegel, R.L.; Miller, K.D.; Jemal, A. Cancer statistics, 2015. *CA Cancer J. Clin.* **2015**, *65*, 5–29. [CrossRef] [PubMed]
2. Tsumori, T.; Nakao, K.; Miyata, M.; Izukura, M.; Monden, Y.; Sakurai, M.; Kawashima, Y.; Nakahara, K. Clinicopathologic study of thyroid carcinoma infiltrating the trachea. *Cancer* **1985**, *56*, 2843–2848. [CrossRef]
3. Takano, T. Fetal cell carcinogenesis of the thyroid. *Endocr. J.* **2004**, *51*, 509–515. [CrossRef]
4. Ito, Y.; Miyauci, A. Prognostic factors and therapeutic strategies for differentiated carcinomas of the thyroid. *Endocr. J.* **2009**, *56*, 177–192. [CrossRef]
5. Czaja, J.M.; McCaffrey, T.V. The surgical management of laryngotracheal invasion by well-differentiated papillary thyroid carcinoma. *Arch. Otolaryngol. Head Neck Surg.* **1997**, *123*, 484–490. [CrossRef] [PubMed]
6. Ishihara, T.; Yamazaki, S.; Kobayashi, K.; Inoue, H.; Fukai, S.; Ito, K.; Mimura, T. Resection of the trachea infiltrated by thyroid carcinoma. *Ann. Surg.* **1982**, *195*, 496–500. [CrossRef]
7. Tuttle, M.R.; Morris, L.F.; Haugen, B.R.; Shah, J.P.; Sosa, J.A.; Rohren, E.; Subramaniam, R.M.; Hunt, J.L.; Perrier, N.D. Thyroid-Differentiated and Anaplastic Carcinoma in AJCC Cancer Staging Manual, 8th ed.; Amin, M.B., Ed.; Springer: Chicago, IL, USA, 2017; pp. 873–890.
8. Avenia, N.; Vannucci, J.; Monacelli, M.; Lucchini, R.; Polistena, A.; Santoprete, S.; Potenza, R.; Andolfi, M.; Puma, F. Thyroid cancer invading the airway: Diagnosis and management. *Int. J. Surg.* **2015**, *28*, S75–S78. [CrossRef]
9. Kato, S.; Demura, S.; Shinmura, K.; Yokogawa, N.; Shimizu, T.; Tsuchiya, H. Current Management of Bone Metastases from Differentiated Thyroid Cancer. *Cancers* **2021**, *13*, 4429. [CrossRef]
10. Davidson, C.D.; Gillis, N.E.; Carr, F.E. Thyroid Hormone Receptor Beta as Tumor Suppressor: Untapped Potential in Treatment and Diagnostics in Solid Tumors. *Cancers* **2021**, *13*, 4254. [CrossRef]
11. Ferrari, C.; Santo, G.; Ruta, R.; Lavelli, V.; Rubini, D.; Mammucci, P.; Sardaro, A.; Rubini, G. Early Predictive Response to Multi-Tyrosine Kinase Inhibitors in Advanced Refractory Radioactive-Iodine Differentiated Thyroid Cancer: A New Challenge for [18F]FDG PET/CT. *Diagnostics* **2021**, *11*, 1417. [CrossRef]
12. Wang, X.; Yin, G.; Zhang, W.; Song, K.; Zhang, L.; Guo, Z. Prostaglandin Reductase 1 as a Potential Therapeutic Target for Cancer Therapy. *Front. Pharmacol.* **2021**, *12*, 717730. [CrossRef] [PubMed]
13. Orlandi, F.; Caraci, P.; Berruti, A.; Puligheddu, B.; Pivano, G.; Dogliotti, L.; Angeli, A. Chemotherapy with dacarbazine and 5-fluorouracil in advanced medullary thyroid cancer. *Ann. Oncol.* **1994**, *5*, 763–765. [CrossRef] [PubMed]

14. Haugen, B.R.; Alexander, E.K.; Bible, K.C.; Doherty, G.M.; Mandel, S.J.; Nikiforov, Y.E.; Pacini, F.; Randolph, G.W.; Sawka, A.M.; Schlumberger, M.; et al. 2015 American Thyroid Association Management Guidelines for Adult Patients with Thyroid Nodules and Differentiated Thyroid Cancer: The American Thyroid Association Guidelines Task Force on Thyroid Nodules and Differentiated Thyroid Cancer. *Thyroid* **2016**, *26*, 1–133. [CrossRef] [PubMed]
15. Cordes, M.; Götz, T.I.; Lang, E.W.; Coerper, S.; Kuwert, T.; Schmidkonz, C. Advanced thyroid carcinomas: Neural network analysis of ultrasonographic characteristics. *Thyroid Res.* **2021**, *14*, 16. [CrossRef] [PubMed]
16. Wang, Z.; Snyder, M.; Kenison, J.E.; Yang, K.; Lara, B.; Lydell, E.; Bennani, K.; Novikov, O.; Federico, A.; Monti, S.; et al. How the AHR Became Important in Cancer: The Role of Chronically Active AHR in Cancer Aggression. *Int. J. Mol. Sci* **2021**, *22*, 387. [CrossRef]
17. Moretti, S.; Nucci, N.; Menicali, E.; Morelli, S.; Bini, V.; Colella, R.; Mandarano, M.; Sidoni, A.; Puxeddu, E. The Aryl Hydrocarbon Receptor Is Expressed in Thyroid Carcinoma and Appears to Mediate Epithelial-Mesenchymal-Transition. *Cancers* **2020**, *12*, 145. [CrossRef]
18. Lian, C.; Guo, Y.; Zhang, J.; Chen, X.; Peng, C. Targeting CD147 is a Novel Strategy for Antitumor Therapy. *Curr. Pharm. Des.* **2017**, *23*, 4410–4421. [CrossRef]
19. Wanga, M.; Zhanga, S. Sunb, Q.; Yanga, X.; Wangc, Y.; Shangd, R.; Zhua, Y.; Yaoe, H.; Li, Y. Dual effects of an anti-CD147 antibody for Esophageal cancer therapy. *Cancer Biol. Ther.* **2019**, *20*, 1443–1452. [CrossRef]
20. Dana, P.; Kariya, R.; Vaeteewoottacharn, K.; Sawanyawisuth, K.; Seubwai, W.; Matsuda, K.; Okada, S.; Wongkham, S. Upregulation of CD147 Promotes Metastasis of Cholangiocarcinoma by Modulating the Epithelial-to-Mesenchymal Transitional Process. *Oncol. Res.* **2017**, *25*, 1047–1059. [CrossRef] [PubMed]
21. Fang, F.; Li, Q.; Wu, M.; Nie, C.; Xu, H.; Wang, L. CD147 promotes epithelial-mesenchymal transition of prostate cancer cells via the Wnt/β-catenin pathway. *Exp. Ther. Med.* **2020**, *20*, 3154–3160. [CrossRef]
22. Tan, H.; Ye, K.; Wang, Z.; Tang, H. CD147 expression as a significant prognostic factor in differentiated thyroid carcinoma. *Transl. Res.* **2008**, *152*, 143–149. [CrossRef]
23. Huang, P.; Mao, L.F.; Zhang, Z.P.; Lv, W.W.; Feng, X.P.; Liao, H.J.; Dong, C.; Kaluba, B.; Tang, X.F.; Chang, S. Down-Regulated miR-125a-5p Promotes the Reprogramming of Glucose Metabolism and Cell Malignancy by Increasing Levels of CD147 in Thyroid Cancer. *Thyroid* **2018**, *28*, 613–623. [CrossRef]
24. Grillo, H.C. (Ed.) Tracheal reconstruction: Anterior approach and extended resection. In *The Surgery of Trachea and Bronchi*; BC Decker Inc.: Toronto, ON, Canada, 2004.
25. Puma, F.; Ceccarelli, S.; Potenza, R.; Italiani, A.; Melis, A.; Cagini, L.; Monacelli, M. Rescue Tracheostomy for Patients with Unresectable Large Growing Neck Masses. *Ann. Thorac. Surg.* **2021**. [CrossRef]
26. Puma, F.; Meattelli, M.; Kolodziejek, M.; Properzi, M.G.; Capozzi, R.; Matricardi, A.; Cagini, L.; Vannucci, J. An Alternative Method for Airway Management with Combined Tracheal Intubation and Rigid Bronchoscope. *Ann. Thorac. Surg.* **2019**, *107*, e435–e436. [CrossRef]
27. Polistena, A.; Vannucci, J.; Monacelli, M.; Lucchini, R.; Sanguinetti, A.; Avenia, S.; Santoprete, S.; Triola, R.; Cirocchi, R.; Puma, F.; et al. Thoracic duct lesions in thyroid surgery: An update on diagnosis, treatment and prevention based on a cohort study. *Int. J. Surg.* **2016**, *28*, S33–S37. [CrossRef]
28. Duan, Z.; Li, Y.; Li, L. Promoting epithelial-to-mesenchymal transition by D-kynurenine via activating aryl hydrocarbon receptor. *Mol. Cell Biochem.* **2018**, *448*, 165–173. [CrossRef] [PubMed]
29. Roman, A.C.; Carvajal-Gonzalez, J.M.; Merino, J.M.; Mulero-Navarro, S.; Fernandez-Salguero, P.M. The aryl hydrocarbon receptor in the crossroad of signalling networks with therapeutic value. *Pharmacol. Ther.* **2018**, *185*, 50–63. [CrossRef] [PubMed]
30. Da, C.; Wu, K.; Yue, C.; Bai, P.; Wang, R.; Wang, G.; Zhao, M.; Lv, Y.; Hou, P. N-cadherin promotes thyroid tumorigenesis through modulating major signaling pathways. *Oncotarget* **2017**, *8*, 8131–8142. [CrossRef] [PubMed]
31. Chetty, R.; Serra, S. Membrane loss and aberrant nuclear localization of E-cadherin are consistent features of solid pseudopapillary tumour of the pancreas. An immunohistochemical study using two antibodies recognizing different domains of the E-cadherin molecule. *Histopathology* **2008**, *52*, 325–330. [CrossRef] [PubMed]
32. Zarca, T.A.; Han, A.C.; Edelson, M.I.; Rosenblum, N.G. Expression of cadherins, p53, and BCL2 in small cell carcinomas of the cervix: Potential tumorsuppressor role for N-cadherin. *Int. J. Gynecol. Cancer* **2003**, *13*, 240–243. [CrossRef]
33. Ali, K.M.; Awny, S.; Ibrahim, D.A.; Metwally, I.H.; Hamdy, O.; Refky, B.; Abdallah, A.; Abdelwahab, K. Role of P53, E-cadherin and BRAF as predictors of regional nodal recurrence for papillary thyroid cancer. *Ann. Diagn. Pathol.* **2019**, *40*, 59–65. [CrossRef]
34. Jensen, K.; Patel, A.; Hoperia, V.; Larin, A.; Bauer, A.; Vasko, V. Dynamic changes in E-caderin gene promoter methylation during metastatic progression in papillary thyroid cancer. *Exp. Ther. Med.* **2010**, *1*, 457–462. [CrossRef] [PubMed]
35. Zhou, C.; Yang, C.; Chong, D. E-cadherin expression is associated with susceptibility and clinicopathological characteristics of thyroid cancer. *Medicine* **2019**, *98*, e16187. [CrossRef]
36. Burandt, E.; Lübbersmeyer, F.; Gorbokon, N.; Büscheck, F.; Luebke, A.M.; Menz, A.; Kluth, M.; Hube-Magg, C.; Hinsch, A.; Höflmayer, D.; et al. E-Cadherin expression in human tumors: A tissue microarray study on 10,851 tumors. *Biomark. Res.* **2021**, *9*, 44. [CrossRef] [PubMed]
37. Guo, W.; Abudumijiti, H.; Xu, L.; Hasim, A. CD147 promotes cervical cancer migration and invasion by up-regulating fatty acid synthase expression. *Int. J. Clin. Exp. Pathol.* **2019**, *12*, 4280–4288.

38. Yu, B.; Zhang, Y.; Wu, K.; Wang, L.; Jiang, Y.; Chen, W.; Yan, M. CD147 promotes progression of head and neck squamous cell carcinoma via NF-kappa B signaling. *J. Cell Mol. Med.* **2019**, *23*, 954–966. [CrossRef]
39. Suzuki, S.; Toyoma, S.; Tsuji, T.; Kawasaki, Y.; Yamada, T. CD147 mediates transforming growth factor-β1-induced epithelial-mesenchymal transition and cell invasion in squamous cell carcinoma of the tongue. *Exp. Ther. Med.* **2019**, *17*, 2855–2860. [CrossRef] [PubMed]
40. Puxeddu, E.; Moretti, S.; Giannico, A.; Martinelli, M.; Marino, C.; Avenia, N.; Cristofani, R.; Farabi, R.; Reboldi, G.; Ribacchi, R.; et al. Ret/PTC activation does not influence clinical and pathological features of adult papillary thyroid carcinomas. *Eur. J. Endocrinol.* **2003**, *148*, 505–513. [CrossRef] [PubMed]

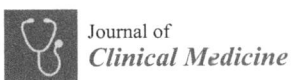

Journal of
Clinical Medicine

Article

Thyroidectomy for Cancer: The Surgeon and the Parathyroid Glands Sparing

Giuliano Perigli [1], Fabio Cianchi [1], Francesco Giudici [1,*], Edda Russo [1], Giulia Fiorenza [1], Luisa Petrone [2], Clotilde Sparano [2], Fabio Staderini [1], Benedetta Badii [1] and Alessio Morandi [1]

[1] Department of Experimental and Clinical Medicine, University of Florence, Largo Brambilla, 6, 50135 Florence, Italy; giuliano.perigli@unifi.it (G.P.); fabio.cianchi@unifi.it (F.C.); edda.russo@unifi.it (E.R.); giulia.fiorenza@yahoo.it (G.F.); fabio.staderini@unifi.it (F.S.); benedettabadii@yahoo.it (B.B.); morandialessio9@gmail.com (A.M.)
[2] Department of Biomedical, Experimental and Clinical Sciences Mario Serio, University of Florence, Largo Brambilla, 6, 50135 Florence, Italy; luisa.petrone@unifi.it (L.P.); clotilde.sparano@unifi.it (C.S.)
* Correspondence: francesco.giudici@unifi.it

Abstract: Background: The diagnosis of thyroid cancer is continuously increasing and consequently the amount of thyroidectomy. Notwithstanding the actual surgical skill, postoperative hypoparathyroidism still represents its most frequent complication. The aims of the present study are to analyze the rate of postoperative hypoparathyroidism after thyroidectomy, performed for cancer by a single first operator, without any technological aid, and to compare the data to those obtained adopting the most recent technological adjuncts developed to reduce the postoperative hypoparathyroidism. Methods: During the period 1997–2020 at the Endocrine Surgery Unit of the Department of Clinical and Experimental Medicine of the University of Florence, 1648 consecutive extracapsular thyroidectomies for cancer (401 with central compartment node dissection) were performed. The percentage of hypoparathyroidism, temporary or permanent, was recorded both in the first period (Group A) and in the second, most recent period (Group B). Total thyroidectomies were compared either with those with central compartment dissection and lobectomies. Minimally invasive procedures (MIT, MIVAT, some transoral) were also compared with conventional. Fisher's exact and Chi-square tests were used for comparison of categorical variables. $p < 0.01$ was considered statistically significant. Furthermore, a literature research from PubMed® has been performed, considering the most available tools to better identify parathyroid glands during thyroidectomy, in order to reduce the postoperative hypoparathyroidism. We grouped and analyzed them by technological affinity. Results: On the 1648 thyroidectomies enrolled for the study, the histotype was differentiated in 93.93 % of cases, medullary in 4% and poorly differentiated in the remaining 2.06%. Total extracapsular thyroidectomy and lobectomy were performed respectively in 95.45% and 4.55%. We recorded a total of 318 (19.29%) cases of hypocalcemia, with permanent hypoparathyroidism in 11 (0.66%). In regard to the literature, four categories of tools to facilitate the identification of the parathyroids were identified: (a) vital dye; (b) optical devices; (c) autofluorescence of parathyroids; and (d) autofluorescence enhanced by contrast media. Postoperative hypoparathyroidism had a variable range in the different groups. Conclusions: Our data confirm that the incidence of post-surgical hypoparathyroidism is extremely low in the high volume centers. Its potential reduction adopting technological adjuncts is difficult to estimate, and their cost, together with complexity of application, do not allow immediate routine use. The trend towards increasingly unilateral surgery in thyroid carcinoma, as confirmed by our results in case of lobectomy, is expected to really contribute to a further reduction of postsurgical hypoparathyroidism.

Keywords: thyroid carcinoma; postoperative complications; hypoparathyroidism; hypocalcemia; parathyroid glands; methylene blue; optical devices; autofluorescence; indocyanine green

Citation: Perigli, G.; Cianchi, F.; Giudici, F.; Russo, E.; Fiorenza, G.; Petrone, L.; Sparano, C.; Staderini, F.; Badii, B.; Morandi, A. Thyroidectomy for Cancer: The Surgeon and the Parathyroid Glands Sparing. *J. Clin. Med.* **2021**, *10*, 4323. https://doi.org/10.3390/jcm10194323

Academic Editors: Giovanni Vitale and Giovanni Conzo

Received: 21 July 2021
Accepted: 18 September 2021
Published: 23 September 2021

Publisher's Note: MDPI stays neutral with regard to jurisdictional claims in published maps and institutional affiliations.

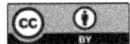

Copyright: © 2021 by the authors. Licensee MDPI, Basel, Switzerland. This article is an open access article distributed under the terms and conditions of the Creative Commons Attribution (CC BY) license (https://creativecommons.org/licenses/by/4.0/).

1. Introduction

The incidence of thyroid carcinoma has more than tripled in recent decades and consequently so have thyroidectomies and their related complications [1,2]. It has long been known that the most frequent of these is postoperative hypocalcaemia from temporary or permanent parathyroid insufficiency due to unavoidable, involuntary removal, thermal or vascular damage of the parathyroids. The incidence increases if total thyroidectomy is associated with central compartment lymph-node dissection, when parathyroid glands are often accidentally or inevitably removed in the pursuit of oncological radicality [3,4]. The temporary form is still frequent and the permanent form is problematic to treat due to the potential negative aspects of prolonged administration of calcium and vitamin D and the unavailability of a replacement hormone [5,6]. Considering earlier diagnosis with smaller size of thyroid carcinoma, the most recent guidelines point towards less aggressive and often unilateral surgical treatment [1–7]. The expected reduction in hypoparathyroidism is not substantial. In fact, total thyroidectomy remains by far the most prevalent intervention due to the presence of concomitant contralateral nodularity or hormonal hyperfunction [8]. Moreover, even in lesions with indication for radiometabolic therapeutic completion, surgical radicality should always be pursued to avoid potential interferences in the humoral and instrumental follow-up of a parenchymal residual. Although hypoparathyroidism is the most common complication after thyroidectomy, the literature reports extremely different incidence and prevalence values, ranging from 1.6% to more than 50%. In literature, the adoption of non-univocal and non-standardized parameters in reporting postoperative complications determines the inclusion in the different case series of very heterogeneous patients, symptomatic or asymptomatic, with mild or severe hypocalcaemia [9–11]. Especially in the case of permanent hypoparathyroidism, which worsens the quality of life due to replacement therapy and undefined controls, the differences are even more marked if one compares the case histories of dedicated surgical centres, general centres and general epidemiological surveys including patients who have escaped specialist controls. In fact, contrary to what has been estimated, the majority of the studies report hypoparathyroidism with percentages of more than 10%, even though these are often mild forms that can be easily controlled with low doses of calcium and vitamin D, which rarely expose the patient to complications such as calcification of the extra-skeletal soft tissues, basal ganglia and kidney, as observed in cases that require much higher doses to compensate for the almost total lack of parathyroid hormone [12–18].

In the face of these unexpected rates of post-surgical hypoparathyroidism revealed by the most recent studies, it is not surprising that surgeons have turned to testing every means of reducing them. In fact, it no longer seemed sufficient to rely solely on the recommendations of good surgical practice and the individual surgeon's experience and ability to detect them with the naked eye aided only by good lighting and optional optical magnification as basically indicated by the most authoritative guidelines [1].

The present paper, with a mainly clinical focus, has two aims: (a) to analyze the rate of postoperative hypoparathyroidism after thyroidectomy performed for cancer by a single first operator without any technological aid; (b) to evaluate if the numerous technological proposals that have emerged in recent years in an attempt to make objective identification of the parathyroids and assessment of their function, overcoming the limits related to the subjective judgement of the individual surgeon, are really useful in reducing the postoperative hypoparathyroidism incidence.

2. Materials and Methods

During the period 1997–2020 at the Endocrine Surgery Unit of the Department of Clinical and Experimental Medicine of the University of Florence, 1648 consecutive extracapsular thyroidectomies for cancer (401 with central compartment node dissection) were performed, and the patients' data prospectively recorded in an electronic database. A prospective study was conducted after approval by the Area Vasta Regione Toscana/AOUC Ethics Committee (N 20534). An informed written consent was obtained from each patient.

For the follow-up we have collaborated with the Endocrinology Unit of the same institution with which this activity has been constantly shared.

These are 1648 consecutive thyroidectomies, in 401 patients with central compartment lymph node dissection, to treat thyroid carcinoma performed almost exclusively by one of the authors (GP) in little more than 20 years and in small part (<10%) by collaborators always in his presence.

The case series was divided into a first period (March 1997–April 2015) (Group A) and a second period (May 2015–December 2020) (Group B), each consisting of 824 consecutive cases. No technological adjunct was adopted in both periods. The thyroidectomy procedure, always extracapsular, was carried out with the naked eye without magnifying glasses or frontal light but only with the operating light.

In addition to demographic data, the percentages of hypoparathyroidism (symptomatic or asymptomatic), temporary or definitive, were recorded calcium and PTH values, tested preoperatively, and at 12, 18 h and 7 days postoperatively lower than normal (respectively 8.5 mg/dL and 1.5 pmol/L in our laboratory) and the need for calcium-vitamin D replacement therapy over six months after surgery for the definitive form.

We also included the 75 lobectomies in which the central compartment had been explored and compared with total extracapsular thyroidectomies.

Total thyroidectomies were compared with those with central compartment and laterocervical lymph-adenectomy (in which we systematically also performed the central dissection); minimally invasive procedures (MIT, MIVAT, some transoral) with conventional ones and the first period of the series with the second one.

For the statistical analysis, Chi-square tests or Fisher's exact, when appropriate, and were used for comparison of categorical variables. $p < 0.01$ was considered statistically significant.

From the literature published in Pub Med® in recent years, we extracted the most suitable experiments to represent the current means available for a better identification of the parathyroid glands during thyroidectomy. We grouped them by technological affinity. The most reliable in terms of potential immediate clinical use experiments were critically revised.

3. Results

3.1. Our Experience

On 5264 thyroidectomies performed from January 1997 to December 2020, we enrolled all the 1648 patients who had undergone thyroidectomy for carcinoma. The histotype was differentiated in 93.93% of cases, medullary in 4% and poorly differentiated in the remaining 2.06%.

In 95.45% of the cases total extracapsular glandular excisions were performed and in 4.55% lobectomy alone was considered oncologically sufficient after negative exploration of the central compartment.

We recorded a total of 318 hypocalcemia (19.29%) of which 11 (0.66%) diagnosed as permanent hypoparathyroidism requiring therapy for more than 6 months. In particular, we found that hypocalcemia affected 316 patients after total thyroidectomy (20.09%), and only 2 patients after lobectomy (2.66%); after total thyroidectomy, 202 patients (25.06%) had hypocalcemia in Period A and 114 (14.86%) in Period B ($p < 0.0001$), while no patient in Period A and 2 patients (3.51%) in Period B suffered this complication after lobectomy ($p < 0.0001$).

Clinical characteristics of patients are described in Figure 1 and Table 1.

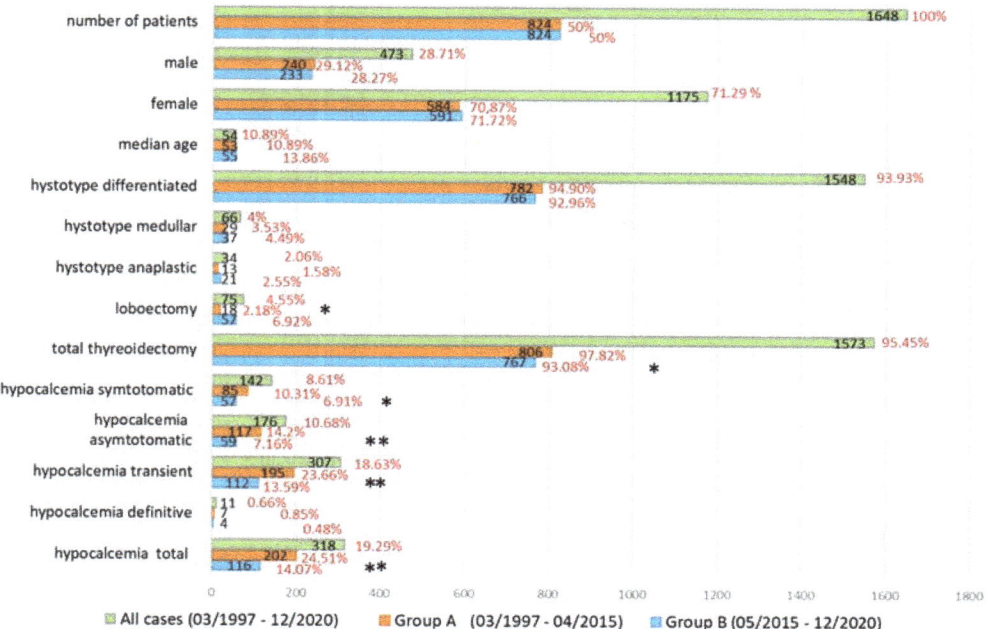

Figure 1. Demographic characteristics of the patients, type of operation and histotype of malignancy, incidences of temporary and permanent hypocalcaemia in the total case series and in the first and second period. Black numbers indicate the number of patients, while red numbers indicate the percentage. Differences between the groups were calculated via the Chi Square, or Fisher's exact test, when appropriate (both 2-tailed); a $p < 0.01$ is considered statistically significant.
* $p < 0.01$, ** $p < 0.0001$.

Table 1. Comparison of conventional and minimally invasive procedures and of patients who received only a total thyroidectomy versus those in whom a central compartment lymphectomy was also performed, whether or not extended to the lateral compartments.

Type of Surgery		Group A		Group B		p Value	Group A		Group B		p Value
		Minimally Invasive					Conventional				
cases		403		257			421		567		
		N.	%	N.	%		N.	%	N.	%	
hypocalcemia	symptomatic	38	9.43	14	5.44	0.0752	47	11.16	43	7.58	0.0577
	asymptomatic	56	13.89	24	9.34	0.0875	61	14.49	35	6.17	<0.0001
	transient	91	22.58	37	14.39	0.01	104	24.7	76	13.4	<0.0001
	definitive	3	0.74	1	0.39	1	4	0.95	2	0.35	0.4106
	total	94	23.32	38	14.78	0.003	108	25.65	78	13.75	<0.0001
Type of Surgery		Cclnd					No Cclnd				
cases		216		185			608		639		
		N.	%	N.	%		N.	%	N.	%	
hypocalcemia	symptomatic	44	20.37	32	17.29	0.4464	45	7.4	28	4.38	0.0293
	asymptomatic	40	18.51	29	15.68	0.5077	73	12.01	27	4.22	<0.0001
	transient	79	36.57	59	31.89	0.3	116	19.08	53	8.29	<0.0001
	definitive	5	2.31	2	1.08	0.4589	2	0.33	2	0.31	1
	total	84	38.88	61	32.97	0.2	118	19.41	55	8.6	<0.0001

Abbreviations: cclnd, central compartment lymph node dissection. Differences between the groups were calculated via the Chi Square, or Fisher's exact test, when appropriate (both two-tailed); a $p < 0.01$ is considered statistically significant.

3.2. Literature Examination

The literature reports four categories of tools that can be used by the surgeon, together with his eyes and experience, to facilitate the identification of the parathyroids (Table 2):

(a) Vital dye such as methylene bleu [19–21].
(b) Optical devices without contrast media and unaffected by ambient light [22–26].
(c) Autofluorescence of parathyroids detected by infrared light or laser stimulation [27–33].
(d) Autofluorescence enhanced by injection of indocyanine green or 5-ALA [34,35].

Table 2. The main original studies evaluating technologies in order to avoid postoperative hypoparathyroidism, from 1971 to 2021.

Reference	Technology	Article Type	Nb pt	Parathyroid Identification	Postoperative Hypo-PTH /Hypoca	Conclusions
Dudley et al. [19] 1971	Intravenous infusion of methylene blue	original/humans	17	41/68	/	Could help to reduce the high incidence of clinical hypoparathyroidism after total thyroidectomy.
Monib et al. [20] 2020	Intraoperative methylene blue spray	original/humans	50	82% accuracy	18%	Safe, feasible, and effective to identify parathyroid glands
Sari et al. [21] 2012	Intraoperative methylene blue spray	original/humans	56	/	5% transient	Identification of parathyroid glands within three minutes and also of recurrent laryngeal nerves and inferior thyroid arteries.
Hu et al. [22] 2021	Dynamic optical contrast imaging (DOCI)	original/animals and humans ex vivo	/	/	/	Facilitates specific parathyroid gland localization
Marsden et al. [23] 2021	Fluorescence lifetime imaging (FLIm)	original/humans	21	100% sensitivity 93% specificity	/	Good sensitivity and specificity for the rapid identification of PG.
Mannoh et al. [24] 2021	Laser speckle contrast imaging (LSCI)	original/humans	72	/	8.3% temporary 1.4% permanent	Promising technique for assessing parathyroid gland vascularity
Kennedy et al. 2021 [25]	Near-infrared molecular Imaging (IMI)	original/humans	5	9/9	1/9 asymptomatic	Accurate and reproducible method of localizing parathyroid glands
Wang et al. [26] 2021	Laser-induced breakdown spectroscopy (LIBS)	original/animals ex vivo	/	/	/	Can discriminate between smear samples of PG and NPG
Paras et al. [27] 2011	Near-infrared (NIR) autofluorescence	original/humans	21	/	/	Parathyroid fluorescence was two to eleven times higher than that of the thyroid tissues with peak fluorescence occurring at 820 to 830 nm.

Table 2. Cont.

Reference	Technology	Article Type	Nb pt	Parathyroid Identification	Postoperative Hypo-PTH /Hypoca	Conclusions
Aoyama et al. [28] 2020	Near-infrared (NIR) autofluorescence	original/humans	2	/	/	The autofluorescence of diseased glands was weaker than that of normal glands, even with the excitation light of NIR.
Akbulut et al. [29] 2021	Near-infrared (NIR) autofluorescence	original/humans	300	25% *	/	Second-generation NIFI (CMOS) displayed higher detection rates and AF intensity.
Kim et al. [30] 2021	Near-infrared (NIR) autofluorescence	original/humans	542	/	4.2% permanent	May reduce temporary hypoparathyroidism and the risk of inadvertent resection of PGs in CND.
Wiseman et al. [31] 2021	Near-infrared (NIR) autofluorescence	original/humans in vivo and ex vivo	/	/	/	Can successfully intraoperatively identify both normal and pathological PGs.
Kiernan et al. [32] 2021	Near-infrared (NIR) autofluorescence	original/humans	83	94.3% accuracy	/	Probe-based NIRAF detection can be a valuable adjunct device to intraoperatively identify PGs.
Mannoh et al. [33] 2021	ParaSPAI a device that combines NIRAF imaging with LSCI	original/humans	/	/	/	Capable of label-free parathyroid gland identification and vascularity assessment through the combination of NIRAF imaging with LSCI.
Suzuki et al. [34] 2011	5-Aminolevulinic Acid	original/humans	13	In all patients at least one	/	Useful to localize the normal parathyroid glands during thyroid surgery
Jin et al. [35] 2018	Indocyanine green	original/humans	26	/	7.69% transient	Safe, easy and effective method to protect the parathyroid and predict postoperative hypoparathyroidism

Abbreviations: / = no available data. Nb pt = number of patients; PG = parathyroid gland; NPG = no parathyroid gland; * = before visual identification of PGs; NIFI = near-infrared fluorescence imaging; CMOS = complementary metal-oxide semiconductor; AF = autofluorescence; CND = central neck dissection; ParaSPAI = parathyroid speckle and autofluorescence imager; LSCI = laser speckle contrast imaging.

4. Discussion

The literature evaluation has enabled us to consolidate certain convictions developed over many years of activity. Firstly, the difficulty of defining hypoparathyroidism due to the variables that characterize it and the clinical manifestations that arise with serum calcium levels, which vary greatly in every single patient [1].

We agree with Sitges-Serra that it is inappropriate and reductive to categorize it clearly between clinical and humoral, temporary and definitive, since functional recovery is a dynamic process that can last up to two years [9].

We have noted a considerable discrepancy in the prevalence of post-surgical hypoparathyroidism, especially permanent, reported in the various case histories according to their origin. The ranges appear almost irreconcilable when comparing the surgical series with the endocrinological or epidemiological ones, and the most common values are around 1–3% in the former and around 12% in the latter [3,8,10,15,36].

There is a unanimous agreement in the literature that the identification and functional preservation of the parathyroids is difficult due to the presence of contiguous similar structures such as thyroid nodules, lymph nodes, adipose lobules or fibrosis from previous operations. Therefore, it is directly related to the sensitivity and experience of the surgeon, even though he strictly adheres to the principles of good surgical practice, which, in addition to anatomical integrity and the number of glands identified, also recommend respect for vascular support [1,37,38]. Recent studies have in fact shown that accidental removal and tissue or vascular damage do not find a remedy in glands autotransplantation [9], and allografting is still not beyond the experimental stage or good hopes for the future [39]. There is evidence that systematic and meticulous research can lead to invisible parathyroids damage and that selective identification is preferable to routine identification. In fact, it would appear that the number of parathyroids actually left 'in situ' is more important than the number of those identified [8,40–43].

Regarding instruments potentially useful in reducing post-surgical hypocalcaemia through better identification and functional preservation of the parathyroids, intraoperative biopsy, rapid PTH dosage on aspirate [44–47] and gamma probe identification [48], which were proposed in the past and are now obsolete because they are invasive, costly, time-consuming and ethically inapplicable as they damage tissue that should ideally be preserved as much as possible, are now rarely used.

The simplest and easiest means of identifying vital parathyroids would be the use of methylene blue. Known for fifty years [19] and appreciated for the identification of pathological glands, it did not provide the same results in the recognition of normal glands during thyroidectomy when injected intravenously. The recent adoption of a spray application directly on the operating field seems to have achieved a high level of accuracy, even avoiding the problem of the potential toxicity [20,21,49].

Looking at the group of instruments based on optical technology such as DOCI (dynamic optical contrast imaging), FLIm (fluorescence lifetime imaging), LSCI (laser speckle contrast imaging), NIMI (near infrared molecular imaging), LIBS (laser induced breakdown spectroscopy), it is immediately evident that, despite the advantage of not using any contrast medium and not being influenced by ambient light, these are still experimental applications and reserved for research centres with strong financial backing, certainly not within the reach of most thyroid surgery centres [22–26,33]. They demonstrate a high level of accuracy in identifying and assessing glandular perfusion, but cannot prevent any iatrogenic damage produced during retrieval, which in any case precedes the test. Due to their complexity, they appear to be far from an imminent clinical application.

Paras et al. were the first in 2011 to discover and describe [27] an autofluorescence of the parathyroids induced by stimulation with high-energy light sources of endogenous fluorophores that reacted by emitting low-energy light. The exploitation of this property, apparently easier to apply and with potentially more immediate advantages, has offered a new opportunity in the attempt to reduce post-surgical hypoparathyroidism [27–33].

The long persistence of autofluorescence in parathyroids even after their removal makes this property unsuitable for perfusion assessment and has necessitated the injection of exogenous fluorophores as contrast agents or dyes (ICG, indocyanine green; 5-ALA, 5-aminolevulinic acid) to enhance natural fluorescence.

There are other commercially available laparoscopic or handheld camera instruments which, although designed for ICG study of other organ perfusion or sentinel node detection, can be used in parathyroid fluorescence detection. Even instruments combining two methods (Niraf and Laser-speckle contrast Imaging), Ref. [33] are not yet fully convincing and in any case not applicable on a large scale.

Solorzano et al., examined in detail all fluorescence-based technology applicable to parathyroid surgery today and compiled a valuable list of possible indications with potential advantages and disadvantages specific to probe-based and chamber-based technology.

Although the literature reports a sensitivity of autofluorescence of 80 to 100%, it is also correctly acknowledged that there are false positives and negatives and that the main limitation of the method lies in its poor tissues penetration power and that it requires the manipulation of parathyroids, exposing to tissue damage. The additional use of ICG improves the power of identification and allows a judgement of perfusion that is not possible with autofluorescence alone. The conclusions are not definitive, so we invite others to further clarify its real cost–benefit [50].

To date, unfortunately only a few studies have demonstrated a direct correlation between visualization and glandular perfusion and a reduction in hypoparathyroidism [30], which is in any case limited to the temporary but not definitive form. Moreover, none of the prevention methods adopted seem to be able to reduce hypocalcaemia [42,49–55].

In summary, alongside with authoritative reviews confirming the feasibility and efficacy of recent parathyroid identification aids [56–58], there are others that urge caution in adopting them too enthusiastically before larger prospective and randomised studies confirm their superiority over surgeon volume and skill [59,60]. For example, the analysis of our case history, while showing values for temporary hypoparathyroidism that are in line with the literature (19.29%), confirms the negligible values of our previous investigations [4,8,18,61,62], for permanent hypoparathyroidism. The strict adoption of the specific principles of thyroid surgery required by the university didactic nature of our hospital and the high volume of cases treated, we believe, is sufficient to justify values much lower than those of other series but not too dissimilar from other Italian multicentric experiences where values of temporary and permanent hypoparathyroidism of 8.3% and 1.7% respectively are reported [3].

In this regard, the comparison between the first and second part of our series seems very expressive: although they are absolutely superimposable in terms of demographic characteristics and the methods adopted, they reveal statistically significant differences for both forms of hypoparathyroidism, confirming the well-known and recently reaffirmed [14] relationship between the surgeon's case-volume and the number of complications.

As expected, and as already noted in our previous experiences, the differences between minimally invasive and conventional surgery in the two groups are not significant [61,62].

In the second group, in accordance with the most recent guidelines, lobectomies increased but hypocalcaemia, which was never definitive, remained negligible, confirming that unilateral surgery, even in the cases we included with exploration of the central compartment, protects against hypocalcaemic complications.

On the other hand, the values are very different in both groups when comparing simple thyroidectomies and those accompanied by lymphectomy of the central compartment, respectively 19.41% vs. 38.8% in Group A and 8.61% vs. 32.97% in Group B. Interestingly, the percentages of hypoparathyroidism remained very similar in the two periods when total thyroidectomy was accompanied by central compartment lymphectomy, 38.88% in Group A and 32.97% in Group B, respectively. Moreover, out of eleven patients with definitive hypoparathyroidism, as many as eight had undergone central compartment lymphectomy, demonstrating that the complication is strictly procedure-dependent and cannot be modified by the surgeon's experience.

In addition, this study also confirms the higher incidence of hypocalcaemia in simple total thyroidectomies for carcinoma compared with total thyroidectomies for benign disease, as previously reported by us and other authors (19.29% vs. 12.99), [4,8,14,63]. However, a recent article from Onder CE et al., 2020, reports that the management of the patients with hypocalcaemia is suboptimal with active vitamin D and cholecalciferol treatment [64].

The limitation common to all the examined tools is that they only record what has already taken place and are not able to modify the intra-operative procedure except to indicate an autotransplant in the event of hypoperfusion, with the possibility to increase the risk of hypocalcaemia [9], therefore, the surgeon remains the one who has to assess the parathyroids site, shape, color (and its possible variations) or, by touch, their consistency.

5. Conclusions

Our findings show that post-surgical hypoparathyroidism is extremely uncommon in high-volume institutions. Its potential decrease through the employment of technical adjuncts is impossible to quantify, and their expense, combined with the complexity of their application, makes them unsuitable for immediate usage. As evidenced by our findings in the case of lobectomy, the trend toward more unilateral thyroid surgery is predicted to lead to a further reduction in postsurgical hypoparathyroidism.

Author Contributions: Conceptualization, G.P. and A.M.; methodology, E.R., C.S.; statistical analysis, E.R.; investigation, F.G., L.P., F.C., F.S., B.B., G.F. writing G.P., A.M., F.G., E.R.; editing, A.M., E.R.; supervision, G.P., F.G., F.C. All authors have read and agreed to the published version of the manuscript.

Funding: This research received no external funding.

Institutional Review Board Statement: The study was conducted according to the guidelines of the Declaration of Helsinki, and approved by the Area Vasta Regione Toscana/AOUC Ethics Committee (N 20534).

Informed Consent Statement: A written informed consent was obtained from each patient.

Acknowledgments: We thank Elisangela Miceli for the English revision.

Conflicts of Interest: The authors declare no conflict of interest.

References

1. Haugen, B.R.; Alexander, E.K.; Bible, K.C.; Doherty, G.M.; Mandel, S.J.; Nikiforov, Y.E.; Pacini, F.; Randolph, G.W.; Sawka, A.M.; Schlumberger, M.; et al. 2015 American Thyroid Association Management Guidelines for Adult Patients with Thyroid Nodules and Differentiated Thyroid Cancer: The American Thyroid Association Guidelines Task Force on Thyroid Nodules and Differentiated Thyroid Cancer. *Thyroid* **2016**, *26*, 1–133. [CrossRef] [PubMed]
2. Pellegriti, G.; Frasca, F.; Regalbuto, C.; Squatrito, S.; Vigneri, R. Worldwide increasing incidence of thyroid cancer: Update on epidemiology and risk factors. *J. Cancer Epidemiol.* **2013**, *2013*, 965212. [CrossRef] [PubMed]
3. Rosato, L.; Avenia, N.; Bernante, P.; De Palma, M.; Gulino, G.; Nasi, P.G.; Pelizzo, M.R.; Pezzullo, L. Complications of thyroid surgery: Analysis of a multicentric study on 14,934 patients operated on in Italy over 5 years. *World J. Surg.* **2004**, *28*, 271–276. [CrossRef]
4. Perigli, G.; Fiorenza, G.; Badii, B.; Skalamera, I.; Foppa, C.; Cianchi, F. Prevenzione e trattamento della ipocalcemia precoce e tardiva dopotiroidectomia. *L'Endocrinologo* **2018**, *19*, 6–9.
5. Bilezikian, J.P.; Brandi, M.L.; Cusano, N.E.; Mannstadt, M.; Rejnmark, L.; Rizzoli, R.; Rubin, M.R.; Winer, K.K.; Liberman, U.A.; Potts, J.T., Jr. Management of Hypoparathyroidism: Present and Future. *J. Clin. Endocrinol. Metab.* **2016**, *101*, 2313–2324. [CrossRef] [PubMed]
6. Allas, S.; Ovize, M.; Culler, M.D.; Geraul, C.; van de Wetering, J.; Mannstadt, M. A Single Administration of AZP-3601, a Novel, Long-Acting PTH Analog, Induces a Significant and Sustained Calcemic Response: Preliminary Data From a Randomized, Double-Blind, PlaceboControlled Phase 1 Study. *J. Endocr. Soc.* **2021**, *5*, A254. [CrossRef]
7. Tuttle, R.M. Controversial Issues in Thyroid Cancer Management. *J. Nucl. Med.* **2018**, *59*, 1187–1194. [CrossRef] [PubMed]
8. Puzziello, A.; Rosato, L.; Innaro, N.; Orlando, G.; Avenia, N.; Perigli, G.; Calo, P.G.; De Palma, M. Hypocalcemia following thyroid surgery: Incidence and risk factors. A longitudinal multicenter study comprising 2631 patients. *Endocrine* **2014**, *47*, 537–542. [CrossRef] [PubMed]
9. Sitges-Serra, A. Etiology and Diagnosis of Permanent Hypoparathyroidism after Total Thyroidectomy. *J. Clin. Med.* **2021**, *10*, 543. [CrossRef]
10. Edafe, O.; Antakia, R.; Laskar, N.; Uttley, L.; Balasubramanian, S.P. Authors' reply: Systematic review and meta-analysis of predictors of post-thyroidectomy hypocalcaemia. *Br. J. Surg.* **2014**, *101*, 883–884. [CrossRef]
11. Raffaelli, M.; De Crea, C.; D'Amato, G.; Moscato, U.; Bellantone, C.; Carrozza, C.; Lombardi, C.P. Post-thyroidectomy hypocalcemia is related to parathyroid dysfunction even in patients with normal parathyroid hormone concentrations early after surgery. *Surgery* **2016**, *159*, 78–84. [CrossRef]

12. Pepe, J.; Colangelo, L.; Biamonte, F.; Sonato, C.; Danese, V.C.; Cecchetti, V.; Occhiuto, M.; Piazzolla, V.; De Martino, V.; Ferrone, F.; et al. Diagnosis and management of hypocalcemia. *Endocrine* 2020, *69*, 485–495. [CrossRef] [PubMed]
13. Yazicioglu, M.O.; Yilmaz, A.; Kocaoz, S.; Ozcaglayan, R.; Parlak, O. Risks and prediction of postoperative hypoparathyroidism due to thyroid surgery. *Sci. Rep.* 2021, *11*, 11876. [CrossRef]
14. Bedi, H.K.; Jedrzejko, N.; Nguyen, A.; Aspinall, S.R.; Wiseman, S.M. Thyroid and parathyroid surgeon case volume influences patient outcomes: A systematic review. *Surg. Oncol.* 2021, *38*, 101550. [CrossRef]
15. Lui, D.T.W.; Fung, M.M.H.; Lee, C.H.; Fong, C.H.Y.; Woo, Y.C.; Lang, B.H.H. A territory-wide assessment of the incidence of persistent hypoparathyroidism after elective thyroid surgery and its impact on new fracture risk over time. *Surgery* 2021. [CrossRef]
16. Lorenz, K.; Raffaeli, M.; Barczynski, M.; Lorente-Poch, L.; Sancho, J. Volume, outcomes, and quality standards in thyroid surgery: An evidence-based analysis-European Society of Endocrine Surgeons (ESES) positional statement. *Langenbecks Arch. Surg.* 2020, *405*, 401–425. [CrossRef] [PubMed]
17. Anneback, M.; Hedberg, J.; Almquist, M.; Stalberg, P.; Norlen, O. Risk of Permanent Hypoparathyroidism After Total Thyroidectomy for Benign Disease: A Nationwide Population-based Cohort Study From Sweden. *Ann. Surg.* 2020. [CrossRef] [PubMed]
18. Marcucci, G.; Cianferotti, L.; Parri, S.; Altieri, P.; Arvat, E.; Benvenga, S.; Betterle, C.; Bondanelli, M.; Boscaro, M.; Camozzi, V.; et al. HypoparaNet: A Database of Chronic Hypoparathyroidism Based on Expert Medical-Surgical Centers in Italy. *Calcif. Tissue Int.* 2018, *103*, 151–163. [CrossRef] [PubMed]
19. Dudley, N.E. Methylene blue for rapid identification of the parathyroids. *Br. Med. J.* 1971, *3*, 680–681. [CrossRef]
20. Monib, S.; Mohamed, A.; Abdelaziz, M.I. Methylene Blue Spray for Identification of Parathyroid Glands During Thyroidectomy. *Cureus* 2020, *12*, e11569. [CrossRef]
21. Sari, S.; Aysan, E.; Muslumanoglu, M.; Ersoy, Y.E.; Bektasoglu, H.; Yardimci, E. Safe thyroidectomy with intraoperative methylene blue spraying. *Thyroid Res.* 2012, *5*, 15. [CrossRef]
22. Hu, Y.; Han, A.Y.; Huang, S.; Pellionisz, P.; Alhiyari, Y.; Krane, J.F.; Shori, R.; Stafsudd, O.; St John, M.A. A Tool to Locate Parathyroid Glands Using Dynamic Optical Contrast Imaging. *Laryngoscope* 2021, *31*, 2391–2397. [CrossRef]
23. Marsden, M.; Weaver, S.S.; Marcu, L.; Campbell, M.J. Intraoperative Mapping of Parathyroid Glands Using Fluorescence Lifetime Imaging. *J. Surg. Res.* 2021, *265*, 42–48. [CrossRef] [PubMed]
24. Mannoh, E.A.; Thomas, G.; Baregamian, N.; Rohde, S.; Solorzano, C.C.; Mahadevan-Jansen, A. Assessing Intraoperative Laser Speckle Contrast Imaging of Parathyroid Glands in Relation to Thyroidectomy Patient Outcomes. *Thyroid* 2021. [CrossRef] [PubMed]
25. Kennedy, G.T.; Azari, F.S.; Newton, A.D.; Bernstein, E.S.; Fraker, D.L.; Wachtel, H.; Singhal, S. Use of Near-Infrared Molecular Imaging for Localizing Visually Occult Parathyroid Glands in Ectopic Locations. *JAMA Otolaryngol. Head Neck Surg.* 2021, *147*, 669–671. [CrossRef] [PubMed]
26. Wang, Q.; Xiangli, W.; Chen, X.; Zhang, J.; Teng, G.; Cui, X.; Idrees, B.S.; Wei, K. Primary study of identification of parathyroid gland based on laser-induced breakdown spectroscopy. *Biomed. Opt. Express* 2021, *12*, 1999–2014. [CrossRef] [PubMed]
27. Paras, C.; Keller, M.; White, L.; Phay, J.; Mahadevan-Jansen, A. Near-infrared autofluorescence for the detection of parathyroid glands. *J. Biomed. Opt.* 2011, *16*, 067012. [CrossRef]
28. Aoyama, M.; Takizawa, H.; Yamamoto, K.; Inui, T.; Miyamoto, N.; Sakamoto, S.; Kobayashi, T.; Uehara, H.; Tangoku, A. Effects of excitation light intensity on parathyroid autofluorescence with a novel near-infrared fluorescence imaging system: Two surgical case reports. *Gland Surg.* 2020, *9*, 1584–1589. [CrossRef]
29. Akbulut, S.; Erten, O.; Gokceimam, M.; Kim, Y.S.; Krishnamurthy, V.; Heiden, K.; Jin, J.; Siperstein, A.; Berber, E. Intraoperative near-infrared imaging of parathyroid glands: A comparison of first- and second-generation technologies. *J. Surg. Oncol.* 2021, *123*, 866–871. [CrossRef]
30. Kim, D.H.; Kim, S.W.; Kang, P.; Choi, J.; Lee, H.S.; Park, S.Y.; Kim, Y.; Ahn, Y.C.; Lee, K.D. Near-Infrared Autofluorescence Imaging May Reduce Temporary Hypoparathyroidism in Patients Undergoing Total Thyroidectomy and Central Neck Dissection. *Thyroid* 2021, *31*, 1400–1408. [CrossRef]
31. Wiseman, S.M.; Saleh, N.; Tootooni, A.; Eshraghi, P.; Jama, R.; Saleh, S. Parathyroid identification during thyroid and parathyroid operations: A pilot study evaluating a novel low cost autofluorescence based device. *Am. J. Surg.* 2021, *221*, 1150–1158. [CrossRef] [PubMed]
32. Kiernan, C.M.; Thomas, G.; Baregamian, N.; Solomicronrzano, C.C. Initial clinical experiences using the intraoperative probe-based parathyroid autofluorescence identification system-PTeye during thyroid and parathyroid procedures. *J. Surg. Oncol.* 2021, *124*, 271–281. [CrossRef] [PubMed]
33. Mannoh, E.A.; Parker, L.B.; Thomas, G.; Solorzano, C.C.; Mahadevan-Jansen, A. Development of an imaging device for label-free parathyroid gland identification and vascularity assessment. *J. Biophotonics* 2021, *14*, e202100008. [CrossRef] [PubMed]
34. Suzuki, T.; Numata, T.; Shibuya, M. Intraoperative photodynamic detection of normal parathyroid glands using 5-aminolevulinic acid. *Laryngoscope* 2011, *121*, 1462–1466. [CrossRef] [PubMed]
35. Jin, H.; Dong, Q.; He, Z.; Fan, J.; Liao, K.; Cui, M. Application of a Fluorescence Imaging System with Indocyanine Green to Protect the Parathyroid Gland Intraoperatively and to Predict Postoperative Parathyroidism. *Adv. Ther.* 2018, *35*, 2167–2175. [CrossRef]

36. Orloff, L.A.; Wiseman, S.M.; Bernet, V.J.; Fahey, T.J., 3rd; Shaha, A.R.; Shindo, M.L.; Snyder, S.K.; Stack, B.C., Jr.; Sunwoo, J.B.; Wang, M.B. American Thyroid Association Statement on Postoperative Hypoparathyroidism: Diagnosis, Prevention, and Management in Adults. *Thyroid* **2018**, *28*, 830–841. [CrossRef] [PubMed]
37. Delbridge, L.W.; Suliburk, J.; Sidhu, S.; Sywak, M. Parathyroid Cancer: Is There an Epidemic? *ANZ J. Surg.* **2009**, *79*, A18. [CrossRef]
38. Park, I.; Rhu, J.; Woo, J.W.; Choi, J.H.; Kim, J.S.; Kim, J.H. Preserving Parathyroid Gland Vasculature to Reduce Post-thyroidectomy Hypocalcemia. *World J. Surg.* **2016**, *40*, 1382–1389. [CrossRef]
39. Mihai, R.; Thakker, R.V. Management of Endocrine Disease: Postsurgical hypoparathyroidism: Current treatments and future prospects for parathyroid allotransplantation. *Eur. J. Endocrinol.* **2021**, *184*, R165–R175. [CrossRef]
40. Chang, Y.K.; Lang, B.H.H. To identify or not to identify parathyroid glands during total thyroidectomy. *G'and Surg.* **2017**, *6*, S20–S29. [CrossRef]
41. Lang, B.H.; Chan, D.T.; Chow, F.C. Visualizing fewer parathyroid glands may be associated with lower hypoparathyroidism following total thyroidectomy. *Langenbecks Arch. Surg.* **2016**, *401*, 231–238. [CrossRef] [PubMed]
42. Antakia, R.; Edafe, O.; Uttley, L.; Balasubramanian, S.P. Effectiveness of preventative and other surgical measures on hypocalcemia following bilateral thyroid surgery: A systematic review and meta-analysis. *Thyroid* **2015**, *25*, 95–106. [CrossRef] [PubMed]
43. Lorente-Poch, L.; Sancho, J.; Munoz, J.L.; Gallego-Otaegui, L.; Martinez-Ruiz, C.; Sitges-Serra, A. Failure of fragmented parathyroid gland autotransplantation to prevent permanent hypoparathyroidism after total thyroidectomy. *Langenbecks Arch. Surg.* **2017**, *402*, 281–287. [CrossRef]
44. Huang, H.Y.; Li, H.; Lin, S.J.; Deng, W.Y.; Li, Q.L.; Chen, Y.F.; Yang, A.K.; Zhang, Q.; Guo, Z.M. Fine-needle aspiration with measurement of parathyroid hormone levels in thyroidectomy. *Zhonghua Er Bi Yan Hou Tou Jing Wai Ke Za Zhi* **2013**, *48*, 934–938. [PubMed]
45. Zou, X.; Shi, L.; Zhu, G.; Zhu, L.; Bao, J.; Fan, J.; Hu, Y.; Zhou, B.; Lv, Z. Fine-needle aspiration with rapid parathyroid hormone assay to identify parathyroid gland in thyroidectomy. *Medicine* **2020**, *99*, e19840. [CrossRef]
46. Xia, W.; Zhang, J.; Shen, W.; Zhu, Z.; Yang, Z.; Li, X. A Rapid Intraoperative Parathyroid Hormone Assay Based on the Immune Colloidal Gold Technique for Parathyroid Identification in Thyroid Surgery. *Front. Endocrinol.* **2020**, *11*, 594745. [CrossRef] [PubMed]
47. Coan, K.E.; Yen, T.W.F.; Carr, A.A.; Evans, D.B.; Wang, T.S. Confirmation of Parathyroid Tissue: Are Surgeors Aware of New and Novel Techniques? *J. Surg. Res.* **2020**, *246*, 139–144. [CrossRef] [PubMed]
48. Grubbs, E.G.; Mittendorf, E.A.; Perrier, N.D.; Lee, J.E. Gamma probe identification of normal parathyroid glands during central neck surgery can facilitate parathyroid preservation. *Am. J. Surg.* **2008**, *196*, 931–935, discussion 935–936. [CrossRef]
49. Patel, H.P.; Chadwick, D.R.; Harrison, B.J.; Balasubramanian, S.P. Systematic review of intravenous methylene blue in parathyroid surgery. *Br. J. Surg.* **2012**, *99*, 1345–1351. [CrossRef]
50. Solorzano, C.C.; Thomas, G.; Berber, E.; Wang, T.S.; Randolph, G.W.; Duh, Q.Y.; Triponez, F. Current state of intraoperative use of near infrared fluorescence for parathyroid identification and preservation. *Surgery* **2021**, *169*, 868–878. [CrossRef]
51. Lavazza, M.; Liu, X.; Wu, C.; Anuwong, A.; Kim, H.Y.; Liu, R.; Randolph, G.W.; Inversini, D.; Boni, L.; Rausei, S.; et al. Indocyanine green-enhanced fluorescence for assessing parathyroid perfusion during thyroidectomy. *Gland Surg.* **2016**, *5*, 512–521. [CrossRef]
52. Di Marco, A.N.; Palazzo, F.F. Near-infrared autofluorescence in thyroid and parathyroid surgery. *Gland Surg.* **2020**, *9*, S136–S146. [CrossRef]
53. Weng, Y.J.; Jiang, J.; Min, L.; Ai, Q.; Chen, D.B.; Chen, W.C.; Huang, Z.H. Intraoperative near-infrared autofluorescence imaging for hypocalcemia risk reduction after total thyroidectomy: Evidence from a meta-analysis. *Head Neck* **2021**, *43*, 2523–2533. [CrossRef]
54. Demarchi, M.S.; Karenovics, W.; Bedat, B.; Triponez, F. Intraoperative Autofluorescence and Indocyanine Green Angiography for the Detection and Preservation of Parathyroid Glands. *J. Clin. Med.* **2020**, *9*, 830. [CrossRef] [PubMed]
55. Goncalves, L.N.; van den Hoven, P.; van Schaik, J.; Leeuwenburgh, L.; Hendricks, C.H.F.; Verduijn, P.S.; van der Bogt, K.E.A.; van Rijswijk, C.S.P.; Schepers, A.; Vahrmeijer, A.L.; et al. Perfusion Parameters in Near-Infrared Fluorescence Imaging with Indocyanine Green: A Systematic Review of the Literature. *Life* **2021**, *11*, 433. [CrossRef] [PubMed]
56. Dip, F.; Falco, J.; Verna, S.; Prunello, M.; Loccisano, M.; Quadri, P.; White, K.; Rosenthal, R. Randomized Controlled Trial Comparing White Light with Near-Infrared Autofluorescence for Parathyroid Gland Identification During Total Thyroidectomy. *J. Am. Coll. Surg.* **2019**, *228*, 744–751. [CrossRef]
57. Thomas, G.; Solorzano, C.C.; Baregamian, N.; Mannoh, E.A.; Gautam, R.; Irlmeier, R.T.; Ye, F.; Nelson, J.A.; Long, S.E.; Gauger, P.G.; et al. Comparing intraoperative parathyroid identification based on surgeon experience versus near infrared autofluorescence detection—A surgeon-blinded multi-centric study. *Am. J. Surg.* **2021**. [CrossRef] [PubMed]
58. Solorzano, C.C.; Thomas, G.; Baregamian, N.; Mahadevan-Jansen, A. Detecting the Near Infrared Autofluorescence of the Human Parathyroid: Hype or Opportunity? *Ann. Surg.* **2020**, *272*, 973–985. [CrossRef] [PubMed]
59. Abbaci, M.; De Leeuw, F.; Breuskin, I.; Casiraghi, O.; Lakhdar, A.B.; Ghanem, W.; Laplace-Builhe, C.; Hartl, D. Parathyroid gland management using optical technologies during thyroidectomy or parathyroidectomy: A systematic review. *Oral Oncol.* **2018**, *87*, 186–196. [CrossRef]
60. Wong, A.; Wong, J.C.Y.; Pandey, P.U.; Wiseman, S.M. Novel techniques for intraoperative parathyroid gland identification: A comprehensive review. *Expert Rev. Endocrinol. Metab.* **2020**, *15*, 439–457. [CrossRef]

61. Perigli, G.; Cortesini, C.; Qirici, E.; Boni, D.; Cianchi, F. Clinical benefits of minimally invasive techniques in thyroid surgery. *World J. Surg.* **2008**, *32*, 45–50. [CrossRef] [PubMed]
62. Perigli, G.; Qirici, E.; Badii, B.; Kokomani, A.; Staderini, F.; Luconi, M.; Crescioli, C.; Mannelli, M.; Maggi, M.; Cianchi, F. Feasibility and safety of minimal-incision thyroidectomy for Graves' disease: A prospective, single-center study. *Head Neck* **2013**, *35*, 1345–1348. [CrossRef] [PubMed]
63. Kim, H.I.; Kim, T.H.; Choe, J.H.; Kim, J.H.; Kim, J.S.; Kim, Y.N.; Kim, H.; Kim, S.W.; Chung, J.H. Surgeon volume and prognosis of patients with advanced papillary thyroid cancer and lateral nodal metastasis. *Br. J. Surg.* **2018**, *105*, 270–278. [CrossRef] [PubMed]
64. Onder, C.E.; Kuskonmaz, S.M.; Koc, G.; Firat, S.F.; Omma, T.; Culha, C. Evaluation of management of patients with postoperative permanent hypoparathyroidism. How close are we to the targets? *Minerva Endocrinol.* **2020**. Online ahead of print. [CrossRef]

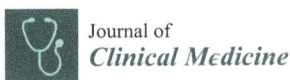

Article

Risk Factors for Low Levels of Parathyroid Hormone after Surgery for Thyroid Cancer: A Single Center Study

Francesca Privitera [1], Rossella Gioco [1], Ileana Fazio [1], Alessio Volpicelli [1], Maria Teresa Cannizzaro [2], Salvatore Costa [1], Matteo Angelo Cannizzaro [1] and Massimiliano Veroux [1,3,*]

1. Department of General Surgery, Azienda Ospedaliera Universitaria Policlinico San Marco 95123 Catania, Italy; f.privitera05@gmail.com (F.P.); rosellagioco1992@gmail.com (R.G.); fazioileana@gmail.com (I.F.); alessiovolpicelli94321@gmail.com (A.V.); salvatore.costa@policlinico.unict.it (S.C.); cannizzaromatteoangelo@yahoo.it (M.A.C.)
2. Radiology Unit, Azienda Ospedaliera Universitaria Policlinico San Marco, 95123 Catania, Italy; maraterex@yahoo.it
3. Department of Medical and Surgical Sciences and Advanced Technologies, University Hospital of Catania, 95123 Catania, Italy
* Correspondence: veroux@unict.it

Citation: Privitera, F.; Gioco, R. Fazio, I.; Volpicelli, A.; Cannizzaro, M.T.; Costa, S.; Cannizzaro, M.A.; Veroux, M. Risk Factors for Low Levels of Parathyroid Hormone after Surgery for Thyroid Cancer: A Single Center Study. *J. Clin. Med.* **2021**, *10*, 4113. https://doi.org/10.3390/jcm10184113

Academic Editors: Giovanni Conzo, Andreas Zielke and Pierpaolo Trimboli

Received: 18 July 2021
Accepted: 8 September 2021
Published: 12 September 2021

Publisher's Note: MDPI stays neutral with regard to jurisdictional claims in published maps and institutional affiliations.

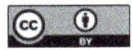

Copyright: © 2021 by the authors. Licensee MDPI, Basel, Switzerland. This article is an open access article distributed under the terms and conditions of the Creative Commons Attribution (CC BY) license (https://creativecommons.org/licenses/by/4.0/).

Abstract: Background: Thyroidectomy is the definitive treatment for most patients with thyroid cancer. Hypoparathyroidism is the most frequent complication of thyroidectomy, and its pathogenesis is multifactorial. The aim of this study is to evaluate the patient- and surgical-related risk factors for hypoparathyroidism after surgery for thyroid cancer. Methods: In this retrospective study, patients referred to surgery for thyroid cancer from 2016 to 2019 were enrolled. Preoperative serum calcium and parathyroid hormone (PTH) and postoperative 24 h PTH and calcium levels were evaluated. Demographic data, type of surgery, incidence of hypoparathyroidism and hypocalcemia were recorded for all the patients. Patients were divided into two groups based on post-operative PTH levels (≤12 and >12 pg/mL). Results: A total of 189 patients were enrolled in this study. There were 146 women (87.3%) and 43 men (22.7%), with a mean age of 51.3 years. A total of 79 patients (41.7%) underwent a neck dissection. A total of 59 patients (31.1%) had a postoperative PTH level < 12 pg/mL. Female sex, neck dissection, the yield of lymph node dissection and incidental parathyroidectomy were significantly associated with postoperative hypoparathyroidism. Incidental parathyroidectomy was reported in 44 (23.2%) patients and was correlated with younger age (<40 years) and neck dissection. There was no difference in the rate of post-operative hypocalcemia between patients with incidental parathyroidectomy and those without. Conclusions: Young patients undergoing neck dissection and with incidental parathyroidectomy have the highest risk of postoperative hypoparathyroidism after surgery for thyroid cancer. However, a large proportion of patients without incidental parathyroidectomy may have temporary hypocalcemia, suggesting that impaired blood supply of parathyroid glands during their identification and dissection may play a relevant role.

Keywords: parathyroid hormone; hypocalcemia; thyroid cancer; incidental parathyroidectomy; parathyroid hormone; female; thyroidectomy; lobectomy; central neck dissection; lymph node

1. Introduction

Thyroid cancer is the most common endocrine tumor and its incidence has significantly increased over the last three decades [1]. Although the prognosis of thyroid cancer is usually good, in most cases a surgical approach is required. Total thyroidectomy is usually recommended for patients with thyroid nodules in which thyroid cancer is suspected in order to improve survival and lower recurrence [2,3]. Total thyroidectomy is one of the most frequently performed endocrine surgical procedures, and it can lead to serious complications, including temporary or permanent cordal palsy or postoperative bleeding, although hypoparathyroidism is the most frequent complication [4–6]. Hypoparathyroidism with hypocalcemia may affect 3–49% of patients undergoing thyroid surgery [4–14]. Many risk factors have been associated with an increased incidence of post-operative hypocalcemia. Post-thyroidectomy hypocalcemia may arise from an incidental parathyroid removal, but the risk is also increased when a larger number of parathyroid glands are left in situ due to a compromised blood supply as a result of their dissection [6,9,13]; this risk could be further increased when a neck dissection is associated with a total thyroidectomy [6,8–11,13]. Parathyroid hormone (PTH) levels are the most frequently evaluated biochemical factor in the development of post-operative hypocalcemia, but the association between PTH levels and postoperative hypocalcemia has been reported with conflicting results [9,15,16]. Moreover, there is no consensus on the most useful predictive cut-off point for post-operative PTH levels and the appropriate time of PTH measurement after surgery: 1 h PTH level after skin closure may be predictive of postoperative hypocalcemia [6,8–11,13], while other studies suggested that a reduction in postoperative PTH of more than 44% [17] or more than 60% [18] is predictive of temporary biochemical hypocalcemia [7,14,19].

In this study, we evaluated the risk factors for low levels of PTH after surgery for thyroid cancer to identify the patient and surgical related factors that could have a significant correlation with the development of hypoparathyroidism.

2. Materials and Methods

All patients who were scheduled for surgical treatment for thyroid cancer between January 2016 and December 2019 were retrospectively reviewed. All patients were diagnosed with thyroid cancer based either on a fine needle aspiration or at final histological examination. Inclusion criteria included the following: normal biochemical results of calcium metabolism, normal serum albumin and total protein and normal thyroid, liver, and kidney functions.

Cases of completed thyroidectomy and patients with diseases or who were taking medications that affect calcium homeostasis were excluded. Each participant received and signed an informed consent form. Total extracapsular excision of the thyroid gland was performed on each patient by the same team of two surgeons. Central neck dissection, bilateral or ipsilateral lymphadenectomy, were performed on suspicious enlarged lymph nodes on the bilateral or ipsilateral sides. No prophylactic unilateral or bilateral lymphadenectomy was performed.

All parathyroids were visualized intraoperatively. In each case, the thyroid was devascularized by selective closure of distal branches of the thyroid arteries to spare the vascular supply of the parathyroids. Biochemical monitoring of mineral homeostasis included the following: serum calcium (Calcium Arsenazo III, Beckman Coulter, Inc., normal range: 8.1–10.2 mmol/L), phosphate (Inorganic Phosphorous, Beckman Coulter, Inc., normal range: 0.81–1.45 mmol/L) and PTH (Access Intact PTH Assay, Beckman Coulter, Inc., normal range: 12–88 pg/mL), measured pre-operatively and 24 h after surgery. Temporary postoperative hypocalcemia was considered for calcium serum levels lower than 8.0 mg/dL, measured 24 h after surgery. Hypoparathyroidism was considered for PTH levels < 12 pg/mL. Patients with biochemical hypocalcemia (<8 mg/dL) or with symptoms associated with serum calcium decrease were given calcium carbonate orally as well as calcium gluconate intravenously, when needed. Symptoms were monitored until discharge and thereafter on an outpatient basis. In case of symptoms of hypocalcemia or serum calcium < 8 mg/dL, an oral supplementation of calcium and calcitriol was administered until resolution of symptoms or normalization of serum calcium levels. Definitive hypocalcemia was defined as the need for treatment with calcium or calcitriol at 6 months after surgery.

Clinical and follow-up data were retrieved from our electronic database and included sex, age, preoperative serum calcium levels, preoperative serum PTH levels, surgical procedures (thyroidectomy/lobectomy) including neck dissection, number of retrieved lymph nodes, thyroid volume, incidental parathyroidectomy, post-operative calcium levels, post-operative PTH levels, definitive histological examination, presence of thyroiditis based on histopathology reports and surgical complications. Pathological staging was based on the tumor/nodes/metastases (TNM) system.

Pathology reports were reviewed for documentation of parathyroids identified in the specimen.

Patients were divided into two groups based on post-operative PTH levels (≤ 12 and >12 pg/mL). Thyroid volume was calculated through the measurements of the depth (d), the width (w) and the length (l) of each lobe, as reported at final histological examination. The volume is calculated by the ellipsoid formula:

$$V (mL) = 0.52 \times d \times w \times l\ (cm)$$

Permanent hypoparathyroidism was considered at PTH levels ≤ 12 pg/mL or clinical symptoms of permanent hypocalcemia at 6-month follow-up [14]. Statistical data analysis was performed using SPSS (version 20.0; SPSS Inc., Chicago, IL, USA). Data are expressed as mean $\pm$ standard deviation (SD). To compare parametric variables, the Pearson chi-square test or Fisher's exact test was used. To compare non-parametric variables, Student T test or Mann–Whitney U test was used. The difference between the two means was calculated using the Wilson test. Odds ratios (OR) were reported with 95% confidence interval (95% CI) and P values The level of statistical significance was determined at $p < 0.05$.

3. Results

A total of 189 patients undergoing thyroid surgery for thyroid cancer between January 2016 and December 2019 were enrolled in this study. There were 146 women (87.3%) and 43 men (22.7%), with a mean age of 51.3 years (range, 19–75). Patients' demographics, operative details, histological findings and postoperative events are reported in Table 1.

Table 1. Patients' characteristics.

Characteristic	N (%)
Age	
Male	43 (22.8)
Female	146 (77.2)
Mean age (years)	51.3 $\pm$ 22.4
Surgical Procedure	
Total Thyroidectomy	183 (96.8)
Lobectomy	6 (3.2)
Histological type	
Papillary	163 (86.2)
Follicular	44 (23.2)
Other (medullary, anaplastic, rare tumors)	7 (3.7)
TNM Classification	
T1	130 (68.7)
T2	10 (5.3)
T3	48 (25.6)
T4	1 (5.4)
Lymph-node metastasis (N+)	12 (6.4)

Table 1. Cont.

Characteristic	N (%)
Unintentional parathyroidectomy	44 (23.3)
Portion of parathyroid	12 (26.3)
One Parathyroid	32 (72.7)
Parathyroid glands identified during surgery	
0	3 (1.5)
1	6 (3.2)
2	45 (23.9)
3	81 (42.9)
4	54 (28.5)
Auto-transplanted parathyroids	20 (10.5)
Post-operative hypocalcemia	69 (36.5%)
Definitive Hypocalcemia	5 (2.6)

Most patients (183, 96.8%) underwent a total thyroidectomy, while six patients underwent a lobectomy (3.2%). A total of 79 patients (41.7%) underwent a neck dissection. Most patients were finally diagnosed with papillary cancer (163, 86.2%) or follicular cancer (44, 23.2%). Post-operative temporary hypocalcemia was present in 69 (36.5%) patients, while only five (2.6%) patients experienced a definitive hypocalcemia. Most patients with hypocalcemia presented with numbness and tingling in their fingertips, toes and the perioral region, while no patients presented convulsions.

A total of 59 patients (31.1%) had a postoperative PTH level < 12 pg/mL (Table 2). Younger female patients were at higher risk of low PTH levels after thyroid surgery. Hypoparathyroidism presented more frequently in female (37.3%) compared to male patients (12.7%, $p < 0.001$). Interestingly, the total thyroidectomy did not increase the risk of low PTH, but the neck dissection significantly increased the risk of parathyroid injury (OR = 2.56 (95% CI 1.36–4.82), $p = 0.004$), and patients with low postoperative PTH had a higher mean number of lymph nodes retrieved compared to patients with higher PTH levels (8.53 vs. 4.12, $p = 0.005$). Low levels of PTH were associated with an increased rate of incidental parathyroidectomy, which was present in 35.6% of the patients; this was associated with an OR of 2.44 (95% CI 1.22–4.88, $p = 0.017$). However, 25 patients (18.4%) with normal post-operative PTH levels had an incidental parathyroidectomy, suggesting that this is not the only factor contributing to the development of post-operative parathyroid dysfunction and hypocalcemia. Indeed, the number of parathyroid glands identified during surgery and auto-transplanted parathyroids did not correlate with the incidence of postoperative hypoparathyroidism.

While there was not a significant difference in pre-operative PTH levels between the two groups, mean postoperative PTH levels were significantly different (4.3 ± 3.63 pg/mL vs. 35.6 ± 17.5 pg/mL, $p < 0.001$). Overall, patients with postoperative hypocalcemia had 70.6% lower PTH levels compared with preoperative levels, and this difference was even more pronounced in patients with postoperative PTH levels < 12 pg/mL (92%). Histological type, cancer volume and thyroid volume did not correlate with post-operative PTH levels.

Table 2. Risk factors for low level of postoperative PTH.

Characteristics	PTH < 12 pg/mL N (%)	PTH > 12 pg/mL N (%)	p Value
Patients	59 (31.1)	130 (68.9)	
Age (mean, years)	48.4 ± 12.2	53.4 ± 11.8	0.011
Age Groups			
<40	16 (27.1)	23 (17.7)	0.008
41–55	29 (49.1)	45 (34.6)	0.849
>55	14 (23.7)	62 (47.6)	0.754
Sex			
Male	6 (10.2)	41 (31.6)	
Female	53 (89.8)	89 (68.4)	<0.001
Surgical Procedure			
Total Thyroidectomy	59 (100)	124 (95)	0.898
Lobectomy	0	6 (5)	
Neck dissection	34 (58)	45 (35)	0.004
Central neck dissection	15 (25.4)	20 (15.3)	0.622
Unilateral Lymphadenectomy	14 (23.7)	20 (15.3)	0.532
Bilateral lymphadenectomy	5 (8.4)	5 (3.8)	0.455
PTH levels (mean)			
Preoperative	53.6 ± 26.9	53.1 ± 20.5	0.884
Postoperative	4.3 ± 3.63	35.6 ± 17.5	<0.001
Incidental Parathyroidectomy			
No	33 (64.4)	107 (82.4)	
Yes	21 (35.6)	23 (17.6)	<0.001
Auto-transplanted parathyroids	3 (6.7)	16 (11.5)	0.312
Parathyroid glands identified during surgery			
0	1 (1.6)	2 (1.5)	0.936
1	2 (3.4)	4 (3)	0.912
2	15 (25.4)	30 (23)	0.726
3	21 (35.6)	60 (46.3)	0.173
4	20 (34)	34 (26.2)	0.275
Histological type			
Papillary	55 (93.2)	108 (83)	0.832
Follicular	11 (18.6)	33 (25.3)	0.651
Other (medullary, anaplastic, rare tumors)	0	7 (5.3)	0.821
Thyroid volume (mean, cm^2)	23.43 ± 26.52	24.9 ± 26.4	0.724
Cancer volume (mean, cm)	0.93 ± 0.6	1.02 ± 0.9	0.654
Number of retrieved lymph nodes (mean)	8.53	4.12	0.005
Postoperative Hypocalcemia			
Temporary	37 (63)	33 (25.4)	<0.05
Definitive	5 (8)	0	
Preoperative/postoperative PTH levels ratio	92%	49.5%	<0.05

Table 2. Cont.

Characteristics	PTH < 12 pg/mL N (%)	PTH > 12 pg/mL N (%)	p Value
TNM Classification			
T1	36 (61)	94 (71.1)	0.120
T2	3 (5)	7 (5.4)	0.622
T3	20 (34)	28 (21.5)	0.070
T4	0	1 (0.9)	
N+	36 (61)	54 (41.5)	**0.012**
6-month Postoperative serum calcium (mean, g/dL)	8.8 ± 0.53	9.3 ± 0.42	0.643
6-month postoperative PTH level (mean, pg/mL)	18.22 ± 8.34	26.3 ± 10.4	0.138

A total of 37 patients (63%) in the group of PTH < 12 pg/mL developed a temporary postoperative hypocalcemia, compared to 33 patients (25.4%, $p < 0.01$) in the group of PTH > 12 pg/mL. Interestingly, five patients (8%) with a postoperative PTH value < 12 pg/mL developed a definitive hypocalcemia, while no patient in the group with postoperative PTH levels > 12 pg/mL developed a definitive hypoparathyroidism. Female sex, age < 55 years and PTH levels < 12 pg/mL were predictive of postoperative temporary hypocalcemia, while the incidental parathyroidectomy did not increase the risk of hypocalcemia (Table 3).

Table 3. Risk factors for temporary hypocalcemia.

Characteristics	OR	95% CI	p Value
Sex			
Male	1		
Female	4.06	1.618–10.228	**<0.05**
Age (ys)			
<40	1.73	0.83–3.59	**<0.01**
41–55	1.82	0.97–3.41	**<0.05**
>55	1		
PTH < 12 pg/mL	4.94	2.55–9.55	**<0.001**
Incidental parathyroidectomy	0.63	0.31–1.25	0.186

All patients who developed a definitive hypocalcemia had a 1-day postoperative PTH level < 1 pg/mL, and a postoperative PTH level < 5 pg/mL was a strong predictive factor for definitive hypoparathyroidism (OR = 24.5 (95% CI 2.83–212.51, $p < 0.0001$). At the 6-month follow-up, serum calcium and PTH levels were similar among the two groups.

A subsequent analysis on risk factors for incidental parathyroidectomy was performed (Table 4). In 19 patients (10%), a parathyroid gland was auto-transplanted, of which only three developed a transient post-operative hypocalcemia. There was no significant difference in the incidence of incidental parathyroidectomy among patients < 55 years compared to those >55 years. However, when stratified for age, younger (<40 years) patients had the higher risk of having an incidental parathyroidectomy (RR 1.8 OR 2.2 (95% CI 1.02–4.88), compared to patients > 41 years (RR 0.9 OR 0.6 (95 CI 0.308–1.157). Patients who underwent neck dissection had an increased risk of incidental parathyroidectomy (OR 3.03 (95% CI 1.50–6.12, $p < 0.001$), with the risk increasing with the number of retrieved lymph nodes, being the highest for > 8 lymph-nodes (OR 1.7, 95% CI 0.58–5.00, $p = 0.044$) retrieved. There was no significant correlation between the number of parathyroid glands identified during surgery and the risk of incidental parathyroidectomy. Patients with unintentional parathyroidectomy had significantly lower postoperative PTH levels (19.3± 19.2

vs. 27.3 ± 23 pg/mL, $p = 0.03$) and, although there was a higher incidence of postoperative biochemical hypocalcemia, this did not reach the statistical significance (45.4% vs. 34.4%, $p = 0.194$). There were no significant differences for gender or histological type.

Table 4. Risk factors for un-intentional parathyroidectomy.

Characteristics	Unintentional Parathyroidectomy	No Parathyroidectomy	
	N (%)	N (%)	p Value
Patients	44 (23.2)	145 (76.7)	
Sex			
Male	11 (25)	35 (24.2)	0.743
Female	33 (75)	110 (75.8)	0.896
Age (years, %)	50.1 ± 14.1	51.7 ± 11.9	0.451
<55	26 (59)	83 (57.2)	
>55	18 (41)	62 (42.8)	0.827
Age Groups			
<40	13 (29.5)	21 (14.5)	**0.015**
41–55	13 (29.5)	63 (43.4)	0.123
>55	18 (41)	61 (42.1)	0.091
Total thyroidectomy/lobectomy	43 (97.7)	140 (96.6)	0.833
Lobectomy	1 (2.3)	5 (4.6)	0.901
Neck dissection	28 (63.6)	51 (35.1)	**0.001**
Number of retrieved lymph nodes			
<4	15	30	OR 1 (95% CI 0.39–2.78)
5–8	2	10	OR 0.3 (95% CI 0.07–1.76)
>8	8	11	OR 1.7 (95% CI 0.58–5.00)
Parathyroid glands identified during surgery			
0	1 (2.2)	2 (1.3)	0.674
1	2 (4.6)	4 (2.8)	0.555
2	13 (29.5)	32 (22)	0.307
3	16 (36.3)	65 (44.8)	0.322
4	12 (27.2)	42 (28.9)	0.215
Preoperative PTH (mean, pg/mL)	55.9 ± 27	52.5 ± 21.3	0.396
Postoperative PTH (mean, pg/mL)	19.3 ± 19.2	27.3 ± 23	**0.03**
PTH < 12 pg/mL	21 (47.7)	39 (26.8)	**0.009**
Temporary Hypocalcemia < 8 mg/dL	20 (45.4)	50 (34.4)	0.194
Definitive Hypocalcemia	4 (10)	1 (2)	0.135
Underlying disease			
Papillary	37 (84.1)	126 (86.9)	0.626
Follicular	12 (27.3)	32 (22.1)	0.435
Hashimoto thyroiditis	6 (13.6)	31 (21.4)	0.201
Others	3 (6.8)	4 (6.8)	0.832
Thyroid volume (mean, cm^3)	16.4 ± 8.45	26.5 ± 28.5	**0.002**
Postoperative serum calcium (mean, mg/dL)	8.1 ± 0.65	8.3 ± 0.6	0.07
6-month Postoperative serum calcium (mean, g/dL)	9.1 ± 0.55	9.6 ± 0.35	0.845

Bold of numbers was for those statistically significant.

4. Discussion

Hypoparathyroidism is the most common complication after thyroid surgery, but the true incidence is debatable due to the heterogeneity in classification and identification of this complication. A recent meta-analysis reported a median incidence of temporary and permanent hypoparathyroidism following thyroidectomy ranging from 19% to 38% and 0% to 3%, respectively, suggesting that a large number of patients undergoing thyroid surgery may suffer from this complication [13].

This study investigated the patient- and surgery-related risk factors associated with low postoperative PTH levels. After thyroidectomy, monitoring of PTH and serum calcium levels is mandatory for identifying the hypoparathyroidism before the development of severe and symptomatic hypocalcemia [20]. Because postoperative calcium levels may be confounded by prophylactic calcium and calcitriol administration, or by low preoperative vitamin D levels, many groups preferred the measuring of intraoperative or postoperative intact PTH levels drawn at various time points in the early post-thyroidectomy period [10,14,20]. A recent statement on hypoparathyroidism of the American Thyroid Association found that the timing of PTH measurements in published studies has ranged from 10 min to 24 h post-thyroidectomy [14], and that a postoperative PTH level < 15 pg/mL is usually predictive of hypocalcemia [6,8–11,13,20,21]. However, serum PTH levels may remain stable within the first days after thyroidectomy and day 1 PTH levels may be accurate enough to predict hypocalcemia and direct the initiation of calcium supplementation [4,21].

In our study, postoperative hypocalcemia developed in 36.5% of patients, while a total of 59 patients (31.1 %) had a postoperative PTH level < 12 pg/mL. PTH levels may be a significant predictive factor for post-operative hypoparathyroidism and hypocalcemia: among the 37 patients with PTH < 12 pg/mL who developed a temporary postoperative hypocalcemia, five patients (8%) developed a definitive hypocalcemia, while no patients with hypocalcemia and PTH levels > 12 pg/mL developed a definitive hypocalcemia.

Postoperative PTH levels are significantly related to postoperative hypocalcemia [22], and a recent systematic review showed that patients with a decrease in post-operative PTH had a 69–100% chance of developing temporary hypocalcemia [13]. Moreover, the accuracy of an absolute PTH level to predict temporary hypocalcemia ranges from 34% to 100%, while the accuracy for a change in PTH ranges from 72% to 100%; however, the development of hypocalcemia despite a normal PTH level is up to 54% for an absolute PTH value and up to 50% for a percentage change in PTH, suggesting that even patients with a normal PTH can develop hypocalcemia [13]. This assumption was further demonstrated by Del Rio et al. [6] who showed that, among the 101 patients presenting with hypocalcemia (serum calcium < 7.5mg/dL) beyond postoperative day 1, only 49 had PTH values less than 12 pg/mL, whereas the others 52 patients had PTH values within the normal range; additionally, there was no statistically significant difference in absolute PTH values in patients with hypocalcemia compared with patients with eucalcemia [6].

This was also confirmed in our study where, although a higher incidence of postoperative hypocalcemia (serum calcium < 8 mg/dL) was observed in patients with a lower postoperative PTH level (<12 pg/mL), there was no significant difference of PTH levels between patients with postoperative hypocalcemia and patients with normocalcemia; this suggests that low PTH levels, although potentially predictive of postoperative temporary hypocalcemia, do not indicate an absolute risk of hypocalcemia, and similarly, a normal PTH value does not guarantee normocalcemia.

The mechanism of hypoparathyroidism after thyroidectomy has not been fully elucidated and is likely to be multifactorial, including surgical technique, parathyroid injury, patient gender, incidental parathyroidectomy and neck dissection [14,20].

Age < 40 years was found to be significantly associated with hypoparathyroidism. In literature, there are conflicting data about the correlation between post-operative hypoparathyroidism and patient age: while temporary hypocalcemia may be associated either with advanced age [16] or younger age [23,24], most studies found no significant association with age [2,10,13]. More recently, a retrospective study on 278 Chinese patients found a significant association between age and postoperative hypocalcemia [5], while Del Rio et al. [6] did not find such association among 2108 patients undergoing thyroid surgery for benign and malignant diseases.

Many studies tried to find an explanation to female predisposition to post-thyroidectomy hypocalcemia [6] and, although the specific mechanism is not certain, the gender disparity may be related to effects of sexual steroids on PTH secretion [25,26]. Female patients were at higher risk of developing postoperative hypoparathyroidism (53/142, 37.3%) compared to male patients (6/47, 12.7%, $p < 0.001$). Female sex and age were found to be significant risk factors for postoperative hypocalcemia with conflicting results: in their retrospective study, Karadeniz and Akcay [27], found that young age (<28.5 years old) and female sex were risk factors for post-operative hypocalcemia; in contrast, Algarni's retrospective analysis [28] found no significant correlation with female sex, probably because of the small sample size of the study (40 patients).

The extent of surgery may influence the rate of postoperative hypoparathyroidism. The number of parathyroids glands identified during surgery and auto-transplanted parathyroids did not influence the rate of post-operative hypocalcemia, as reported in many studies [9]. It should be noted that in patients with thyroid cancer, parathyroid glands may be not easily identified since they could be confounded with enlarged lymph-nodes or with the fat tissue surrounding the thyroid; this could partially explain the higher rate of incidental parathyroidectomy in patients with thyroid cancer.

In our study, patients who underwent neck dissection had an increased risk of parathyroid injury. Moreover, patients with low post-operative PTH levels had a higher mean number of lymph-nodes retrieved compared to patients with higher PTH levels. Total thyroidectomy is seen to have an equivocal association with symptomatic hypocalcemia, with little evidence suggesting an association with either temporary or permanent hypocalcemia [10]. However, neck dissection demonstrates a significant association with hypoparathyroidism [5,16,23,26], but a recent meta-analysis demonstrated that the addition of neck dissection to total thyroidectomy shows an association only with symptomatic and permanent hypocalcemia, but not with temporary biochemical hypocalcemia [10].

No significant correlation was found between histological type, cancer volume and thyroid volume and postoperative hypoparathyroidism, as reported in other studies [27]. In contrast, Mo et al. [4], in their study investigating the risk for temporary hypocalcemia in 176 patients undergoing total thyroidectomy for papillary thyroid carcinoma, found that tumor diameter was a risk factor for temporary hypocalcemia in female patients, while histological diagnosis of papillary cancer may be related to an increased incidence of postoperative hypocalcemia [26].

Incidental parathyroidectomy was present in 44 (23.2%) patients, and it correlated significantly with low postoperative PTH levels. This was consistent with data reported in literature, where incidental parathyroidectomy was identified in 4%–28% of thyroid specimens [21,27,29–33]. In this study, incidental parathyroidectomy was correlated with younger age (<40 years) and with neck dissection with higher lymph-node yield, while total thyroidectomy and histological findings did not increase the incidence of incidental parathyroidectomy. Malignancy and neck dissection, together with the surgeon's experience have been identified as the strongest risk factors associated with incidental parathyroidectomy [26,27,29–33]. In their study, Barrios et al. [30], among 1114 thyroidectomies and 396 concurrent central neck dissections performed across seven surgeons, found that central neck dissection, either prophylactic or therapeutic, but not the yield of lymphadenectomy, increased the risk of incidental parathyroidectomy (OR 2.68 and 4.44, respectively). In contrast, the surgeon's experience had a protective role, suggesting that high-volume surgeons could safely perform more extensive central neck dissections with lower incidences of complications [30]. The extent of thyroid surgery is not necessarily associated with increased risk of incidental parathyroidectomy [26,27,29–33], as reported in our experience. Interestingly, incidental parathyroidectomy was associated with a higher risk of temporary hypoparathyroidism and with permanent hypocalcemia, although not statistically significant, but not with temporary hypocalcemia. This apparent paradox may be correlated to the function of the remaining parathyroid glands [34]. However, the 26.8% and the 34.4% of patients without incidental parathyroidectomy experienced temporary postoperative hypoparathyroidism and hypocalcemia, respectively, suggesting that extensive identification and dissection of parathyroids may compromise their blood supply and, therefore, their function [9,30,35].

The main limitations of this study are the retrospective nature and the relatively small sample size. However, surgical procedures were performed by the same surgical team in a high-volume center, and this could reduce the bias caused by different surgeon experience.

In conclusion, surgery for thyroid cancer may be associated to an increased risk of postoperative hypoparathyroidism and hypocalcemia. While neck dissection and incidental parathyroidectomy may increase the rate of postoperative hypoparathyroidism, a large proportion of patients without incidental parathyroidectomy may experience postoperative hypocalcemia, suggesting that a careful surgical technique is recommended for reducing the risk of post-operative complications.

Author Contributions: Conceptualization, F.P., M.A.C. and M.V.; methodology, M.A.C. and M.V.; formal analysis, F.P., I.F. and M.V.; investigation, F.P., M.T.C., M.A.C. and M.V.; data curation, F.P., R.G., I.F., A.V. and S.C.; writing—original draft preparation, F.P., I.F. and M.V.; writing—review and editing, M.V. All authors have read and agreed to the published version of the manuscript.

Funding: The acknowledged funders/supporters played no role in the study design, collection, analysis, interpretation of data, manuscript writing, or decision to submit the report for publication. This study was funded by the School in General Surgery of the University of Catania.

Institutional Review Board Statement: The study was conducted in accordance with the principles of the 1975 Declaration of Helsinki and the Ethical Committee of the University Hospital of Catania ruled that no formal ethical approval was required in this particular case, as it conforms to normal clinical practice.

Informed Consent Statement: All patients signed an informed consent detailing all the procedures.

Data Availability Statement: It is possible for de-identified data to be made available upon reasonable request.

Conflicts of Interest: The authors declare no conflict of interest.

References

1. Davies, L.; Welch, H.G. Increasing incidence of thyroid cancer in the United States, 1973–2002. *JAMA* **2006**, *295*, 2164–2167. [CrossRef] [PubMed]
2. Carling, T.; Udelsman, R. Thyroid cancer. *Annu. Rev. Med.* **2014**, *65*, 125–137. [CrossRef] [PubMed]
3. Wilson, C. Surgery: Benign thyroid disease-total or subtotal thyroidectomy? *Nat. Rev. Endocrinol.* **2011**, *8*, 4. [CrossRef] [PubMed]
4. Mo, K.; Shang, J.; Wang, K.; Gu, J.; Wang, P.; Nie, X.; Wang, W. Parathyroid Hormone Reduction Predicts Transient Hypocalcemia after Total Thyroidectomy: A Single-Center Prospective Study. *Int. J. Endocrinol.* **2020**, *2020*, 4. [CrossRef] [PubMed]
5. Wang, Y.H.; Bhandari, A.; Yang, F.; Zhang, W.; Xue, L.J.; Liu, H.G.; Zhang, X.H.; Chen, C.Z. Risk factors for hypocalcemia and hypoparathyroidism following thyroidectomy: A retrospective Chinese population study. *Cancer Manag. Res.* **2017**, *9*, 627–635. [CrossRef]
6. Del Rio, P.; Rossini, M.; Montana, C.M.; Viani, L.; Pedrazzi, G.; Loderer, T.; Cozzani, F. Postoperative hypocalcemia: Analysis of factors influencing early hypocalcemia development following thyroid surgery. *BMC Surg.* **2019**, *18*, 25. [CrossRef] [PubMed]
7. Puzziello, A.; Gervasi, R.; Orlando, G.; Innaro, N.; Vitale, M.; Sacco, R. Hypocalcaemia after total thyroidectomy: Could intact parathyroid hormone be a predictive factor for transient postoperative hypocalcemia? *Surgery* **2015**, *157*, 344–348. [CrossRef] [PubMed]
8. De Carvalho, G.B.; Diamantino, L.R.; Schiaveto, L.F.; Forster, C.H.Q.; Shiguemori, É.H.; Hirata, D.; Kohler, H.F.; Lira, R.B.; Vartanian, J.G.; Matieli, J.E.; et al. Identification of secondary predictive factors for acute hypocalcemia following thyroidectomy in patients with low postoperative parathyroid hormone levels without overt calcium deficiency: A cohort study. *Am. J. Otolaryngol.* **2021**, *42*, 103115. [CrossRef]
9. McMurran, A.E.L.; Blundell, R.; Kim, V. Predictors of post-thyroidectomy hypocalcaemia: A systematic and narrative review. *J. Laryngol. Otol.* **2020**, *134*, 541–552. [CrossRef]
10. Wang, X.; Zhu, J.; Liu, F.; Gong, Y.; Li, Z. Preoperative vitamin D deficiency and postoperative hypocalcemia in thyroid cancer patients undergoing total thyroidectomy plus central compartment neck dissection. *Oncotarget* **2017**, *8*, 78113–78119. [CrossRef]

11. Godlewska, P.; Benke, M.; Stachlewska-Nasfeter, E.; Gałczyński, J.; Puła, B.; Dedecjus, M. Risk factors of permanent hypoparathyroidism after total thyroidectomy and central neck dissection for papillary thyroid cancer: A prospective study. *Endokrynol. Pol.* **2020**, *71*, 126–133. [CrossRef]
12. Azadbakht, M.; Emadi-Jamali, S.M.; Azadbakht, S. Hypocalcemia following total and subtotal thyroidectomy and associated factors. *Ann. Med. Surg.* **2021**, *66*, 102417. [CrossRef]
13. Edafe, O.; Antakia, R.; Laskar, N.; Uttley, L.; Balasubramanian, S.P. Systematic review and meta-analysis of predictors of post-thyroidectomy hypocalcaemia. *Br. J. Surg.* **2014**, *101*, 307–320. [CrossRef] [PubMed]
14. Orloff, L.A.; Wiseman, S.M.; Bernet, V.J.; Fahey, T.J., 3rd; Shaha, A.R.; Shindo, M.L.; Snyder, S.K.; Stack, B.C.; Sunwoo, J.B.; Wang, M.B. American Thyroid Association Statement on Postoperative Hypoparathyroidism: Diagnosis, Prevention, and Management in Adults. *Thyroid* **2018**, *28*, 830–841. [CrossRef] [PubMed]
15. Calò, P.G.; Conzo, G.; Raffaeli, M.; Medas, F.; Gambardella, C.; de Crea, C.; Gordini, L.; Patrone, R.; Sessa, L.; Erdas, E.; et al. Total thyroidectomy alone versus ipsilateral versus bilateral prophylactic central neck dissection in clinically node-negative differentiated thyroid carcinoma. A retrospective multicenter study. *Eur. J. Surg. Oncol.* **2017**, *43*, 126–132. [CrossRef]
16. Docimo, G.; Ruggiero, R.; Casalino, G.; Del Genio, G.; Docimo, L.; Tolone, S. Risk factors for postoperative hypocalcemia. *Updates Surg.* **2017**, *69*, 255–260. [CrossRef] [PubMed]
17. Chapman, D.B.; French, C.C.; Leng, X.; Browne, J.D.; Waltonen, J.D.; Sullivan, C.A. Parathyroid hormone early percent change: An individualized approach to predict postthyroidectomy hypocalcemia. *Am. J. Otolaryngol.* **2012**, *33*, 216–220. [CrossRef] [PubMed]
18. Lecerf, P.; Orry, D.; Perrodeau, E.; Lhommet, C.; Charretier, C.; Mor, C.; Valat, C.; Bourlier, P.; de Calan, L. Parathyroid hormone decline 4 hours after total thyroidectomy accurately predicts hypocalcemia. *Surgery* **2012**, *152*, 863–868. [CrossRef]
19. Caglià, P.; Puglisi, S.; Buffone, A.; Bianco, S.L.; Okatyeva, V.; Veroux, M.; Cannizzaro, M.A. Post-thyroidectomy hypoparathyroidism, what should we keep in mind? *Ann. Ital. Chir.* **2017**, *6*, 371–381.
20. Gafni, R.I.; Collins, M.T. Hypoparathyroidism. *N. Engl. J. Med.* **2019**, *380*, 1738–1747. [CrossRef]
21. Selberherr, A.; Scheuba, C.; Riss, P.; Niederle, B. Postoperative hypoparathyroidism after thyroidectomy: Efficient and cost-effective diagnosis and treatment. *Surgery* **2015**, *157*, 349–353. [CrossRef]
22. Eismontas, V.; Slepavicius, A.; Janusonis, V.; Zeromskas, P.; Beisa, V.; Strupas, K.; Dambrauskas, Z.; Gulbinas, A.; Martinkenas, A. Predictors of postoperative hypocalcemia occurring after a total thyroidectomy: Results of prospective multicenter study. *BMC. Surg.* **2018**, *18*, 55. [CrossRef] [PubMed]
23. White, M.G.; James, B.C.; Nocon, C.; Nagar, S.; Kaplan, E.L.; Angelos, P.; Grogan, R.H. One-hour PTH after thyroidectomy predicts symptomatic hypocalcemia. *J. Surg. Res.* **2016**, *201*, 473–479. [CrossRef]
24. Kaleva, A.I.; Hone, R.W.; Tikka, T.; Al-Lami, A.; Balfour, A.; Nixon, I.J. Predicting hypocalcaemia post-thyroidectomy: A retrospective audit of results compared to a previously published nomogram in 64 patients treated at a district general hospital. *Clin. Otolaryngol.* **2017**, *42*, 442–446. [CrossRef] [PubMed]
25. Sands, N.B.; Payne, R.J.; Côté, V.; Hier, M.P.; Black, M.J.; Tamilia, M. Female gender as a risk factor for transient post-thyroidectomy hypocalcemia. *Otolaryngol. Head Neck Surg.* **2011**, *145*, 561–564. [CrossRef] [PubMed]
26. Coimbra, C.; Monteiro, F.; Oliveira, P.; Ribeiro, L.; de Almeida, M.G.; Condé, A. Hypoparathyroidism following thyroidectomy: Predictive factors. *Acta. Otorrinolaringol. Esp.* **2017**, *68*, 106–111. [CrossRef]
27. Karadeniz, E.; Akcay, M.N. Risk Factors of Incidental Parathyroidectomy and its Relationship with Hypocalcemia after Thyroidectomy: A Retrospective Study. *Cureus* **2019**, *11*, e5920. [CrossRef]
28. Algarni, M.; Alzahrani, R.; Dionigi, G.; Hadi, A.H.; AlSubayea, H. Parathyroid hormone and serum calcium levels measurements as predictors of postoperative hypocalcemia in total thyroidectomy. *Gland Surg.* **2017**, *6*, 428–432. [CrossRef] [PubMed]
29. Du, W.; Fang, Q.; Zhang, X.; Cui, M.; Zhao, M.; Lou, W. Unintentional parathyroidectomy during total thyroidectomy surgery: A single surgeon's experience. *Medicine* **2017**, *96*, e6411. [CrossRef]
30. Barrios, L.; Shafqat, I.; Alam, U.; Ali, N.; Patio, C.; Filarski, C.F.; Bankston, H.; Mallen-St Clair, J.; Luu, M.; Zumsteg, Z.S.; et al. Incidental parathyroidectomy in thyroidectomy and central neck dissection. *Surgery* **2021**, *169*, 1145–1151. [CrossRef]
31. Sitges-Serra, A.; Gallego-Otaegui, L.; Suarez, S.; Lorente-Poch, L.; Munne, A.; Sancho, J.J. Inadvertent parathyroidectomy during total thyroidectomy and central neck dissection for papillary thyroid carcinoma. *Surgery* **2017**, *161*, 712–719. [CrossRef]
32. Bai, B.; Chen, Z.; Chen, W. Risk factors and outcomes of incidental parathyroidectomy in thyroidectomy: A systematic review and meta-analysis. *PLoS ONE* **2018**, *13*, e0207088. [CrossRef]
33. Lin, Y.S.; Hsueh, C.; Wu, H.Y.; Yu, M.C.; Chao, T.C. Incidental parathyroidectomy during thyroidectomy increases the risk of postoperative hypocalcemia. *Laryngoscope* **2017**, *127*, 2194–2200. [CrossRef]
34. Promberger, R.; Ott, J.; Kober, F.; Karik, M.; Freissmuth, M.; Hermann, M. Normal parathyroid hormone levels do not exclude permanent hypoparathyroidism after thyroidectomy. *Thyroid* **2011**, *21*, 145–150. [CrossRef] [PubMed]
35. Chew, C.; Li, R.; Ng, M.K.; Chan, S.T.F.; Fleming, B. Incidental parathyroidectomy during total thyroidectomy is not a direct cause of post-operative hypocalcaemia. *ANZ J. Surg.* **2018**, *88*, 158–161. [CrossRef]

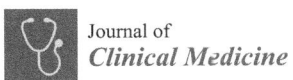

Article

Expression and Clinical Utility of Transcription Factors Involved in Epithelial–Mesenchymal Transition during Thyroid Cancer Progression

Enke Baldini [1,†], Chiara Tuccilli [1,†], Daniele Pironi [1], Antonio Catania [1], Francesco Tartaglia [1], Filippo Maria Di Matteo [1], Piergaspare Palumbo [1], Stefano Arcieri [1], Domenico Mascagni [1], Giorgio Palazzini [1], Domenico Tripodi [1], Alessandro Maturo [1], Massimo Vergine [1], Danilo Tarroni [1], Eleonora Lori [1], Iulia Catalina Ferent [1], Corrado De Vito [2], Poupak Fallahi [3], Alessandro Antonelli [3], Simona Censi [4], Matteo D'Armiento [5], Susy Barollo [1], Caterina Mian [4], Aldo Morrone [5], Vito D'Andrea [1], Salvatore Sorrenti [1,†] and Salvatore Ulisse [1,*,†]

1 Department of Surgical Sciences, Sapienza University of Rome, 00161 Rome, Italy; enke.baldini@uniroma1.it (E.B.); chiara.tuccilli@gmail.com (C.T.); daniele.pironi@uniroma1.it (D.P.); antonio.catania@uniroma1.it (A.C.); francesco.tartaglia@uniroma1.it (F.T.); filippomaria.dimatteo@uniroma1.it (F.M.D.M.); piergaspare.palumbo@uniroma1.it (P.P.); stefano.arcieri@uniroma1.it (S.A.); domenico.mascagni@uniroma1.it (D.M.); giorgio.palazzini@uniroma1.it (G.P.); domenico.tripodi@uniroma1.it (D.T.); alessandro.maturo@uniroma1.it (A.M.); massimo.vergine@uniroma1.it (M.V.); danilo.tarroni@uniroma1.it (D.T.); eleonora.lori@uniroma1.it (E.L.); Iulia.ferent@uniroma1.it (I.C.F.); vito.dandrea@uniroma1.it (V.D.); salvatore.sorrenti@uniroma1.it (S.S.)
2 Department of Public Health and Infectious Diseases, Sapienza University of Rome, 00161 Rome, Italy; corrado.devito@uniroma1.it
3 Department of Clinical and Experimental Medicine, University of Pisa, 56126 Pisa, Italy; poupak.fallahi@med.unipi.it (P.F.); alessandro.antonelli@med.unipi.it (A.A.)
4 Department of Medicine, University of Padua, 35128 Padua, Italy; simona.censi@unipd.it (S.C.); susibarollo@yahoo.it (S.B.); caterina.mian@unipd.it (C.M.)
5 Scientific Direction, IRCCS San Gallicano Dermatological Institute, 00144 Rome, Italy matteo.darmiento@ifo.gov.it (M.D.); aldo.morrone@ifo.gov.it (A.M.)
* Correspondence: salvatore.ulisse@uniroma1.it
† The first and the last two authors provided an equal contribution.

Abstract: The transcription factors involved in epithelial–mesenchymal transition (EMT-TFs) silence the genes expressed in epithelial cells (e.g., E-cadherin) while inducing those typical of mesenchymal cells (e.g., vimentin). The core set of EMT-TFs comprises Zeb1, Zeb2, Snail1, Snail2, and Twist1. To date, information concerning their expression profile and clinical utility during thyroid cancer (TC) progression is still incomplete. We evaluated the EMT-TF, E-cadherin, and vimentin mRNA levels in 95 papillary TC (PTC) and 12 anaplastic TC (ATC) tissues and correlated them with patients' clinicopathological parameters. Afterwards, we corroborated our findings by analyzing the data provided by a case study of the TGCA network. Compared with normal tissues, the expression of E-cadherin was found reduced in PTC and more strongly in ATC, while the vimentin expression did not vary. Among the EMT-TFs analyzed, Twist1 seems to exert a prominent role in EMT, being significantly associated with a number of PTC high-risk clinicopathological features and upregulated in ATC. Nonetheless, in the multivariate analysis, none of the EMT-TFs displayed a prognostic value. These data suggest that TC progression is characterized by an incomplete EMT and that Twist1 may represent a valuable therapeutic target warranting further investigation for the treatment of more aggressive thyroid cancers.

Keywords: thyroid cancers; epithelial–mesenchymal transition; transcription factors; Twist1; Snail; Zeb; E-cadherin; vimentin; prognosis

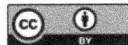

1. Introduction

Epithelial–mesenchymal transition (EMT) indicates a physiological path by means of which a well-polarized epithelial cell gradually loses its cell–cell contacts and acquires the morphological and functional capabilities of a mesenchymal cell [1,2]. Three different types of EMT have been described: type I takes place during the embryogenesis and morphogenesis of organs, type II occurs during tissue regeneration, as well as the fibrotic process, and type III is responsible for cancer metastasis [2–4]. It is worth noting that the conversion from an epithelial to a mesenchymal cell embraces a variety of cellular modifications, not all of which are realized during the EMT. Actually, regarding type III EMT, there is evidence indicating that tumor cells infrequently undertake a complete EMT, whereby they acquire some mesenchymal characteristics while conserving epithelial features [2–6]. The ability of a cancer cell to acquire a mixed epithelial–mesenchymal phenotype, together with its capability to move along the epithelial–mesenchymal spectrum, is now recognized as the epithelial–mesenchymal plasticity (EMP) [7]. The extent of EMT is thought to impact on the metastatization approach adopted by tumor cells, whereby those showing a partial EMT migration as a multicellular cluster, while those with a complete EMT are likely to migrate as single cells [8].

Different factors associated with the microenvironment of tumors are thought to play a role in EMT [3]. These include: (i) cellular and humoral components of inflammation, which have been shown to be potent inducers of EMT in tumor cells [9,10]; (ii) hypoxia and the induction of hypoxia-inducible factors (HIFs) [11,12]; and extracellular matrix components, such as laminins, fibronectin, and collagens [13–19]. In addition, Wnt by binding to its frizzled receptor, along with a number of growth factors, including the epidermal growth factor (EGF), the fibroblast growth factor (FGF), the insulin growth factor (IGF), the platelet-derived growth factor (PDGF), and the transforming growth factor β (TGFβ), by binding with their cognate tyrosine kinase receptors, have been shown to modulate the EMT process [3,4]. All the above-mentioned factors have been shown to upregulate the expression of the so-called EMT transcription factors (EMT-TFs) of the Zeb, Snail (also known as Slug), and Twist families [3]. The latter include Zeb1 and Zeb2, Snail1 and Snail2, and Twist1, which function as repressors of the expression of E-cadherin, claudin, occludin, and other genes involved in the epithelial phenotype while inducing the expression of genes typical of the mesenchymal phenotype, including N-cadherin, vimentin, catenin and others [3]. Experimental evidence accumulated over the last few years indicates that the role of EMT-TFs is not limited to the regulation of cancer cell invasion and metastatization but embraces additional important roles among cell fate specification, cancer stem cell plasticity, malignant transformation and tumor initiation, cancer cell survival in response to therapy, and immune evasion [20]. As a consequence, EMT-TFs have been recognized as potential targets for anticancer therapy.

Follicular thyroid cancers (TC) represent the most common endocrine malignancy and the fifth-most common cancer in women [21–23]. Its annual incidence, about 3% of all cancers, has increased over the last decades due to the improved ability to diagnose malignant transformations in small thyroid nodules [22,23]. Differentiated (DTC) papillary (PTC) and follicular (FTC) thyroid carcinomas represent the majority of thyroid cancers, which may dedifferentiate to form the more aggressive and poorly differentiated TC (PDTC) and the highly aggressive and incurable anaplastic thyroid carcinomas (ATC) [24,25]. Even if derived from the same cell type, the different TC histotypes show peculiar histological features, biological behaviors, and degrees of differentiation as a result of different genetic alterations [24,26]. In PTC, which account for 85–90% of all TC, more than 96% of the underlying driver mutations have been identified [25]. Among these, the BRAF^{V660E} mutation is particularly frequent in PTC, as it is present in about half of all PTCs [26–28].

In the present study, we evaluated the expression level of Twist1, Snai1, Snai2, Zeb1, and Zeb2 in 95 PTC and 12 ATC tissues compared, respectively, with their normal matched tissues or a pool of normal thyroid tissues. The expression levels of the different EMT transcription factors were then correlated with the patients' clinicopathological parameters.

The same was also evaluated in over 350 PTC patients from the TGCA network and available in the public cBioPortal website [26,29].

2. Materials and Methods

2.1. Tissue Samples, Histology, and Patient Staging

Normal and matched PTC tissues were obtained from surgical specimens of 95 patients (19 males and 76 females, age range 11–83 years, median 44 years) who underwent total thyroidectomy for papillary thyroid cancer (PTC) at the Department of Surgical Sciences, "Sapienza" University of Rome (38 patients) or at the Department of Medicine, University of Padua (57 patients) enrolled from 2009 to 2016. ATC tissues were collected from surgical specimens of 12 patients (4 males and 8 females, age range 57–79 years, median 69 years) who had surgery at the Department of Medicine, University of Padua (7 patients) or at the Department of Clinical and Experimental Medicine of Pisa (5 patients). All the patients gave their informed consent, and the study was approved by the local ethical committee (Protocol No. 2615). The tissue samples were collected, quickly frozen in liquid nitrogen, and stored at $-80\,^\circ$C until use. Patients older than 45 years of age underwent total thyroidectomy with dissection of the lymph nodes of the central compartment (level VI). Patients younger than 45 years of age had total thyroidectomy with dissection of the lymph nodes of the central compartment limited to patients with nodal disease. Surgical resection of the lymph nodes from the lateral neck compartments (levels II–V) was performed in patients with nodal disease diagnosed by preoperative ultrasound-guided fine-needle aspiration (FNA) cytology and/or thyroglobulin (Tg) measurements in the FNA washout. Of the 95 PTC patients, 72 (75.8%) exhibited the classical form, 18 (18.9%) the follicular, 2 (2.1%) the tall-cell, and 2 (2.1%) the oncocytic variants. The histological diagnoses were carried out independently by two different histopathologists according to the World Health Organization's classification [24]. At the time of surgery lymph node metastases were found in 39 (41.1%) patients. Following TNM staging, 59 (62.1%) patients were classified as stage I, 1 (1.1%) as stage II, 29 (30.5%) as stage III, and 6 (6.3%) as stage IV. Approximately 40–50 days after the operation, all of the patients underwent radioiodine therapy followed by thyroid hormone replacement therapy. The disease-free status was checked 4 to 5 months later by means of neck ultrasound and serum Tg assay. Recurrences were diagnosed by measuring the serum Tg levels either in basal conditions or following recombinant human TSH stimulation, the determination of FNA cytology and/or Tg in the FNA wash-out from lymph nodes, ^{131}I whole-body scan, and a histological analysis following surgical resection of the lesion [30]. The follow-up included 79 patients (mean 57.1 ± 36.7 months, range 5–141 months), 52 (54.7%) of whom were at TNM stage I. During the follow-up, 16 recurrences were recorded, 12 being cervical lymph nodes and 4 being lung metastases. As regards ATC patients, they all died from the disease (survival time range 1–25 months, median 6 months). In parallel, we analyzed analogous clinical and molecular data obtained from a previous study by The Cancer Genome Atlas (TGCA) network on 496 PTC patients; for 396 of whom, data on the follow-up were available [26,29]. These data were downloaded from the cBioPortal website [29].

2.2. Determination of BRAF^{V600E} Mutation

The BRAF status was determined on 76 tumor tissue samples. The small amount of tissue did not allow for determining the BRAF status on the remaining tissue samples. Genomic DNA was extracted from the frozen tissues using the DNeasy Blood and Tissues kit (QIAGEN, Milan, Italy) following the manufacturer's protocol. The BRAF status of exon 15 was assessed by both direct sequencing and mutant allele-specific PCR amplification for the T to A substitution at the nucleotide 1799 (V600E), using the procedure previously described [31].

2.3. Extraction and Analysis of mRNA

Frozen normal and tumor thyroid tissues were homogenized with the ultra-turrax and total RNA extracted by applying the acid guanidinium thiocyanate–phenol–chloroform method [32]. The first cDNA strand was synthesized from 5 µg of RNA with M-MLV reverse transcriptase and anchored oligo(dT)23 primers (Merk Life Science, Milan, Italy). Parallel controls for DNA contamination were carried out by omitting the reverse transcriptase. The templates thus obtained were used for quantitative PCR amplifications of TWIST1; SNAI1; SNAI2; ZEB1; ZEB2; CDH1; VIMENTIN; and three different housekeeping genes (GAPDH, RPL13A, and SDHA) employing the LightCycler instrument (Roche Diagnostics, Mannheim, Germany), the SYBR Premix Ex Taq II (TliRNase H Plus) (Takara, Otsu, Shiga, Japan), and the specific primers listed in Table 1. Negative controls were performed by preparing the samples with the same procedure without reverse transcriptase. Amplicon specificities were checked by automated DNA sequencing (Bio-Fab Research, Rome, Italy), an evaluation of the melting temperatures, and electrophoresis on 2% agarose gel containing ethidium bromide.

Table 1. Sequences, genomic positions, and amplicon sizes of the primers used in qRT-PCR for the target and reference genes. GAPDH, glyceraldehyde-3-phosphate dehydrogenase; RPL13a, ribosomal protein L13a; SDHA, succinate dehydrogenase complex, subunit A; Twist1, twist basic helix-loop-helix transcription factor 1; Snail1, snail family zinc finger 1; Snail2, snail family zinc finger 2; Zeb1, zinc finger E-box binding homeobox 1; Zeb2, zinc finger E-box-binding homeobox 2.

Gene	Primer Sequence	Exons	Amplicon Length
GAPDH	F: 5′-ATCATCAGCAATGCCTCCTG-3′ R: 5′-GGCCATCCACAGTCTTCTG-3′	6 to 7 8	136 bp
RPL13a	F: 5′-ACCGTGCGAGGTATGCTG-3′ R: 5′-TAGGCTTCAGACGCACGAC-3′	4 to 5 6	148 bp
SDHA	F: 5′-GCATAAGAACATCGGAACTGC-3′ R: 5′-GGTCGAACGTCTTCAGGTG-3′	12 13	147 bp
Twist1	F: 5′-ATGTCATTGTTTCCAGAGAAGG-3′ R: 5′-CCACGCCCTGTTTCTTTG-3′	16 17	137 bp
Snail1	F: 5′-ACCCACACTGGCGAGAAG-3′ R: 5′-CAGGGACATTCGGGAGAAG-3′	19 20	150 bp
Snail2	F: 5′-GGTTGCTTCAAGGACACATTAG-3′ R: 5′-TGGAGAAGGTTTTGGAGCAG-3′	12 13	162 bp
Zeb1	F: 5′-ACCACCCTTGAAAGTGATCC-3′ R: 5′-CTGATTCTACACCGCCCAAA-3′	2 3	115 bp
Zeb2	F: 5′-CCCTTCTGCGACATAAATACG-3′ R: 5′-CGAGTGAAGCCTTGAGTGC-3′	1 2	113 bp
E-cadherin	F:5′-CATTCTGGGGATTCTTGGAG-3′ R: 5′-CCGCCTCCTTCTTCATCATA-3′	1 2	156 bp
Vimentin	F:5′-GAGAGAGGAAGCCGAAAACAC-3′ R: 5′-TCCACTTTGCGTTCAAGGTC-3′	1 2	90 bp

Standard curves for all the genes were created using five-fold dilutions of a cDNA mix. Data for the PTC was calculated with the Relative Expression Software Tool (REST 2009) using the geometric media of the 3 housekeeping genes as the normalization factor, whose expression was proven to be stable among the normal, PTC, and ATC tissues during the preliminary experiments [33–35]. The fold changes in the gene expression were calculated between each PTC tissue and its normal counterpart, while the ATC samples, for which the normal matched tissues were not available, were compared to a pool of 10 normal thyroid tissues. A data analysis was performed with the Relative Expression Software Tool (REST 2009) using as the normalization factor the geometric mean of the above-mentioned housekeeping genes, whose expression was proven to be stable among the normal, PTC, and ATC tissues in the preliminary experiments. In the latter, to compare the gene expressions between ATC and PTC, the ΔCt of each gene was calculated using the geometric mean of the above-mentioned housekeeping genes, while the ΔΔCt was obtained by comparing the samples ΔCt with that of samples showing the lowest gene expression.

2.4. Western Blot

Frozen tissue fragments from normal and tumor tissues were ground using a mortar and pestle in liquid nitrogen, then lysed in a RIPA buffer with an added fresh protease inhibitor cocktail, sonicated, and centrifuged at 13,000 rpm for 20 min. The protein concentrations were determined by the Bradford assay. Protein aliquots of 30 µg were separated by SDS-PAGE and transferred onto nitrocellulose membranes, which were washed with TBS-T (50-mM Tris-HCl, pH 7.4, 150-mM NaCl, and 0.05% Tween-20); saturated with 5% low fat milk in TBS-T; and then incubated at +4 °C overnight with antibodies against E-cadherin 1:1000 (#3195 Cell Signaling Technology, Danvers, MA, USA), vimentin 1:1000 (#5741 Cell Signaling Technology), or GAPDH 1:10,000 (ab8245 Abcam, Cambridge, UK) in TBS-T. After washing, the membranes were incubated with the appropriate horseradish peroxidase-conjugated secondary antibodies against mouse or rabbit IgG (1:20,000) in TBS-T and developed using the LiteAblot EXTEND chemiluminescent substrate (Euroclone, Milan, Italy). Densitometric analyses were carried out using ImageJ software from the National Institutes of Health (Bethesda, MD, USA).

2.5. Statistical Analysis

The Shapiro–Wilk test was used to evaluate the distribution shape of the data. Differences in the mRNA or protein levels between PTC tissues and their normal matched tissues were analyzed by means of the Wilcoxon signed-rank test, while the Mann–Whitney U test was employed to calculate the statistical significance of the differences in the expression levels of the target genes in female vs. male patients, in the classical PTC variant vs. other variants, in $BRAF^{V600E}$-mutated vs. BRAF wild-type ($BRAF^{wt}$) PTC, in metastatic (N1) vs. nonmetastatic (N0) PTC, in T_{1-2} vs. T_{3-4} tumor sizes, in TNM_{I-II} vs. TNM_{III-IV} stages, in the presence or absence of recurrence, and in normal thyroid tissues vs. ATC. The correlations among each mRNA and between the mRNA levels and patient ages or thyroid differentiation scores (TDS) were evaluated using Spearman's Rho test. The TDS, elaborated by the Cancer Genome Atlas Research Network, was calculated by evaluating the mRNA expression levels of sixteen thyroid function genes, which included DIO1, DIO2, DUOX1, DUOX2, FOXE1, GLIS3, NKX2-1, PAX8, SLC26A4, SLC5A5, SLC5A8, TG, THRA, THRB, TPO, and TSHR [26]. The strength of the correlation was interpreted, considering a correlation coefficient value (r): $0 < r < 0.19$ very weak, $0.20 < r < 0.39$ weak, $0.40 < r < 0.59$ moderate, $0.60 < r < 0.79$ strong, and $0.80 < r < 1.00$ very strong [36]. Finally, Cox regression was performed to quantify the hazard ratio (HR) of several explanatory variables, both continuous and categorical. All available covariates were included in the analysis after the assessment of the proportional hazard assumption and absence of multicollinearity. The backwards stepwise approach was used for the model selection. All the statistical analyses were carried out using SPSS software (IBM, Armonk, NY, USA), and the results were considered significantly different if the pertaining p-values were lower than 0.05.

3. Results

Analyses of the five EMT-TFs mRNA levels of the 95 PTC tissues, compared to their normal matched tissues, revealed that all of them were deregulated in the majority of cancer tissues, as shown in panel A of Figure 1. With the exception of Twist1, which showed a minimal, but significant, increment in the median value, all the other EMT-TFs showed a significant reduction in their medians compared to the normal matched tissues (Figure 1). A very similar outcome emerged from the analysis of a case study from The

Cancer Genome Atlas (TGCA) network comprising 505 PTCs, as reported in panels B–F of Figure 1 [26,29]. It has to be mentioned that, while, in our analyses, the mRNA levels of the different EMT-TFs in PTC tissues were compared with the normal matched tissues, in the TGCA study, the EMT-TF expressions found in 505 PTC tissues were compared with those found in 59 unmatched normal tissues [26].

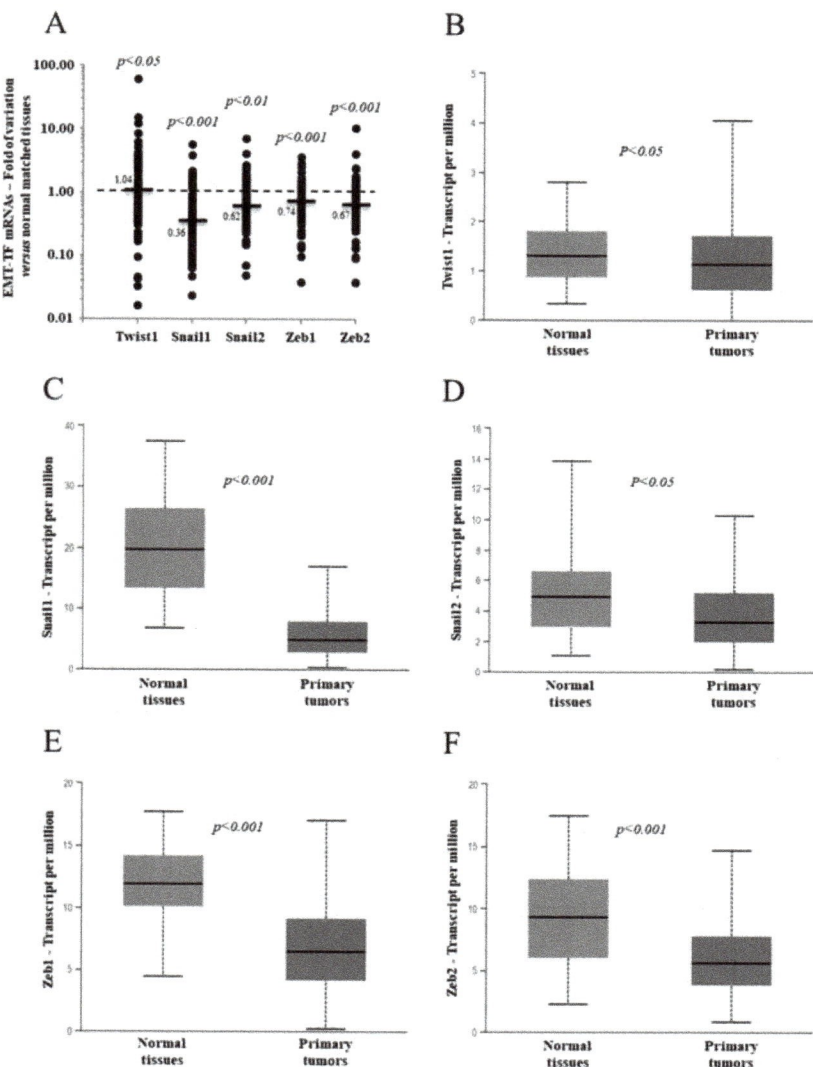

Figure 1. Expression level of the EMT transcription factors (EMT-TFs) in 95 papillary thyroid cancer (PTC) tissues compared with the normal matched tissues from our case study (**A**) or from The Cancer Genome Atlas network (**B–F**) case study consisting of 59 normal tissues and 505 PTC tissues. (**A**) The small bars represent the median with the values indicated. The dotted line represents the expression level for the normal matched tissues. (**B–F**) The data are presented as a box plot reporting the median value (small bar) and the first (lower box limit) and third (upper box limit) quartiles and range of the values observed for each gene.

Additionally, we also analyzed the expression at the mRNA level of E-cadherin and vimentin, well-known EMT markers whose gene transcriptions are modulated by the EMT-TFs under investigation [1–3]. In our case study, a trend toward a reduction of E-cadherin mRNA and the protein level was observed, but it did not achieve statistical significance. Vimentin, on the other hand, was found slightly but significantly reduced at the mRNA level but not at the protein level (Figure 2).

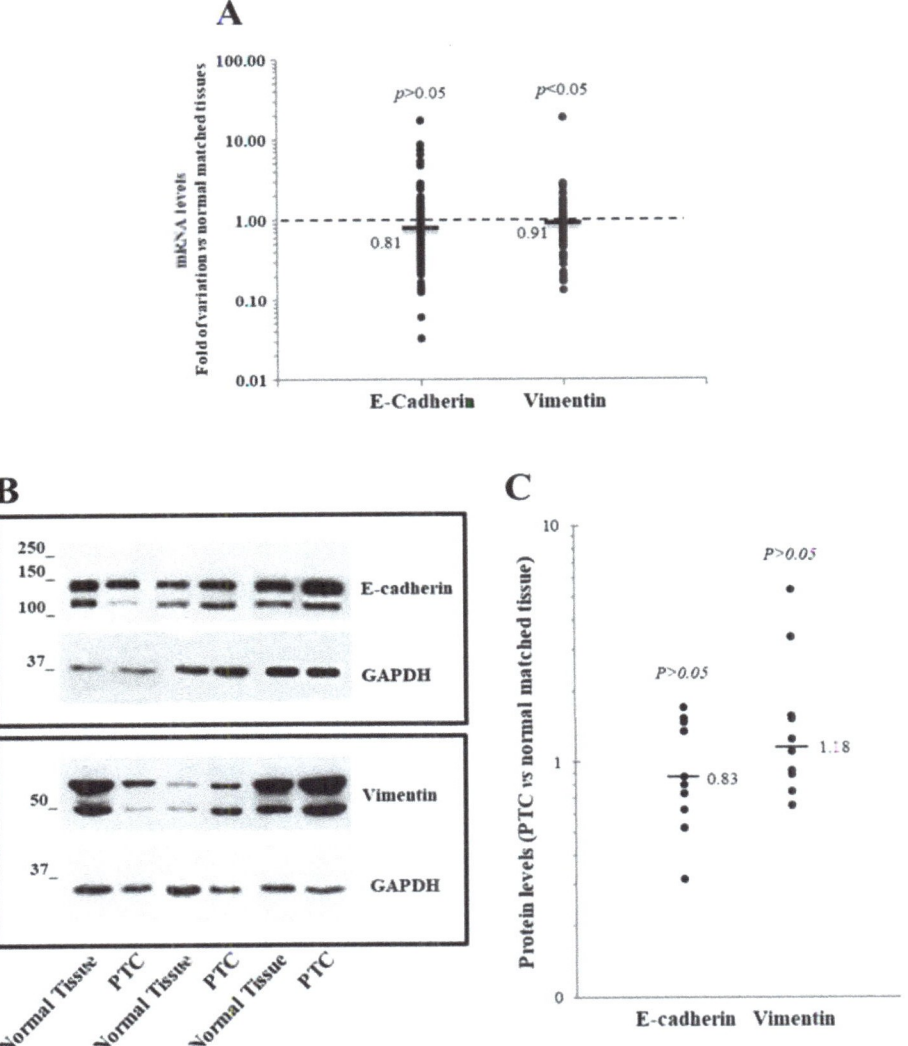

Figure 2. Expression level of the E-cadherin and vimentin in 95 papillary thyroid cancer (PTC) tissues compared with the normal matched tissues. (**A**) The E-cadherin and vimentin mRNA levels are reported. The small bars represent the median, with the values indicated. The dotted line represents the expression levels for the normal matched tissues. (**B**,**C**) The E-cadherin and vimentin Western blot results obtained on 10 PTC tissues and their normal counterparts. (**B**) A representative Western blot image shows three PTC, and the normal matched tissue are shown. (**C**) A densitometric analysis of the 10 PTC tissues analyzed is reported.

The analysis of the mRNA data from the TGCA case study (Figure 3) indicated a significant reduction of the E-cadherin expression in PTC tissues, while that of vimentin was not significantly affected.

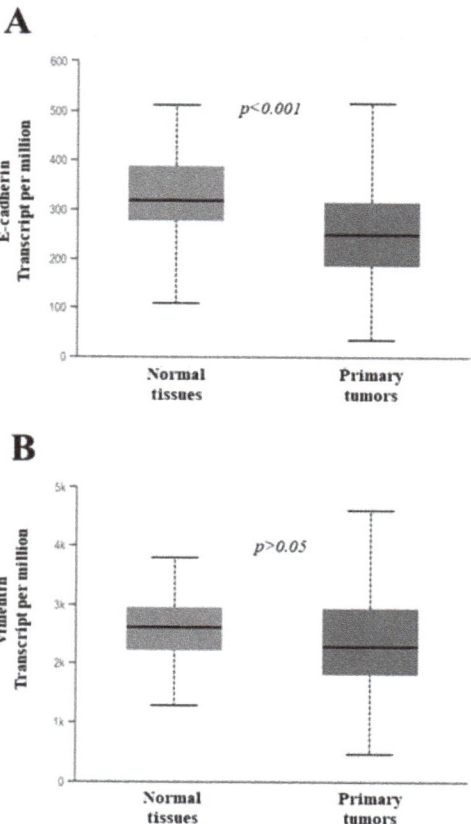

Figure 3. Expression level of the E-cadherin gene and vimentin from The Cancer Genome Atlas network case study consisting of 59 normal tissues and 505 PTC tissues. (**A,B**) The data are presented as a box plot reporting the median value (small bar) and the first (lower box limit) and third (upper box limit) quartiles and the range of the values observed for each gene.

We also evaluated the presence of any correlations among all the mRNAs. The results, reported in Table 2, showed several positive correlations between the different EMT-TFs. In particular, a strong correlation was found both in our case series and in that from the TGCA between Zeb1 and Zeb2, while a strong-to-moderate correlation was evident between Zeb2 and Snai2, Zeb2 and Twist1, Zeb1 and Snai2, and Snai2 and Twist1. E-cadherin and vimentin showed only weak or very weak correlations between each other and the other EMT-TFs (Table 2).

Table 2. Correlation analysis among the expression levels of the EMT transcription factor, E-cadherin, and vimentin from the present case study consisting of 95 PTCs (A) or from the TGCA case study consisting of 388 PTCs (B). Correlations among all the mRNAs were evaluated using the Spearman's Rho test.

(A) Correlation Coefficient							
	Twist1	Snail1	Snail2	Zeb1	Zeb2	E-Cadherin	Vimentin
Twist1	1.000	0.120	0.448	0.464	0.360	−0.155	0.128
p-value	-	0.246	<0.001	<0.001	<0.001	0.133	0.220
Snail1		1.000	0.339	0.378	0.369	0.376	0.393
p-value		-	<0.001	<0.001	<0.001	<0.001	<0.001
Snail2			1.000	0.581	0.552	−0.007	0.335
p-value			-	<0.001	<0.001	0.943	0.001
Zeb1				1.000	0.745	0.005	0.330
p-value				-	<0.001	0.961	0.001
Zeb2					1.000	−0.089	0.343
p-value					-	0.392	0.001
E-Cadherin						1.000	0.292
p-value						-	0.004
Vimentin							1.000
p-value							-
(B) Correlation Coefficient							
	Twist1	Snail1	Snail2	Zeb1	Zeb2	E-Cadherin	Vimentin
Twist1	1.000	0.249	0.694	0.291	0.502	−0.181	0.265
p-value	-	<0.001	<0.001	<0.001	<0.001	<0.001	<0.001
Snail1		1.000	0.321	0.235	0.192	0.276	0.264
p-value		-	<0.001	<0.001	<0.001	<0.001	<0.001
Snail2			1.000	0.552	0.697	−0.019	0.256
p-value			-	<0.001	<0.001	0.714	<0.001
Zeb1				1.000	0.720	−0.095	0.076
p-value				-	<0.001	0.061	0.135
Zeb2					1.000	−0.060	0.343
p-value					-	0.242	<0.05
E-Cadherin						1.000	0.096
p-value						-	0.060
Vimentin							1.000
p-value							-

In the present study, the expression of the five EMT-TFs, E-cadherin, and vimentin detected in the PTC tissues was also compared with that observed in the 12 ATC tissues. Figure 4 shows that the level of Twist1 mRNA appears to be considerably increased in ATC compared to PTC, while the mRNA levels of all the other EMT-TFs are not significantly modulated.

Regarding the two EMT markers, we found that the expression of E-cadherin strongly decreased in ATC, while that of vimentin was not significantly modulated (Figure 5).

Next, we performed a univariate analysis to evaluate the association among the EMT-TF expressions and several clinicopathological parameters, including age at the moment of diagnosis, gender, tumor histology, BRAF status, size (T), lymph node metastases (N), stage, and recurrences. Since some categories of tumor sizes and stages were poorly represented, it was necessary to combine them in order to avoid the inclusion of overly small groups in the statistics. As shown in Table 3, in our case study, none of the EMT-TFs analyzed were significantly associated with the patient clinicopathological parameters, except for the Snai2 with BRAF status. Furthermore, Twist1 showed an increased trend in association with the BRAF^{V600E} mutation ($p = 0.06$).

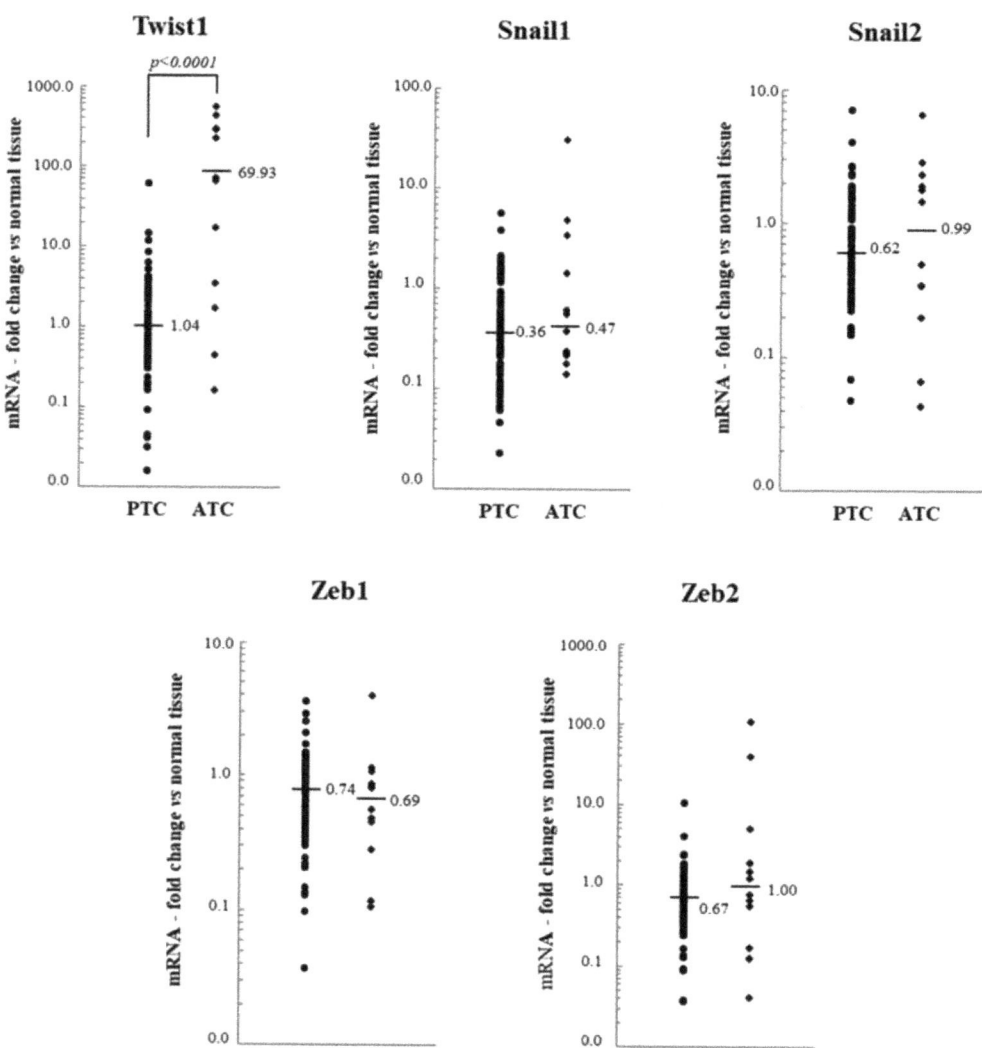

Figure 4. Expression level of the EMT transcription factors (EMT-TFs) in 95 papillary thyroid cancer (PTC) and 12 anaplastic thyroid cancer (ATC) tissues. The small bars represent the median with the values indicated. The dotted line represents the expression level in normal tissues.

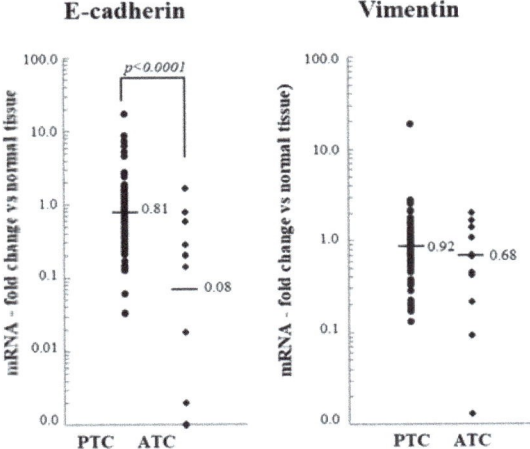

Figure 5. The E-cadherin and vimentin mRNA levels of 95 papillary thyroid cancer (PTC) and 12 anaplastic thyroid cancer (ATC) tissues. The small bars represent the median with the values indicated. The dotted line represents the expression levels in normal tissues.

Table 3. A univariate analysis of the EMT transcription factor expression and the clinicopathological features of 95 PTC patients. In parentheses is the number of patients. The median values of the mRNA fold change between PTC tissue and its normal counterpart are listed for each category of clinical parameters, except for patients' ages, for which the correlation coefficients are reported. pT, tumor size; pN, lymph node metastasis: TNM, Tumor, Node, Metastasis staging system.

	Twist1	p	Snail1	p	Snail2	p	Zeb1	p	Zeb2	p
Gender										
Male ($n = 19$)	0.94	0.42	0.38	0.72	0.58	0.72	0.60	0.21	0.56	0.38
Female ($n = 76$)	1.21		0.36		0.69		0.77		0.68	
Age (year) Corr. Coeff.	−0.124	0.23	−0.111	0.29	−0.088	0.40	−0.076	0.47	−0.022	0.84
Histology										
Classical Variant ($n = 72$)	1.14	0.70	0.37	0.82	0.60	0.50	0.72	0.40	0.66	0.65
Other Variants ($n = 23$)	0.97		0.32		0.82		0.84		0.79	
BRAF										
Wild Type ($n = 38$)	0.68	0.06	0.55	0.09	0.53	0.04	0.66	0.69	0.56	0.85
V600E ($n = 38$)	1.35		0.31		0.84		0.66		0.73	
pT										
T_{1-2} ($n = 39$)	1.04	0.88	0.42	0.15	0.68	0.75	0.80	0.33	0.55	0.42
T_{3-4} ($n = 56$)	1.09		0.33		0.62		0.60		0.78	
pN										
N_0 ($n = 56$)	1.14	0.40	0.34	0.58	0.69	0.90	0.79	0.31	0.72	0.73
N_1 ($n = 39$)	0.98		0.36		0.61		0.58		0.66	
TNM Stage										
I–II ($n = 60$)	1.25	0.36	0.37	0.50	0.66	0.98	0.78	0.61	0.58	0.31
III–IV ($n = 35$)	0.79		0.36		0.61		0.72		0.79	
Recurrences										
No ($n = 63$)	0.79	0.47	0.39	0.58	0.69	0.71	0.72	0.45	0.64	0.60
Yes ($n = 16$)	1.40		0.32		0.70		0.58		0.49	

However, when this type of analysis was performed on the data available from the TCGA database, several associations emerged between the expressions of the EMT-TFs and patient clinicopathological parameters represented in Table 4. Specifically, Twist1 was found to correlate with the thyroid differentiation score (TDS) and to associate with the histological variants, BRAF/RAS phenotype, tumor size, lymph node metastasis, and TNM stage. Additionally, Snai1 and Zeb2 correlated significantly with the TDS. Snai2 was found to associate with the gender, histological variants, BRAF/RAS phenotype, and lymph node metastases, while Zeb1 was found to be associated significantly with the histological variants, BRAF phenotype, tumor size, and disease recurrences. On the contrary, Zeb2 did not associate or correlate with any of the clinicopathological parameters (Table 4).

Table 4. Univariate analysis of the EMT-TF expressions and clinicopathological features of over 350 PTC patients from the TGCA database. In parentheses is the number of patients. TDS, Thyroid Differentiation Score. Median values of the mRNA Z-scores in PTC tissues are listed for each category of clinical parameters, except the patient's age and TDS, for which correlation coefficients are reported.

	Twist1	p	Snai1	p	Snai2	p	Zeb1	p	Zeb2	p
Gender										
Male (n = 93)	−0.326	0.07	−0.305	0.41	−0.153	0.04	−0.105	0.69	−0.132	0.26
Female (n = 271)	−0.329		−0.235		−0.278		−0.168		−0.257	
Age (year) Corr. Coeff.	0.016	0.76	−0.054	0.30	0.066	0.21	−0.016	0.76	−0.016	0.76
Histological variants										
Classical (n = 249)	−0.320	<0.001	−0.219	0.56	−0.226	0.02	−0.206	0.001	−0.209	0.68
Follicular (n = 81)	−0.401		−0.285		−0.426		0.273		−0.269	
Tall cell (n = 28)	0.099		−0.311		−0.106		−0.682		−0.127	
BRAF/RAS status										
BRAF-like (n = 272)	−0.239	<0.001	−0.278	0.12	−0.163	<0.001	−0.209	<0.001	−0.155	0.08
RAS-like (n = 116)	−0.441		−0.179		−0.441		0.205		−0.310	
TDS Corr. Coeff.	−0.245	<0.001	0.245	<0.001	−0.071	0.16	0.327	<0.001	0.046	0.37
pT										
T$_{1-2}$ (n = 231)	−0.359	<0.01	−0.231	0.36	−0.306	0.40	−0.045	0.02	−0.230	0.33
T$_{3-4}$ (n = 131)	−0.242		−0.309		−0.153		−0.313		−0.282	
pN										
N$_0$ (n = 172)	−0.357	<0.01	−0.289	0.44	−0.338	0.02	−0.086	0.81	−0.199	0.83
N$_1$ (n = 153)	−0.239		−0.221		−0.138		−0.164		−0.240	
TNM Stage										
I–II (n = 231)	−0.350	<0.01	−0.232	0.19	−0.299	0.28	−0.095	0.05	−0.233	0.43
III–IV (n = 131)	−0.261		−0.315		−0.129		−0.307		−0.252	
Recurrences										
No (n = 301)	−0.311	0.48	−0.288	0.68	−0.207	0.07	−0.142	0.02	−0.230	0.40
Yes (n = 22)	−0.394		−0.337		−0.500		−0.548		−0.377	

As regards E-cadherin and vimentin expression, no significant correlations or associations with the clinicopathological parameters were observed in our case study (panel A of Table 5). The same analysis performed on the TGCA database revealed that a higher expression of E-cadherin was associated with the classical histological variants and the BRAF/RAS phenotype (panel B of Table 5). A higher vimentin expression was found to correlate inversely with age and to associate with the male gender, BRAF phenotype, and lymph node metastases (panel B of Table 5).

Table 5. A univariate analysis of the E-cadherin and vimentin expressions and clinicopathological features of PTC patients from the present case study (**A**) or from the TGCA database (**B**). In parentheses is the number of patients. TDS, Thyroid Differentiation Score.

(A)	E-cadherin	p	Vimentin	p
Gender				
Male ($n = 19$)	1.05	0.153	0.83	0.309
Female ($n = 76$)	0.78		0.92	
Age (year) Corr. Coeff.	0.022	0.835	−0.173	0.096
PTC histology				
Classical Variant ($n = 72$)	0.85	0.262	0.92	0.758
Other Variants ($n = 23$)	0.76		0.97	
BRAF				
Wild Type ($n = 38$)	0.84	0.905	0.90	0.767
V600E ($n = 38$)	0.94		0.92	
pT				
T_{1-2} ($n = 39$)	0.95	0.104	0.95	0.161
T_{3-4} ($n = 56$)	0.73		0.90	
pN				
N_0 ($n = 56$)	0.80	0.256	0.92	0.478
N_1 ($n = 39$)	0.81		0.90	
TNM Stage				
I–II ($n = 60$)	0.80	0.814	0.92	0.274
III–IV ($n = 35$)	0.81		0.90	
Recurrence				
No ($n = 63$)	0.94	0.102	0.90	0.282
Yes ($n = 16$)	0.73		0.84	
(B)	E-cadherin	p	Vimentin	p
Gender				
Male ($n = 93$)	0.158	0.625	0.092	0.021
Female ($n = 271$)	−0.074		−0.206	
Age (year) Corr. Coeff.	−0.065	0.216	−0.165	0.002
PTC histology				
Classical variant ($n = 249$)	0.074		−0.150	
Follicular variant ($n = 81$)	−0.300	0.012	−0.167	0.203
Tall cell variant ($n = 28$)	−0.177		−0.318	
BRAF-like vs. RAS-like				
BRAF-like ($n = 272$)	−0.00005	0.048	−0.100	0.028
RAS-like ($n = 116$)	−0.145		−0.241	
TDS	0.029	0.564	0.008	0.871
pT				
T_{1-2} ($n = 231$)	−0.029	0.757	−0.194	0.260
T_{3-4} ($n = 131$)	−0.024		−0.091	
pN				
N_0 ($n = 172$)	−0.025	0.919	−0.239	0.021
N_1 ($n = 153$)	−0.079		−0.044	
TNM Stage				
I–II ($n = 250$)	0.065	0.054	−0.153	0.667
III–IV ($n = 112$)	−0.154		−0.149	
Recurrence				
No ($n = 301$)	−0.097	0.222	−0.133	0.539
Yes ($n = 22$)	0.169		−0.237	

We finally created some Cox regression models to predict the probability of DFI as a function of the predictor variables (reported in Tables 3 and 4) for our case study and for that of the TGCA network, respectively. In both settings, the EMT-TFs and E-cadherin and vimentin mRNA levels were included among the predictor variables, but none of them emerged as significant DFI predictors. The only independent prognostic factor for recurrence was lymph node metastasis, with a hazard ratio of 21.0 (95% CI 2.7–161.0, $p < 0.01$) in our case study and of 5.8 (95% CI 1.7–20.1, $p < 0.01$) in the TGCA case study.

4. Discussion

Epithelial–mesenchymal transition (EMT) represents a hallmark of cancer progression, because it is required for the invasion and metastatization of cancer cells [37,38]. During this process, a pivotal role is played by a number of transcription factors (EMT-TFs), including Zeb1 and Zeb2, Snail1 and Snail2, and Twist1, which function as repressors of the genes of the epithelial phenotype (i.e., E-cadherin) while inducing the expression of genes typical of the mesenchymal phenotype (i.e., vimentin) [3]. Consistent with their role in cancer progression and dissemination, higher expressions of EMT-TFs have been demonstrated to associate with a poor prognosis, anticancer drug resistance, and tumor radiosensitivity in different human cancers, including thyroid carcinomas [39–44]. In recent years, new therapeutic strategies have been investigated to pharmacologically inhibit EMT-TFs to tackle cells that have undergone EMT or to reverse the EMT process selectively [42]. Based on this evidence, the present study sought to verify the expression and the possible clinical utility of all the above-mentioned EMT-TFs in papillary thyroid carcinoma (PTC), the most frequent type of thyroid cancer, and in invariably fatal anaplastic thyroid carcinomas (ATC). In fact, although different reports described the expression of single EMT-TFs in thyroid cancer, to the best of our knowledge, only one study, from the TGCA research network, analyzed the expression of all the EMT-TFs in a single case study [26]. The data obtained from our case series were compared with those available from the study reporting the genomic landscape of 496 PTC, 396 of which had follow-ups [26].

The expression profile of the EMT-TFs in our PTC case study showed a significant reduction of the Snail1, Snail2, Zeb1, and Zeb2 mRNA levels both in our own case study and in that of the TGCA [29]. However, the results diverged regarding the Twist1 mRNA, because a slight although significant increase was observed in our PTC samples, while a slightly significant reduction was evident in those from the TGCA. It is worth mentioning that this discrepancy, like others encountered, might be a reflection of the different sizes of the two case series or the different normalization approaches employed to evaluate the variations in the mRNA level of the genes investigated. The analyses were performed against normal matched tissues in the present study and against unmatched normal tissues in the TGCA study [26]. Weak-to-moderate positive correlations were observed among each of the mRNAs of all the EMT-TFs analyzed in both studies. E-cadherin showed a tendentially reduced expression both at the mRNA and protein levels in our PTC samples. The mRNA scores detected by the TGCA analysis also reflected this trend. The only variation found for vimentin was the reduction of the mRNA levels in our PTCs, which, however, were not reproduced by the protein amounts and not even by the mRNA data obtained from the TGCA. Although a more complete characterization is needed, on the whole, these results suggest that EMT is not particularly evident in PTC, because the downregulation of E-cadherin—one of the main initiation events of EMT—occurs, but the vimentin expression remains unchanged, and the EMT-TFs are even reduced [7]. Nevertheless, in the univariate analysis, a higher vimentin expression was associated with the male gender, BRAF phenotype, and lymph node metastases, features linked to increased tumor aggressiveness. This is in line with the current understanding about the role played by the EMT in thyroid cancer progression, which becomes more relevant when the tumor evolves from a differentiated to an anaplastic phenotype [45]. Our study provided evidence substantiating this pattern, since the ATC tissues examined displayed a remarkable increase in the Twist1 mRNA level and a strong reduction in the E-cadherin mRNA. These results corroborate previous reports showing a high expression of Twist1 and a reduced expression of E-cadherin in aggressive follicular carcinomas and ATC tissues [46–49]. All told, these findings appear to suggest a prominent role of Twist1 in the formation of more aggressive thyroid cancers. Unlike what was observed here for the Snail1 and Snail2 mRNAs, a previous study reported that both Snail1 and Snail2 proteins were not detectable in immunohistochemistry (IHC) experiments performed on normal human thyroid tissues or cell lines but expressed at very high levels in human thyroid carcinoma tissues and ATC-derived cell lines [50]. In a different immunohistochemistry study, Buehler and colleagues reported that all normal thyroids, follicular adenomas, and papillary and follicular thyroid carcinomas were negative for Snail2, while the ATC tissues showed a strong nuclear immunoreactivity [47]. Similarly, by means of immunohistochemistry, Wu and colleagues demonstrated that Snail1 expression was higher in widely invasive FTC, PTC, and ATC tissues, though lower in follicular adenoma and minimally invasive FTC tissues [46]. This kind of discrepancy between the expression at the mRNA and protein levels of Snail1 and Snail2 in thyroid cancer remains to be elucidated. One possible explanation is that post-transcriptional mechanism(s) play a major role in regulating Snail1 and Snail2 expressions in thyroid tissues.

Activation of the BRAF oncogene has been indicated as a driving force of EMT in malignant cells. The univariate analysis yielded a higher expression of Snail2 associated with the presence of a $BRAF^{V600E}$ mutation for our PTC samples, which was even more evident in the broader TGCA case series. In the latter, the BRAF-like status was also associated significantly with a reduced Zeb1 mRNA and increased Twist1 mRNA. However, the connection between the $BRAF^{V600E}$ mutation and upregulation of Twist1 has not been elucidated. A previous study, using the non-transformed rat thyroid epithelial cell line PCCL3 conditionally expressing the $BRAF^{V600E}$ protein in a doxycycline-dependent manner, failed to demonstrate any upregulation of the Twist1 protein following the induction of $BRAF^{V600E}$ [49,51]. On the contrary, Puli and colleagues demonstrated that, in the human PTC cell line KTC1, that $BRAF^{V600E}$ induced a Twist1 expression via the ETV5 transcription factor, a downstream effector of the MAPK pathway [52]. Thus, the molecular mechanisms underlying the BRAF mutation/Twist1 expression relation need to be elucidated further. Several researchers also attempted to clarify the association between the BRAF mutations and Snail/E-cadherin expression [53]. In particular, Baquero and colleagues reported that $BRAF^{V600E}$ was capable of promoting thyroid cancer cell invasiveness by reducing E-cadherin expression through a Snail-dependent mechanism [54]. Similar conclusions were made by Ma and colleagues on a murine model of thyroid papillary carcinoma bearing $BRAF^{V600E}$ [55].

EMTs in cancer are linked to cell dedifferentiation, and therefore, one would expect to observe a negative correlation of the thyroid differentiation score (TDS) with the EMT-TFs and EMT markers. Actually, we noticed an inverse relationship between the TDS and Twist1 but a direct correlation between the TDS and Snail1 or Zeb1. Since all PTCs retain a fairly differentiated phenotype, this data would seem to indicate that Twist1 is the factor that comes into play earliest in the dedifferentiative transformation of the tumor. Moreover, the Twist1 expression was greater in the tall-cell PTC variant, which had the lowest TDS and was associated with more advanced stages and higher recurrence risks, while the classical variant, with an intermediate TDS, had an intermediate Twist1 expression, while the follicular variant, characterized by a high level of TDS, had the lowest Twist1 level [26]. In addition, the Twist1 expression was associated significantly with the PTC histological variant. In particular, its expression was the highest in the tall-cell tumors showing the lowest TDS and associated with more advanced stages and higher risks, while the classical variant, with an intermediate TDS, had intermediate Twist1 expression and the follicular variant, characterized by a high level of TDS, had the lowest expression of Twist1 [26]. Twist1 upregulation was also associated with a larger tumor size and higher TNM stage and with lymph node metastases. These data further reinforced the idea that Twist1 is an important modulator of EMT and a major player in the progression of thyroid cancer toward the most aggressive phenotypes. This assumption is further corroborated by the reported ability of the Twist1/miR-584/TUSC2 pathway to induce a resistance to apoptosis of thyroid cancer cells [56]. Besides, the increased Snail2 expression appears to contribute to this process, as it is significantly associated with the tall-cell variant of PTC and lymph node metastases. An opposite kind of behavior was recorded for Zeb1 expression, with higher expression levels in PTC that share a Ras-like phenotype, and in the less aggressive classical and follicular variants. Finally, the multivariate analysis demonstrated that none of the molecular parameters analyzed represented an independent prognostic factor for DFI. In agreement with our previous observations, in this analysis, only lymph node metastasis was capable of a significant prediction of the DFI both in our case study and that of the TGCA network, with a hazard ratio, respectively, of 21.0 and 5.8 [54,57,58].

5. Conclusions

In conclusion, the data reported here show a low expression of E-cadherin, unchanged level of vimentin, and reduction of the majority of EMT-TFs in PTC compared to normal thyroid tissues, which would suggest that thyroid cancer progression is characterized by an incomplete EMT. A more prominent reduction of the E-cadherin mRNA in ATC appears to confirm the assumption that EMT attains major significance in the case of progression from DTC towards the more aggressive PDTCs and ATC. Among all the EMT-TFs analyzed, Twist1 seems to play the most prominent role in the partial kind of EMT occurring in PTC, as it is significantly associated with several PTC high-risk clinicopathological features and is strongly upregulated in ATC tissues and inversely correlated with the expression of E-cadherin. Although, from the multivariate analysis, its prognostic value did not emerge, Twist1 might represent a valuable therapeutic target, warranting further investigation for the treatment of more aggressive thyroid cancers.

Author Contributions: Conceptualization, E.B., C.T., S.S. and S.U.; Data curation, E.B., C.T., C.D.V., M.D., A.M. (Aldo Morrone), S.S. and S.U.; Investigation, E.B., C.T., D.P., A.C., F.T., F.M.D.M., P.P., S.A., D.M., G.P., A.M. (Alessandro Maturo), M.V., D.T. (Danilo Tarroni), E.L., I.C.F., P.F., A.A., S.C., S.B., C.M., V.D., S.S. and S.U.; Methodology, D.T. (Domenico Tripodi); Writing—original draft, E.B., S.S. and S.U.; and Writing—review and editing, E.B., C.T., D.P., A.C., F.T., F.M.D.M., P.P., S.A., D.M., G.P., D.T. (Domenico Tripodi), A.M.(Alessandro Maturo), M.V., D.T. (Danilo Tarroni), E.L., I.C.F., C.D.V., P.F., A.A., S.C., M.D., S.B., C.M., A.M. (Aldo Morrone), V.D., S.S. and S.U. All authors have read and agreed to the published version of the manuscript.

Funding: This research was funded by a grant from the "Sapienza" University of Rome (grant number RM11715C3465FB63).

Institutional Review Board Statement: The study was conducted according to the guidelines of the Declaration of Helsinki and approved by the Sapienza University of Rome/Umberto I Hospital Review Board (Protocol approval number 2615 on 17 January 2013).

Informed Consent Statement: Informed consent was obtained from all the subjects involved in the study.

Data Availability Statement: The data supporting the reported results are available on request.

Acknowledgments: The authors are grateful to Renzo Mocini for the English revision of the manuscript.

Conflicts of Interest: The authors declare no conflict of interest.

References

1. Thiery, J.P.; Sleeman, J.P. Complex networks orchestrate epithelial-mesenchymal transitions. *Nat. Rev. Mol. Cell Biol.* **2006**, *7*, 131–142. [CrossRef]
2. Thiery, J.P.; Acloque, H.; Huang, R.Y.; Nieto, M.A. Epithelial-mesenchymal transitions in development and disease. *Cell* **2009**, *139*, 871–890. [CrossRef]
3. Gaponova, A.V.; Rodin, S.; Mazina, A.A.; Volchkov, P.V. Epithelial-mesenchymal transition: Role in cancer progression and the perspectives of antitumor treatment. *Acta Nat.* **2020**, *12*, 4–23. [CrossRef] [PubMed]

4. Liu, Q.L.; Luo, M.; Huang, C.; Chen, H.N.; Zhou, Z.G. Epigenetic regulation of epithelial to mesenchymal transition in the cancer metastatic cascade: Implications for cancer therapy. *Front. Oncol.* **2021**, *11*, 657546. [CrossRef]
5. Burger, G.A.; Danen, E.H.J.; Beltman, J.B. Deciphering Epithelial-Mesenchymal Transition Regulatory Networks in Cancer through Computational Approaches. *Front. Oncol.* **2017**, *7*, 162. [CrossRef] [PubMed]
6. Grigore, A.D.; Jolly, M.K.; Jia, D.; Farach-Carson, M.C.; Levine, H. Tumor budding: The name is EMT. Partial EMT. *J. Clin. Med.* **2016**, *5*, 51. [CrossRef] [PubMed]
7. Yang, J.; Antin, P.; Berx, G.; Blanpain, C.; Brabletz, T.; Bronner, M. Guidelines and definitions for research on Epithelial-Mesenchymal Transition. *Nat. Rev. Mol. Cell Biol.* **2020**, *21*, 341–352. [CrossRef]
8. Aiello, N.M.; Maddipati, R.; Norgard, R.J.; Balli, D.; Li, J.; Yuan, S.; Yamazoe, T.; Black, T.; Sahmoud, A.; Furth, E.E.; et al. EMT subtype influences epithelial plasticity and mode of cell migration. *Dev. Cell* **2018**, *45*, 681–695. [CrossRef]
9. Suarez-Carmona, M.; Lesage, J.; Cataldo, D.; Gilles, C. EMT and inflammation: Inseparable actors of cancer progression. *Mol. Oncol.* **2017**, *11*, 805–823. [CrossRef]
10. Revilla, G.; Corcoy, R.; Moral, A.; Escolà-Gil, J.C.; Mato, E. Cross-Talk between Inflammatory Mediators and the Epithelial Mesenchymal Transition Process in the Development of Thyroid Carcinoma. *Int. J. Mol. Sci.* **2019**, *20*, 2466. [CrossRef]
11. Daly, C.S.; Flemban, A.; Shafei, M.; Conway, M.E.; Qualtrough, D.; Dean, S.J. Hypoxia modulates the stem cell population and induces EMT in the MCF-10A breast epithelial cell line. *Oncol. Rep.* **2018**, *39*, 483–490. [CrossRef]
12. Joseph, J.P.; Harishankar, M.K.; Pillai, A.A.; Devi, A. Hypoxia induced EMT: A review on the mechanism of tumor progression and metastasis in OSCC. *Oral Oncol.* **2018**, *80*, 23–32. [CrossRef] [PubMed]
13. Horejs, C.M.; Serio, A.; Purvis, A.; Gormley, A.J.; Bertazzo, S.; Poliniewicz, A.; Wang, A.J.; DiMaggio, P.; Hohenester, E.; Stevens, M.M. Biologically-active laminin-111 fragment that modulates the epithelial-to-mesenchymal transition in embryonic stem cells. *Proc. Natl. Acad. Sci. USA* **2014** *111*, 5908–5913. [CrossRef] [PubMed]
14. Chen, Q.K.; Lee, K.; Radisky, D.C.; Nelson, C.M. Extracellular matrix proteins regulate epithelial-mesenchymal transition in mammary epithelial cells. *Differentiation* **2013**, *86*, 126–132. [CrossRef] [PubMed]
15. Akhavan, A.; Griffith, O.L.; Soroceanu, L.; Leonoudakis, D.; Luciani-Torres, M.G.; Daemen, A.; Gray, J.W.; Muschler, J.L. Loss of cell-surface laminin anchoring promotes tumor growth and is associated with poor clinical outcomes. *Cancer Res.* **2012**, *72*, 2578–2588. [CrossRef] [PubMed]
16. Giannelli, G.; Bergamini, C.; Fransvea, E.; Sgarra, C.; Antonaci, S. Laminin-5 with transforming growth factor-beta1 induces epithelial to mesenchymal transition in hepatocellular carcinoma. *Gastroenterology* **2005**, *129*, 1375–1383. [CrossRef]
17. Peng, D.H.; Ungewiss, C.; Tong, P.; Byers, L.A.; Wang, J.; Canales, J.R.; Villalobos, P.A.; Uraoka, N.; Mino, B.; Behrens, C.; et al. ZEB1 induces LOXL2-mediated collagen stabilization and deposition in the extracellular matrix to drive lung cancer invasion and metastasis. *Oncogene* **2017**, *36*, 1925–1938. [CrossRef]
18. Petrini, I.; Barachini, S.; Carnicelli, V.; Galimberti, S.; Modeo, L.; Boni, R.; Sollini, M.; Erba, P.A. ED-B fibronectin expression is a marker of epithelial-mesenchymal transition in translational oncology. *Oncotarget* **2017**, *8*, 4914–4921. [CrossRef]
19. Zhang, J.; Tian, X.J.; Xing, J. Signal Transduction Pathways of EMT Induced by TGF-β, SHH, and WNT and Their Crosstalks. *J. Clin. Med.* **2016**, *5*, 41. [CrossRef]
20. Goossens, S.; Vandamme, N.; Van Vlierberghe, P.; Berx, G. EMT transcription factors in cancer development re-evaluated: Beyond EMT and MET. *Biochim. Biophys. Acta Rev. Cancer* **2017**, *1868*, 584–591. [CrossRef] [PubMed]
21. National Cancer Institute. 2019 SEER Cancer Statistics Review, 1975–2016. 2020. Available online: https://seer.cancer.gov/csr/1975_2016/ (accessed on 16 May 2021).
22. Siegel, R.L.; Miller, K.D.; Jemal, A. Cancer statistics. *CA Cancer J. Clin.* **2019**, *69*, 7–34. [CrossRef] [PubMed]
23. Bray, F.; Ferlay, J.; Soerjomataram, I.; Siegel, R.L.; Torre, L.A.; Jemal, A. Global cancer statistics 2018: GLOBOCAN estimates of incidence and mortality worldwide for 36 cancers in 185 countries. *CA Cancer J. Clin.* **2018**, *68*, 394–424. [CrossRef] [PubMed]
24. Nikiforov, Y.E.; Biddinger, P.W.; Thompson, L.D.R. *Diagnostic Pathology and Molecular Genetics of the Thyroid*; Lippincott Williams & Wilkins: Philadelphia, PA, USA, 2009.
25. Haugen, B.R.; Alexander, E.K.; Bible, K.C.; Doherty, G.M.; Mandel, S.J.; Nikiforov, Y.E.; Pacini, F.; Randolph, G.W.; Sawka, A.M.; Schlumberger, M.; et al. 2015 American Thyroid Association management guidelines for adult patients with thyroid nodules and differentiated thyroid cancer: The American Thyroid Association guidelines task force on thyroid nodules and differentiated thyroid cancer. *Thyroid* **2016**, *26*, 1–133. [CrossRef] [PubMed]
26. The Cancer Genome Atlas Research Network. Integrated genomic characterization of papillary thyroid carcinoma. *Cell* **2014**, *159*, 676–690. [CrossRef] [PubMed]
27. Kimura, E.T.; Nikiforova, M.N.; Zhu, Z.; Knauf, J.A.; Nikiforov, Y.E.; Fagin, J.A. High prevalence of BRAF mutations in thyroid cancer: Genetic evidence for constitutive activation of the RET/PTC-RAS-BRAF signaling pathway in papillary thyroid carcinoma. *Cancer Res.* **2003**, *63*, 1454–1457.
28. Soares, P.; Trovisco, V.; Rocha, A.S.; Lima, J.; Castro, P.; Preto, A.; Máximo, V.; Botelho, T.; Seruca, R.; Sobrinho Simões, M. BRAF mutations and RET/PTC rearrangements are alternative events in the etiopathogenesis of PTC. *Oncogene* **2003**, *22*, 4578–4580. [CrossRef]
29. Gao, J.; Aksoy, B.A.; Dogrusoz, U.; Dresdner, G.; Gross, B.; Sumer, S.O.; Sun, Y.; Jacobsen, A.; Sinha, R.; Larsson, E.; et al. Integrative analysis of complex cancer genomics and clinical profiles using the cBioPortal. *Sci. Signal* **2013**, *6*, pl1. [CrossRef]

30. Baldini, E.; Sorrenti, S.; Di Gioia, C.; De Vito, C.; Antonelli, A.; Gnessi, L.; Carbotta, G.; D'Armiento, E.; Miccoli, P.; De Antoni, E.; et al. Cervical lymph node metastases from thyroid cancer: Does thyroglobulin and calcitonin measurement in fine needle aspirates improve the diagnostic value of cytology? *BMC Clin. Pathol.* **2013**, *13*, 7. [CrossRef] [PubMed]
31. Baldini, E.; Tuccilli, C.; Arlot-Bonnemains, Y.; Chesnel, F.; Sorrenti, S.; De Vito, C.; Catania, A.; D'Armiento, E.; Antonelli, A.; Fallahi, P.; et al. Deregulated expression of VHL mRNA variants in papillary thyroid cancer. *Mol. Cell Endocrinol.* **2017**, *443*, 121–127. [CrossRef]
32. Chomczynsky, P.; Sacchi, P. Single step method of RNA isolation by guanidinium thiocyanate-phenol-chloroform extraction. *Anal. Biochem.* **1987**, *162*, 156–159. [CrossRef]
33. Vandesompele, J.; De Preter, K.; Pattyn, F.; Poppe, B.; Van Roy, N.; De Paepe, A.; Speleman, F. Accurate normalization of real-time quantitative RT-PCR data by geometric averaging of multiple internal control genes. *Genome Biol.* **2002**, *3*, RESEARCH0034. [CrossRef] [PubMed]
34. Ulisse, S.; Baldini, E.; Sorrenti, S.; Barollo, S.; Prinzi, N.; Catania, A.; Nesca, A.; Gnessi, L.; Pelizzo, M.R.; Mian, C.; et al. In papillary thyroid carcinoma BRAFV600E is associated with increased expression of the urokinase plasminogen activator and its cognate receptor, but not with disease-free interval. *Clin. Endocrinol.* **2012**, *77*, 780–786. [CrossRef] [PubMed]
35. Ulisse, S.; Baldini, E.; Sorrenti, S.; Barollo, S.; Gnessi, L.; Catania, A.; Pellizzo, M.R.; Nardi, F.; Mian, C.; De Antoni, E.; et al. High expression of the urokinase plasminogen activator and its cognate receptor associates with advanced stages and reduced disease-free interval in papillary thyroid carcinoma. *J. Clin. Endocrinol. Metab.* **2011**, *96*, 504–508. [CrossRef] [PubMed]
36. Evans, J.D. *Straightforward Statistics for the Behavioral Sciences*; Brooks/Cole Publishing Company: Pacific Grove, CA, USA, 1996.
37. Senga, S.S.; Grose, R.P. Hallmarks of cancer-the new testament. *Open Biol.* **2021**, *11*, 200358. [CrossRef]
38. Hanahan, D.; Weinberg, R.A. Hallmarks of cancer: The next generation. *Cell* **2011**, *144*, 646–674. [CrossRef]
39. Imani, S.; Hosseinifard, H.; Cheng, J.; Wei, C.; Fu, J. Prognostic Value of EMT-inducing transcription factors (EMT-TFs) in metastatic breast cancer: A systematic review and meta-analysis. *Sci. Rep.* **2016**, *6*, 28587. [CrossRef] [PubMed]
40. Ahmadiankia, N.; Khosravi, A. Significance of epithelial-to-mesenchymal transition inducing transcription factors in predicting distance metastasis and survival in patients with colorectal cancer: A systematic review and meta-analysis. *J. Res. Med. Sci.* **2020**, *25*, 60. [CrossRef]
41. Seo, J.; Ha, J.; Kang, E.; Cho, S. The role of epithelial-mesenchymal transition-regulating transcription factors in anti-cancer drug resistance. *Arch. Pharm. Res.* **2021**, *44*, 281–292. [CrossRef]
42. Ashrafizadeh, M.; Mirzaei, S.; Hashemi, F.; Zarrabi, A.; Zabolian, A.; Saleki, H.; Sharifzadeh, S.O.; Soleymani, L.; Daneshi, S.; Hushmandi, K.; et al. New insight towards development of paclitaxel and docetaxel resistance in cancer cells: EMT as a novel molecular mechanism and therapeutic possibilities. *Biomed. Pharmacother.* **2021**, *141*, 111824. [CrossRef] [PubMed]
43. Assani, G.; Zhou, Y. Effect of modulation of epithelial-mesenchymal transition regulators Snail1 and Snail2 on cancer cell radiosensitivity by targeting of the cell cycle, cell apoptosis and cell migration/invasion. *Oncol. Lett.* **2019**, *17*, 23–30. [CrossRef]
44. Hombach-Klonisch, S.; Natarajan, S.; Thanasupawat, T.; Medapati, M.; Pathak, A.; Ghavami, S.; Klonisch, T. Mechanisms of therapeutic resistance in cancer (stem) cells with emphasis on thyroid cancer cells. *Front. Endocrinol.* **2014**, *5*, 37. [CrossRef]
45. Shakib, H.; Rajabi, S.; Dehghan, M.H.; Mashayekhi, F.J.; Safari-Alighiarloo, N.; Hedayati, M. Epithelial-to-mesenchymal transition in thyroid cancer: A comprehensive review. *Endocrine* **2019**, *66*, 435–455. [CrossRef]
46. Wu, J.; Zhang, Y.; Cheng, R.; Gong, W.; Ding, T.; Zhai, Q.; Wang, Y.; Meng, B.; Sun, B. Expression of epithelial-mesenchymal transition regulators TWIST, SLUG and SNAIL in follicular thyroid tumours may relate to widely invasive, poorly differentiated and distant metastasis. *Histopathology* **2019**, *74*, 780–791. [CrossRef] [PubMed]
47. Buehler, D.; Hardin, H.; Shan, W.; Montemayor-Garcia, C.; Rush, P.S.; Asioli, S.; Chen, H.; Lloyd, R.V. Expression of epithelial-mesenchymal transition regulators SNAI2 and TWIST1 in thyroid carcinomas. *Mod. Pathol.* **2013**, *26*, 54–61. [CrossRef]
48. Di Maro, G.; Orlandella, F.M.; Bencivenga, T.C.; Salerno, P.; Ugolini, C.; Basolo, F.; Maestro, R.; Salvatore, G. Identification of targets of Twist1 transcription factor in thyroid cancer cells. *J. Clin. Endocrinol. Metab.* **2014**, *99*, E1617–E1626. [CrossRef] [PubMed]
49. Salerno, P.; Garcia-Rostan, G.; Piccinin, S.; Bencivenga, T.C.; Di Maro, G.; Doglioni, C.; Basolo, F.; Maestro, R.; Fusco, A.; Santoro, M.; et al. TWIST1 plays a pleiotropic role in determining the anaplastic thyroid cancer phenotype. *J. Clin. Endocrinol. Metab.* **2011**, *96*, E772–E781. [CrossRef]
50. Hardy, R.G.; Vicente-Dueñas, C.; González-Herrero, I.; Anderson, C.; Flores, T.; Hughes, S.; Tselepis, C.; Ross, J.A.; Sánchez-García, I. Snail family transcription factors are implicated in thyroid carcinogenesis. *Am. J. Pathol.* **2007**, *171*, 1037–1046. [CrossRef] [PubMed]
51. Mitsutake, N.; Knauf, J.A.; Mitsutake, S.; Mesa, C., Jr.; Zhang, L.; Fagin, J.A. Conditional BRAFV600E expression induces DNA synthesis, apoptosis, dedifferentiation, and chromosomal instability in thyroid PCCL3 cells. *Cancer Res.* **2005**, *65*, 2465–2473. [CrossRef] [PubMed]
52. Puli, O.R.; Danysh, B.P.; McBeath, E.; Sinha, D.K.; Hoang, N.M.; Powell, R.T.; Danysh, H.E.; Cabanillas, M.E.; Cote, G.J.; Hofmann, M.C. The Transcription Factor ETV5 Mediates BRAFV600E-Induced Proliferation and TWIST1 Expression in Papillary Thyroid Cancer Cells. *Neoplasia* **2018**, *20*, 1121–1134. [CrossRef] [PubMed]
53. Mitchell, B.; Dhingra, J.K.; Mahalingam, M. BRAF and Epithelial-Mesenchymal Transition: Lessons from Papillary Thyroid Carcinoma and Primary Cutaneous Melanoma. *Adv. Anat. Pathol.* **2016**, *23*, 244–271. [CrossRef]

54. Baquero, P.; Sánchez-Hernández, I.; Jiménez-Mora, E.; Orgaz, J.L.; Jiménez, B.; Chiloeches, A. (V600E)BRAF promotes invasiveness of thyroid cancer cells by decreasing E-cadherin expression through a Snail-dependent mechanism. *Cancer Lett* **2013**, *335*, 232–241. [CrossRef] [PubMed]
55. Ma, R.; Bonnefond, S.; Morshed, S.A.; Latif, R.; Davies, T.F. Stemness is derived from thyroid cancer cells. *Front. Endocrinol.* **2014**, *5*, 114. [CrossRef] [PubMed]
56. Orlandella, F.M.; Di Maro, G.; Ugolini, C.; Basolo, F.; Salvatore, G. TWIST1/miR-584/TUSC2 pathway induces resistance to apoptosis in thyroid cancer cells. *Oncotarget* **2016**, *7*, 70575–70588. [CrossRef]
57. Wieczorek-Szukala, K.; Lewinski, A. The Role of Snail-1 in Thyroid Cancer-What We Know So Far. *J. Clin. Med.* **2021**, *10*, 2324. [CrossRef]
58. Sorrenti, S.; Carbotta, G.; Di Matteo, F.M.; Catania, A.; Pironi, D.; Tartaglia, F.; Tarroni, D.; Gagliardi, F.; Tripodi, D.; Watanabe, M.; et al. Evaluation of Clinicopathological and Molecular Parameters on Disease Recurrence of Papillary Thyroid Cancer Patient: A Retrospective Observational Study. *Cancers* **2020**, *12*, 3637. [CrossRef] [PubMed]

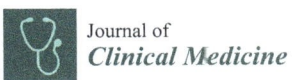

Article

Perioperative Management of Pheochromocytoma: From a Dogmatic to a Tailored Approach

Salvatore Buscemi [1], Giuseppe Di Buono [1], Rocco D'Andrea [2], Claudio Ricci [3,4,*], Laura Alberici [3], Lorenzo Querci [4], Saverio Selva [3], Francesco Minni [3,4], Roberto Citarrella [5], Giorgio Romano [1] and Antonino Agrusa [1]

1. Department of Surgical, Oncological and Oral Sciences (Di.Chir.On.S.), University of Palermo, 90127 Palermo, Italy; salvatore.buscemi02@unipa.it (S.B.); giuseppe.dibuono@unipa.it (G.D.B.); giorgio.romano@unipa.it (G.R.); antonino.agrusa@unipa.it (A.A.)
2. Division of Anaestesioloigist, IRCCS Azienda Ospedaliero-Universitaria Di Bologna, Via Albertoni 15-Italia, 40121 Bologna, Italy; rocco.dandrea@aosp.bo.it
3. Division of Pancreatic Surgery, IRCCS Azienda Ospedaliero-Universitaria Di Bologna, Via Albertoni 15-Italia, 40121 Bologna, Italy; lau.alberici@gmail.com (L.A.); saverio.selva@aosp.bo.it (S.S.); francesco.minni@unibo.it (F.M.)
4. Department of Internal Medicine and Surgery (DIMEC), Alma Mater Studiorum University of Bologna, 40121 Bologna, Italy; querci.lorenzo@gmail.com
5. Department of Health Promotion Sciences Maternal and Infantile Care, Internal Medicine and Medical Specialties (PROMISE), University of Palermo, 90127 Palermo, Italy; roberto.citarrella@unipa.it
* Correspondence: claudio.ricci6@unibo.it; Tel.: +39-051-341541; Fax: +39-051-341483

Abstract: Background: Perioperative management of pheochromocytoma (PCC) remains under debate. Methods: A bicentric retrospective study was conducted, including all patients who underwent laparoscopic adrenalectomy for PCC from 2000 to 2017. Patients were divided into two groups: Group 1 treated with alpha-blockade, and Group 2, without alfa-blockers. The primary end point was the major complication rate. The secondary end points were: the need for advanced intra-operative hemostasis, the admission to the intensive care unit (ICU), the length of stay (LOS), systolic (SBP), and diastolic blood pressure (DBP) Univariate and multivariate analysis was conducted. A p-value < 0.05 was considered statistically significant. Results: Major postoperative complications were similar ($p = 0.49$). Advanced hemostatic agents were 44.9% in Group 1 and 10% in Group 2 ($p < 0.001$). In Group 2, no patients were admitted to the ICU, while only 73.5% of Group 1 ($p < 0.001$) were admitted. The median length of stay was larger in Group 1 than in Group 2 ($p = 0.026$). At the induction, SBP was 130 mmHg in Group 1, and 115 mmHg ($p < 0.001$). The pre-surgery treatment was the only almost statistically significant variable at the multivariate analysis of DBP at the end of surgery. Conclusion: The preoperative use of alfa-blockers should be considered not a dogma in PCC.

Keywords: pheochromocytoma; alfa-blockers; perioperative management

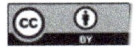

1. Introduction

Pheochromocytoma (PCC) is a neuroendocrine tumor originating from the chromaffin cell in the adrenal medulla that secretes the catecholamine. It has a low incidence of 0.8 per 100,000 individuals/year, occurring in 0.1–0.6% in the hypertensive population [1,2].

The secreted catecholamines explain all the clinical manifestations of this type of tumor. Because the release of catecholamine by PCC is unpredictable, the clinical presentation includes headaches, sweating, tachycardia, palpitation, and hypertension and can range from clinically asymptomatic to life-threatening hypertensive crises [3].

To date, surgical resection is the only cure. Although laparoscopic resection was once considered not indicated in PCC, several studies in the last twenty years have demonstrated that laparoscopic adrenalectomy is associated with less pain, less morbidity, and quick recovery. It is considered the gold standard compared to open adrenalectomy [4–6].

However, general anesthesia induction, abdominal pressure fluctuations, and direct tumor handing could increase catecholamine release, triggering intraoperative hypertensive crisis and increasing the risk for major morbidity [7].

Improvement of operative and anesthetic techniques, such as laparoscopy and new anesthetic drugs, and preoperative medical preparation, has decreased the risk of perioperative hemodynamic instability. The perioperative management includes alpha-receptor blockade, suitable drugs for anesthesia, volume expansion, and postoperative care [8,9]. Historically, the most critical factor that has drastically reduced these patients' perioperative morbidity and mortality is meticulous preoperative preparation. However, no clear guidelines exist about the ideal drug for preoperative preparation, and the evidence from a randomized controlled clinical trial is unavailable [10,11]. The optimal alpha-blockade strategy achieves a seated blood pressure (BP) < 130/80 mmHg, withstanding systolic BP > 90 mmHg. Traditionally, the long-acting, irreversible, non-selective alpha-blocker phenoxybenzamine is initiated 7–14 days preoperatively, and patients present side effects such as nasal congestion, preoperative orthostatic hypotension, and postoperative hypotension [11]. Short-acting, selective alpha-blockers, as doxazosin, have been promoted as alternatives, and they are associated with less preoperative orthostatic hypotension and shorter postoperative hypotension duration than phenoxybenzamine [10]. However, competitive inhibition can be overcome by high levels of catecholamines, and the antihypertensive effect of selective alpha-blockade may not be as potent [9].

Despite the preoperative preparation, 27.3% of the patients experienced hemodynamic instability intraoperatively, which must be promptly and carefully managed intraoperatively [12]. Short-acting drugs with an established safety profile (sodium nitroprusside, nitroglycerine, magnesium, and esmolol) permit good intraoperative blood pressure and heart rate management. The most common complication after tumor removal is hypotension, which may require fluid therapy and vasopressor support. Postoperative management usually requires intensive care or high dependency unit admission [13]. Although the recommendation from many reports suggested that patients with hormonally functional PCC should receive proper adrenoceptor blockade [14], in one recent series, up to one-third did not receive pre-adrenalectomy alpha-blockade [15]. In a recent series, preoperative selective alpha-adrenoceptor antagonist had no benefit in maintaining intraoperative hemodynamic stability in patients with normotensive PCC.

Moreover, they increased the use of vasoactive drugs and colloid infusion compared to PCC, which received no alpha-blockers preoperatively. Whether normotensive PCC patients truly benefit from alpha-adrenergic antagonist preparation remains uncertain [16]. These data suggest that alpha-blockade may sometimes be deemed "unnecessary" in PCC associated with normotension/postural hypotension or apparently "non-functional", not according to recent recommendations and society's guidelines. We performed a multicentric retrospective case-control study of patients undergoing adrenalectomy for PCC from 2000 to 2017 at two University Hospitals.

2. Materials and Methods

We conducted a multicentric retrospective study at St. Orsola-Malpighi Hospital (Bologna) and AOUP "P.Giaccone" Hospital (Palermo). Patients undergoing laparoscopic adrenalectomy for pheochromocytoma from 2000 to 2017 were included in the study. All patients included in the study have a preoperative positive catecholamine test with high levels of plasma-free metanephrines or 24 h urinary fractionated metanephrine). We included both symptomatic and asymptomatic patients.

The first team performed preoperative blood pressure management with alfa-antagonist and beta-antagonist drugs, while the second team did not. Both institutions collected data of patients in a prospectively maintained adrenal database. We performed per-protocol analysis, including only patients with a final pathological diagnosis of PCC. Planned open and bilateral adrenalectomies were excluded from our analysis. Patients with missing anesthetic records were excluded. Patients were divided into two groups based on preoperative alpha-blockade strategy: patients in Group 1 were treated with alpha-blockade, non-selectively with phenoxybenzamine, or blocked selectively with doxazosin ($n = 49$), while patients in Group 2 did not receive alpha-blockade preoperatively ($n = 14$) but only miscellaneous, on-demand, antihypertensive drugs during the crisis. Preoperative data included patient age, sex, Body Mass Index (BMI), comorbidities such as heart vascular disease and hypertension, presence of typical symptoms of PCC (headaches, sweating, tachycardia, palpitation, and hypertensive crisis), dimension of the lesion at CT scan and duration of preoperative treatment in patients receiving alpha-blockade. In the group of patients treated preoperatively with alpha-blockers, both selective and non-selective were used. Patients treated with phenoxybenzamine ($n = 37$) started 2–7 days before hospital admission. Following admission, they received an additional 5–10 days of alpha-blockade with phenoxybenzamine in the hospital. A preoperative high-sodium diet and fluid intake were encouraged to reverse catecholamine-induced blood volume contraction. A beta-blocker was added in cases of tachycardia. The remaining patients were treated with doxazosin ($n = 12$). The starting dose of doxazosin was 1 milligram daily and was titrated in 1-milligram increments to the desired effect. Patients were considered adequately blocked when they achieved a blood pressure below 140/90 mmHg. Patients of Group 2 received daily blood pressure monitoring until the operation and continued their chronic cardiovascular therapy. All patients underwent a cardiac evaluation through a thorough history and physical examination; complete blood count, basic metabolic panel, electrocardiogram, and echocardiogram were performed in all patients. A radial artery line was routinely inserted in both groups to monitor intraoperative hemodynamics. Intraoperative systolic blood pressure (SBP) and diastolic blood pressure (DBP) were measured every 5 min. The anesthesiologists established access with at least two peripheral intravenous lines or the positioning of central access. Anesthesia methods were similar for both groups: propofol was used for induction, and vecuronium bromide thymopeptides was as a muscle relaxant, isoflurane and fentanyl were also used during anesthesia maintenance. Intraoperative data included SBP at induction of anesthesia and pneumoperitoneum. Furthermore, SBP and DBP were monitored at the end of the surgery. In all patients, laparoscopic adrenalectomy was performed, and no conversions occurred; in every hospital, all procedures were performed by the same surgeon with experience in laparoscopic adrenalectomy. No Intraoperative complications were recorded. All patients were treated by using hemostatic agents at the end of the operation. Anesthesiologists determined the thresholds for treating patient hemodynamics and decided whether to use fluid or vasoactive drugs (sodium nitroprusside, nitroglycerine and esmolol). We included in our variables the admission to the intensive care unit (ICU), the length of stay (LOS), postoperative complications, and mortality. Data, which were collected using Excel software, were analyzed by R Studio version 1.1.419 software. For synthesis and variability measurements of continuous values, we chose median and interquartile range (IQR). Univariate inference analysis was conducted using the non-parametric Wilcoxon test for non-normal distribution and the Student's t test for the normal one as well as the Shapiro–Wilk test for continuous variables and Chi-square for proportion. Multivariate analysis was conducted using linear regression models. The values were considered significant when p-value < 0.05.

3. Results

Demographics and preoperative variables are presented in Table 1.

Table 1. Basal characteristics of the two groups.

Variable	Preoperative Anti-Hypertensive Management (n = 49)	Not Preoperative Anti-Hypertensive Management (n = 14)	p-Value
Age (years)	56.00 (IQR 49.00–70.25)	57.00 (IQR 44.00–70.00)	0.5627
Female sex	26 (53.06%)	10 (71.4%)	0.3583
BMI (kg/m^2)	24.00 (IQR 21.25–26.75)	27.00 (IQR 24.00–28.00)	0.0006
Heart disease	11 (22.45%)	0 (0.00%)	0.1147
Hypertension	8 (16.33%)	3 (21.43%)	0.3288
Symptomatic	28 (57.14%)	10 (71.43%)	0.5132
Alpha-blocker	49 (100.00%)		
Beta-blocker	28 (57.14%)		
Calcium channel blocker	2 (4.08%)		
CT-dimension (cm max)	3.2 (IQR 2.38–8.70)	4.5 (IQR 3.63–5.88)	0.0008
Duration of preoperative treatment (days)	10.00 (8.00–18.00)		

BMI: Body Mass Index; IQR: interquartile range.

The age and sex were comparable, whereas a trend was seen for a more significant proportion of women in both groups. Overall, the median age was 56 years in Group 1 and 57 years in Group 2, while 53% and 71.4% were women, respectively, and no statistical differences were detected in the two groups. The BMI of the patients in Group 2 was significantly greater (median 27, IQR 24.00–28.00, and median 24, IQR 21.25–26.75, p-value 0.0006).

There was no statistical difference in comorbidity, such as heart vascular disease and hypertension, in the two groups, even if many patients in Group 1 had preoperative major cardiovascular disease.

Dimension of the lesion detected at the CT scan was larger in patients of Group 2 (median 4.5 cm, IQR 3.63–5.88, median 3.2, IQR 2.38–8.70 respectively, p-value 0.0008), even if in Group 1, laparoscopic adrenalectomy was also performed for lesions larger than 6 cm. All patients in Group 1 were treated using alpha-blockers preoperatively, while only 28 patients (57.14%) needed beta-blockers during preparation. Intraoperative and postoperative results are summarized in Table 2.

Table 2. Results of univariate analysis.

Variables	Preoperative Anti-Hypertensive Management (n = 49)	Not Preoperative Anti-Hypertensive Management (n = 14)	p-Value
Major complications	5 (10.20%)	0 (0.00%)	0.4933
Need for advance intra-operative haemostasis	22 (44.89%)	14 (100.00%)	<0.001
ICU admission	36 (73.47%)	0 (0.00%)	<0.001
Length of stay (days)	5 (IQR 4–6)	4 (IQR 4–4)	0.0260
SBP induction (mmHg)	130 (IQR 120–150)	115 (IQR 110–125)	<0.001
SBP pneumoperitoneum (mmHg)	120 (IQR 100–128.8)	110 (IQR 110–120)	0.3570
SBP end surgery (mmHg)	110 (IQR 100–120)	117.5 (IQR 110–120)	0.0513
DBP end surgery (mmHg)	60 (IQR 50–70)	60 (IQR 60–63.75)	0.6291

ICU: intensive care unit; SBP: systolic blood pressure; DBP: diastolic blood pressure.

Major postoperative complications were observed in 8.5% ($n = 5$) of patients in Group 1, while no major complications were detected in Group 2 ($n = 0$, p-value 0.49). The complications were two cases of pneumonia, two postoperative fluid collections in the surgical site, and one postoperative hematoma in the trocar site.

Moreover, no mortality was reported in either group. The use of advanced hemostatic agents was observed in 44.9% ($n = 22$) of patients in Group 1 and 100% ($n = 14$) of patients in Group 2 (p-value < 0.001). No Group 2 patients were admitted to the ICU, while 73.5% of Bologna patients were transferred to the ICU, resulting in an increase of one day in the median of the length of stay (p-value 0.026). Patients in Group 2 were readmitted to the ward after a few hours of observation and semi-intensive hemodynamic monitoring in the operating complex. During hospitalization in the ward, all patients of both groups were monitored hemodynamically with non-invasive methods. At the induction of anesthesia, SBP was 130 (IQR 120–150) mmHg in Group 1, while in Group 2, a lower SBP (median 115 mmHg, IQR 110–125, p-value 0.001) was detected. Instead, during the induction of pneumoperitoneum, SBP was 120.00 (IQR 100.0–128.8) mmHg for Group 1 and 110 (IQR 110.0–120.0) mmHg for Group 2, with no statistical difference (p-value 0.3570). At the end of the surgery, patients in group 1 had an SBP of about 110.0 (IQR 100.0–120.0) mmHg, while in Group 2, this was about 117.5 (110.0–120.0) mmHg. This difference has a low significance with a p-value of about 0.051. Moreover, DBP at the end of surgery was similar in both groups, with no statistical difference at univariate analysis. We analyzed the difference in SBP at induction and DBP at the end of surgery through multivariate analysis. The pre-surgery treatment was the only almost statistically significant variable at the multivariate analysis of DBP at the end of surgery (Table 3).

Table 3. Results for difference in diastolic blood pressure at end of surgery (multivariate analysis).

Variables	Beta	p-Value
Pre-surgery treatment	9.74801	0.058068
Age	0.01569	0.901548
Sex female	0.97157	0.742060
BMI	−0.22330	0.651397
Hypertension	−2.72738	0.432634
Heart Didease	−3.62446	0.363887
Diabete	−5.99645	0.153887
ASA score	0.39027	0.901152
Symptoms	−4.11863	0.291716
Incidentaloma	−1.28322	0.754422
CT Dimension	0.7616	0.846408

BMI: Body Mass Index; ASA: American Society of Anesthesiologists.

4. Discussion

Adrenalectomy for pheochromocytoma is reported with mortality close to zero in recent studies. The dogma of preoperative fluid and hypotensive drug administrations is widely applied in patients scheduled for pheochromocytoma removal and is assumed to benefit operative outcomes. This paradigm is only based on historical studies of non-standardized practices and criteria for efficacy, with no control group [1,12,15]. With advancements in surgical and anesthetic techniques, severe morbidity and mortality associated with the surgery are low in high-volume centers [2]. The dogma of preoperative blood pressure management is assumed to have a beneficial effect on operative outcomes, but this paradigm is only based on historical studies of non-standardized practices. Recent improvements in anesthetic management could permit an intraoperative reasonable blood pressure control without preoperative treatment, reducing postoperative hypotension. Better knowledge of the disease, efficiency of available intravenous short-acting vasoactive drugs, and careful intraoperative handling of the tumor make it possible to omit preoperative preparation in most patients scheduled for pheochromocytoma removal. Ulchaker et al. [17] reported that 30% of patients received no medication 24 h before surgery. Intraoperative mean blood pressure levels were similar in patients who were not treated preoperatively with antihypertensive medications [17]. Boutros et al. compared 31 patients receiving alpha-blockade preparation with 29 patients who did not receive any hypotensive drugs, and no difference in perioperative mortality or morbidity was found. However, intraoperative blood pressure rise was a little higher in the untreated group [18]. Shao et al. compared pheochromocytoma receiving preparation with doxazosin with a group of patients who did not receive any medication [16]. The intraoperative blood pressure and heart rate were similar in the two groups, whereas the intraoperative colloid transfusion was significantly greater in patients receiving doxazosin. DBP intraoperatively tended to be higher in patients without preoperative a-blockade but was not significant [16]. No severe hypertension/hypotension or tachycardia/bradycardia was detected during surgery in both groups. However, a1-blockade preparation increased the use of vasoactive drugs and intraoperative colloid fluid to maintain their blood pressure stability [16].

Furthermore, the use of noncompetitive a-adrenergic antagonist phenoxybenzamine leads to longer-lasting intraoperative hypotension that requires greater use of vasopressors [19]. Our series preoperative administration of a-adrenergic blockade did not improve the SBP during the operation compared to cases without preoperative antihypertensive management. No severe cardiovascular complications were detected during surgery in both groups. Increased knowledge of the disease, continuous arterial pressure monitoring, fast-acting vasoactive agents, and improvement of the surgical approach have dramatically improved the outcome of patients undergoing adrenalectomy for pheochromocytoma [8,19]. The anesthetic possibilities have transformed, and perhaps the time is ripe to change the management of these patients reducing waiting times for surgery and the risk of postoperative hypotension. Routine preoperative administration of fluids and hypotensive drugs is not supported by any evidence-based study [11]. There are only a few studies on this topic in literature due to the rarity of this disorder. A randomized prospective trial with a greater number of cases is required to confirm whether the a-adrenergic blockade is necessary or not as preoperative management for pheochromocytoma. This study has some limitations: first, the sample size for the group without preoperative treatment was small; second, the bicentric design could introduce some bias producing significant differences in the results, such as those in the use of hemostatic agents or postoperative intensive care; third, the difference in BMI and the size of the tumor could impact the results.

5. Conclusions

In conclusion, this is a small retrospective study and does not attempt, in any way, to influence the perioperative management habits of patients undergoing pheochromocytoma adrenalectomy surgery. In our experience, careful surgical handling of tumor tissue during laparoscopic resection, limited intraabdominal pressure, adequate depth of anesthesia and muscular relaxation, and fast-acting vasoactive agents are the only proven means to avoid intraoperative hypertension. Preoperative strict blood pressure control is possibly a dogma today.

Author Contributions: Conceptualization, S.B. and C.R.; Methodology, S.B., R.D. and C.R.; Software, R.D. and G.D.B.; Validation, S.B. and C.R.; Formal Analysis, R.D.; Investigation, L.A., L.Q., S.S., F.M. and R.C.; Resources, L.A., L.Q., S.S., F.M., R.C., G.R. and A.A.; Data Curation, L.A., L.Q., S.S., F.M., R.C., G.R. and A.A.; Writing—Original Draft Preparation, S.B., G.D.B. and C.R.; Writing—Review and Editing, G.R. and A.A.; Visualization, G.R. and A.A. All authors have read and agreed to the published version of the manuscript.

Funding: This research received no external funding.

Institutional Review Board Statement: Data were extrapolated from prospectively collected databases and managed according to institutional rules.

Informed Consent Statement: Generic informed consent for non-interventional studies was obtained from all subjects involved in the study at the time of surgery or during follow-up.

Data Availability Statement: The data can be requested by contacting the corresponding author.

Conflicts of Interest: The authors declare no conflict of interest.

References

1. Prys-Roberts, C. Phaeochromocytoma—Recent progress in its management. *Br. J. Anaesth.* **2000**, *85*, 44–57. [CrossRef] [PubMed]
2. Lenders, J.W.; Eisenhofer, G.; Mannelli, M.; Pacak, K. Phaeochromocytoma. *Lancet* **2005**, *366*, 665–675. [CrossRef]
3. Challis, B.G.; Casey, R.T.; Simpson, H.L.; Gurnell, M. Is there an optimal preoperative management strategy for phaeochromocytoma/paraganglioma? *Clin. Endocrinol.* **2017**, *86*, 163–167. [CrossRef] [PubMed]
4. Carr, A.A.; Wang, T.S. Minimally Invasive Adrenalectomy. *Surg. Oncol. Clin.* **2016**, *25*, 139–152. [CrossRef] [PubMed]
5. Agrusa, A.; di Buono, G.; Chianetta, D.; Sorce, V.; Citarrella, R.; Galia, M.; Vernuccio, L.; Romano, G.; Gulotta, G. Three-dimensional (3D) versus two-dimensional (2D) laparoscopic adrenalectomy: A case-control study. *Int. J. Surg.* **2015**, *28*, S114–S117. [CrossRef] [PubMed]
6. Agrusa, A.; Romano, G.; Frazzetta, G.; Chianetta, D.; Sorce, V.; Di Buono, G.; Gulotta, G. Laparoscopic adrenalectomy for large adrenal masses: Single team experience. *Int. J. Surg.* **2014**, *12*, S72–S74. [CrossRef] [PubMed]
7. Brunaud, L.; Nguyen-Thi, P.L.; Mirallie, E.; Raffaelli, M.; Vriens, M.; Theveniaud, P.E.; Boutami, M.; Finnerty, B.M.; Vorselaars, W.M.; Rinkes, I.B.; et al. Predictive factors for postoperative morbidity after laparoscopic adrenalectomy for pheochromocytoma: A multicenter retrospective analysis in 225 patients. *Surg. Endosc.* **2016**, *30*, 1051–1059. [CrossRef] [PubMed]
8. Bruynzeel, H.; Feelders, R.A.; Groenland, T.H.; van den Meiracker, A.H.; van Eijck, C.H.; Lange, J.F.; de Herder, W.W.; Kazemier, G. Risk Factors for Hemodynamic Instability during Surgery for Pheochromocytoma. *J. Clin. Endocrinol. Metab.* **2010**, *95*, 678–685. [CrossRef] [PubMed]
9. Kinney, M.A.; Narr, B.J.; Warner, M.A. Perioperative management of pheochromocytoma. *J. Cardiothorac. Vasc. Anesth.* **2002**, *16*, 359–369. [CrossRef] [PubMed]
10. van der Zee, P.A.; de Boer, A. Pheochromocytoma: A review on preoperative treatment with phenoxybenzamine or doxazosin. *Neth. J. Med.* **2014**, *72*, 190–201. [PubMed]
11. Lentschener, C.; Gaujoux, S.; Tesniere, A.; Dousset, B. Point of controversy: Perioperative care of patients undergoing pheochromocytoma removal-time for a reappraisal? *Eur. J. Endocrinol.* **2011**, *165*, 365–373. [CrossRef] [PubMed]
12. Livingstone, M.; Duttchen, K.; Thompson, J.; Sunderani, Z.; Hawboldt, G.; Sarah Rose, M.; Pasieka, J. Hemodynamic Stability During Pheochromocytoma Resection: Lessons Learned Over the Last Two Decades. *Ann. Surg. Oncol.* **2015**, *22*, 4175–4180. [CrossRef] [PubMed]
13. Naranjo, J.; Dodd, S.; Martin, Y.N. Perioperative Management of Pheochromocytoma. *J. Cardiothorac. Vasc. Anesth.* **2017**, *31*, 1427–1439. [CrossRef] [PubMed]
14. Lenders, J.W.; Duh, Q.Y.; Eisenhofer, G.; Gimenez-Roqueplo, A.P.; Grebe, S.K.; Murad, M.H.; Naruse, M.; Pacak, K.; Young, W.F., Jr.; Endocrine, S. Pheochromocytoma and paraganglioma: An endocrine society clinical practice guideline. *J. Clin. Endocrinol. Metab.* **2014**, *99*, 1915–1942. [CrossRef] [PubMed]
15. Luiz, H.V.; Tanchee, M.J.; Pavlatou, M.G.; Yu, R.; Nambuba, J.; Wolf, K.; Prodanov, T.; Wesley, R.; Adams, K.; Fojo, T.; et al. Are patients with hormonally functional phaeochromocytoma and paraganglioma initially receiving a proper adrenoceptor blockade? A retrospective cohort study. *Clin. Endocrinol.* **2016**, *85*, 62–69. [CrossRef] [PubMed]
16. Shao, Y.; Chen, R.; Shen, Z.J.; Teng, Y.; Huang, P.; Rui, W.B.; Xie, X.; Zhou, W.L. Preoperative alpha blockade for normotensive pheochromocytoma: Is it necessary? *J. Hypertens.* **2011**, *29*, 2429–2432. [CrossRef] [PubMed]
17. Ulchaker, J.C.; Goldfarb, D.A.; Bravo, E.L.; Novick, A.C. Successful outcomes in pheochromocytoma surgery in the modern era. *J. Urol.* **1999**, *161*, 764–767. [CrossRef]
18. Boutros, A.R.; Bravo, E.L.; Zanettin, G.; Straffon, R.A. Perioperative management of 63 patients with pheochromocytoma. *Cleve. Clin. J. Med.* **1990**, *57*, 613–617. [CrossRef] [PubMed]
19. Weingarten, T.N.; Cata, J.P.; O'Hara, J.F.; Prybilla, D.J.; Pike, T.L.; Thompson, G.B.; Grant, C.S.; Warner, D.O.; Bravo, E.; Sprung, J. Comparison of two preoperative medical management strategies for laparoscopic resection of pheochromocytoma. *Urology* **2010**, *76*, e6–e11. [CrossRef] [PubMed]

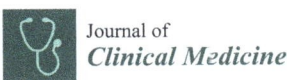

Article

Total Tumor Diameter and Unilateral Multifocality as Independent Predictor Factors for Metastatic Papillary Thyroid Microcarcinoma

Liviu Hîțu [1], Paul-Andrei Ștefan [1,2,3,*] and Doina Piciu [1,4]

1. Doctoral School, Iuliu Hațieganu University of Medicine and Pharmacy, 400012 Cluj-Napoca, Romania; Liviu.Hitu@umfcluj.ro (L.H.); doina.piciu@gmail.com (D.P.)
2. Anatomy and Embryology, Morphological Sciences Department, "Iuliu Hațieganu" University of Medicine and Pharmacy, Victor Babes Street 8, 400012 Cluj-Napoca, Romania
3. Radiology and Imaging Department, County Emergency Hospital, Clinicilor Street 5, 400006 Cluj-Napoca, Romania
4. Department of Endocrine Tumors and Nuclear Medicine, Institute of Oncology "Prof. Dr. Ion Chiricuță", 400015 Cluj-Napoca, Romania
* Correspondence: stefan_paul@ymail.com; Tel.: +40-743957206

Simple Summary: Papillary thyroid microcarcinoma is currently the most frequent endocrine cancer at this time. Usually, this form of cancer is indolent, but there are situations in which it metastasizes. The current classification guidelines are rather simplistic and do not comprehend the whole disease spectrum. Studies that have addressed this issue have evaluated various stages of papillary thyroid carcinoma, considering the scarcity of studies based on European demographic data. We aim to further investigate whether total tumor diameter and multifocality are directly correlated with metastatic forms of papillary thyroid microcarcinoma. The results of this study could validate the confidence with which current guidelines are used or could open new avenues in using the total tumor diameter instead of the size of the largest tumor.

Abstract: The purpose of this study was to assess whether total tumor diameter (TTD) and multifocality are predictors for metastatic disease in papillary thyroid microcarcinomas (PTMC). Eighty-two patients with histologically proven PTMC were retrospectively included. Patients were divided according to the presence of metastatic disease in the metastatic ($n = 41$) and non-metastatic ($n = 41$) demographic-matched group. The morphological features of PTMCs (primary tumor diameter, multifocality, TTD, number of foci, and tumor site) were compared between groups using univariate, multivariate, and receiver operating characteristic analyses. TTD ($p = 0.026$), TTD > 10 mm ($p = 0.036$), and Unilateral Multifocality (UM) ($p = 0.019$) statistically differed between the groups. The combination of the two independent predictors (TTD and UM) was able to assess metastatic risk with 60.98% sensitivity and 75.61% specificity. TTD and UM can be used to predict metastatic disease in PTMC, which may help to better adapt the RAI therapy decision. We believe that TTD and multifocality are tumor features that should be considered in future guidelines.

Keywords: papillary thyroid microcarcinoma; PTMC; total tumor diameter; TTD; unilateral multifocality; metastatic disease; independent predictors

Citation: Hîțu, L.; Ștefan, P.-A.; Piciu, D. Total Tumor Diameter and Unilateral Multifocality as Independent Predictor Factors for Metastatic Papillary Thyroid Microcarcinoma. *J. Clin. Med.* **2021**, *10*, 3707. https://doi.org/10.3390/jcm10163707

Academic Editors: Giovanni Conzo and Renato Patrone

Received: 19 July 2021
Accepted: 18 August 2021
Published: 20 August 2021

Publisher's Note: MDPI stays neutral with regard to jurisdictional claims in published maps and institutional affiliations.

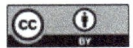

Copyright: © 2021 by the authors. Licensee MDPI, Basel, Switzerland. This article is an open access article distributed under the terms and conditions of the Creative Commons Attribution (CC BY) license (https:// creativecommons.org/licenses/by/ 4.0/).

1. Introduction

Papillary thyroid microcarcinoma (PTMC) is defined as a malignant epithelial tumor with evidence of follicular differentiation and a series of specific nuclear features [1], with the maximum size of the tumor ≤ 1 cm [2]. The incidence of PTMC is increasing due to improved diagnostic methods such as ultrasound (US) with targeted fine-needle aspiration biopsy (FNAB) [2] and is estimated to account for more than 50% of new cases of thyroid cancer [3].

Although PTMC is considered to be the most indolent form of thyroid cancer, lymph node metastases (LNM) and local recurrence are frequently encountered [4]. The incidence rate of central LNM (CLNM) in PTMC is approximately 23–64.1%, and the incidence rate of lateral LNM (LLNM) in PTMC is approximately 3.7–44.5% [5–7].

Regardless of how comprehensive the content of the guidelines is, certain therapeutic settings are still limited. The Updated AJCC/TNM (American Joint Committee on Cancer/Union for International Cancer) Staging System for Differentiated and Anaplastic Thyroid Cancer (8th edition) defines primary tumor's category only by the size of the greatest dimension [8]. The 2015 American Thyroid Association (ATA) places all intrathyroidal PTMCs, whether unifocal or multifocal, in the low-risk category. Only multifocal PTMCs with extrathyroidal extension (ETE) are considered to be in the intermediate-risk group [2]. Other international guidelines regarding thyroid cancer management do not have recommendations regarding PTMC treatment: National Comprehensive Cancer Network (NCCN) 2018 [9], European Thyroid Association (ETA) 2019 [1], and European Society for Medical Oncology (ESMO) 2019 [10].

Several studies show that multifocality/total tumor diameter (TTD) can better assess the aggressiveness of the tumor in PTMC [4,11–16]. Another study claims that calculating TTD in multifocal PTMC to evaluate adverse biological behavior is insufficient and limited [17]. Most research studies addressing the present topic of interest lack demographic data from Europe. Another essential point to note is that TTD has previously been assessed as a risk factor by comparing tumor size between different T stages of PTC (papillary thyroid carcinoma).

Our study aimed to find whether multifocality and TTD can function as predictors for metastatic disease in PTMC.

2. Materials and Methods

2.1. Conceptualization

TTDs' impact on the development of metastatic disease in PTMC in the eastern European population was the focus of our research. This was possible by comparing a target group of metastatic PTMCs with a control group of PTMCs that did not have metastatic disease. To exclude as many aspects as possible that could bias the compared results, the non-metastatic group was chosen to have epidemiological characteristics as near as possible to the target group.

2.2. Study Design and Population

This retrospective study was approved by the Ethical Committee of "Iuliu Hatieganu" University of Medicine and Pharmacy, Cluj-Napoca (number 4458) and of "Prof. Dr. Ion Chiricuță" Institute of Oncology, Cluj-Napoca (number 175/5). The data collection was done retrospectively including all patients treated in our regional oncological center between January 2008 and March 2021 that met the following criteria: initial surgical management of the thyroid, total thyroidectomy associated with central neck dissection, full clinicopathological information available, and final pathological diagnosis of PTMC. Patients with coexisting malignancies, previous history of radiotherapy to the head and neck region, and incomplete data were excluded. All patients have signed the institutional informed consent on participation in scientific studies.

2.3. Data Collection

We conducted a search in our institution database using the keywords: papillary+ thyroid + microcarcinoma + metastasis. After applying the selection criteria, 41 patients with metastatic PTMC were identified. Using the metastatic group's demographic data, we found another 41 patients with PTMC who underwent lymph node dissection but did not have metastatic disease and had demographic parameters that were as close to the metastatic group as possible.

Data collection regarding demographic characteristics, the diagnosis, and the therapeutic protocol was retrieved from the patient medical file. The histopathological information was extracted from the original pathology report. Papillary tumors measuring 1 cm or less in diameter were defined as PTMCs. TNM grading was performed according to the 8th edition of the TNM classification introduced by the American Joint Committee on Cancer [8]. The pathologic features examined were central and lateral nodal metastasis, microscopic and gross extrathyroidal extension (ETE), lymphovascular invasion (LVI), and distant metastasis. A tumor was defined as multifocal if at least 2 foci were found. Multifocality/Unifocality was divided into four separate entities: Unilateral Multifocality (2 or more foci in the same lobe); Bilateral Multifocality (more than 1 focus in both lobes); Bilateral Unifocality (1 focus in each lobe) and Unilateral Unifocality (unique focus). For multifocal lesions, the sum of the maximal diameter of each tumor foci was used to calculate TTD. Patients were divided into two age groups according to age at the time of diagnosis, <55 years and older.

2.4. Statistical Analysis

The metastatic group characteristics were compared with the non-metastatic group. For categorical variables, the Chi-square test and Fisher test were used. For continuous variables, the distribution was tested through the Kolmogorov–Smirnov Test of Normality. For normal distributed continuous variables- independent samples t-test was used, and for non-normal distributed continuous variables—Mann–Whitney U-test. Multivariate regression analyses were performed to identify independent risk factors for metastases. A p-value < 0.05 was considered statistically significant.

We investigated which of the parameters that showed statistically significant results at the univariate analysis are also independent predictors of metastases. In this regard, a multivariate regression analysis (using the "enter" input model) was conducted, with the computation of the coefficient of determination (R-squared) and the variance inflation factor (VIF). Since a high VIF value is an indicator of multicollinearity, features that recorded a VIF of $\geq 10^4$ were excluded from further analysis. The predicted values were saved and subsequently used in a receiver operating characteristics (ROC) analysis to assess the diagnostic power of the entire prediction model. The ROC analysis was also used to determine the diagnostic power of features independently associated with metastases, along with the calculation of the area under the curve (AUC), sensitivity and specificity, with 95% confidence intervals (CIs). Optimal cut-off values were chosen using a common optimization step that maximized the Youden index for predicting patients with metastatic disease. Sensitivity (Se) and specificity (Sp) were computed from the same data, without further adjustments. Statistical analysis was performed by an independent statistician, using The Statistical Package for Social Sciences software (SPSS, version 22.0, Chicago, IL, USA) and MedCalc version 14.8.1 (MedCalc Software, Mariakerke, Belgium).

3. Results

3.1. Baseline and Tumoral Characteristics

Baseline clinicopathological characteristics of the 82 patients who underwent thyroidectomy due to PTMC are presented in Table 1. Mean age of the study participants was 45.5 years with a standard deviation (SD) of 14.0; among these patients 60 (73.2%) were women. Patients younger than 55 years old had a mean age of 37.8 years with a SD of 9.6, while those older than 55 years old had a mean age of 62.0 years with a SD of 4.9. Regarding pN staging, 42 patients (51.2%) were staged N0, 29 patients (35.4%) were N1a staged and 11 patients (13.4%) were staged N1b. Of all patients included in the study, there was only one case of distant metastasis (1.2%)—in the left gluteus muscle. The number of patients in each TNM stage was as follows: 69 (84.2%) in stage I, 12 (14.6%) in stage II, and 1 (1.2%) in stage IVb.

Table 1. Clinicopathological characteristics and the univariate analysis.

	No Metastatic Disease	Metastatic Disease	Total	p-Value
gender, n (%)				
male	11 (26.8%)	11 (26.8%)	22 (26.8%)	1
female	30 (73.2%)	30 (73.2%)	60 (73.2%)	
age at diagnosis (years)				
mean ± SD	46.5 ± 13.5	44.5 ± 14.7	45.5 ± 14.0	0.524
age group, (years)				
<55 (mean ± SD)	39.1 ± 8.9	36.5 ± 10.3	37.8 ± 9.6	0.310
≥55 (mean ± SD)	62.3 ± 5.8	61.7 ± 3.9	62.0 ± 4.9	0.754
pN stage, n (%)				
N0	41 (100%)	1 (2.4%)	42 (51.2%)	
N1a	0	29 (70.7%)	29 (35.4%)	**0.0001**
N1b	0	11 (26.8%)	11 (13.4%)	
M stage, n (%)				
M0	41 (100%)	40 (97.6%)	81 (98.8%)	**0.0001**
M1	0	1 (2.4%)	1 (1.2%)	
AJCC TNM staging, n (%)				
I	41 (100%)	28 (68.3%)	69 (84.2%)	
II	0	12 (29.3%)	12 (14.6%)	**0.0001**
IVb	0	1 (2.4%)	1 (1.2%)	
PTMC subtype, n (%)				
Conventional	25 (61.0%)	27 (65.9%)	52 (63.4%)	
Follicular variant	12 (29.3%)	11 (26.9%)	23 (28.1%)	
Oncocytic	3 (7.3%)	1 (2.4%)	4 (4.9%)	0.532
Diffuse sclerosing	0	1 (2.4%)	1 (1.2%)	
Solid/Trabecular	0	1 (2.4%)	1 (1.2%)	
Columnar cell	1 (2.4%)	0	1 (1.2%)	
lymphatic invasion, n (%)				
presence	5 (12.2%)	8 (19.5%)	13 (15.9%)	0.364
absence	36 (87.8%)	33 (80.5%)	69 (84.1%)	
vascular invasion, n (%)				
presence	3 (7.3%)	5 (12.2%)	8 (9.8%)	1
absence	38 (92.7%)	36 (87.8%)	74 (90.2%)	
perineural invasion, n (%)				
presence	2 (4.9%)	3 (7.3%)	5 (6.1%)	0.712
absence	39 (95.1%)	38 (92.7%)	77 (93.9%)	
microscopic capsular invasion, n (%)				
presence	12 (29.3%)	12 (29.3%)	24 (29.3%)	1
absence	29 (70.7%)	29 (70.7%)	58 (70.7%)	

n—data expressed as patients number (%); pN—pathologic lymph node stage; M—distant metastasis; AJCC TNM—American Joint Committee on Cancer Classification of Malignant Tumors; PTMC—papillary thyroid microcarcinoma. A statistically significant difference was defined as $p < 0.05$; bold values are statistically significant.

Analyzing the distribution of PTMC subtypes, 52 patients (63.4%) had conventional PTMC, the second most common subtype being the follicular variant-23 patients (28.1%). Four patients (4.9%) had oncocytic variant, one (1.2%) for diffuse sclerosing, one (1.2%) for solid variant and one (1.2%) for columnar cell variant.

The lymphatic invasion was present for 13 patients (15.9%), vascular invasion for 8 patients (9.8%), and perineural invasion was observed for only 5 patients (6.1%). A microscopic capsular invasion was found in 24 patients (29.3%). Table 2 shows the focal and dimensional features. The median value for primary tumor diameter (PTD) was 5.0 mm with an interquartile range (IQR) of 5.3 mm. The mean value for PTD less than 5 mm was 4.0 with an IQR of 1.5, whereas the mean value for PTD 6–10 mm was 9.0 with a 2.5 IQR.

Table 2. Focal and dimensional characteristics and the univariate analysis results.

	No Metastatic Disease	Metastatic Disease	Total	p-Value
primary tumor diameter (mm)				
median ± IQR	4.0 ± 4.5	6.0 ± 5.0	5.0 ± 5.3	0.061
≤5 mm	3.2 ± 2.0	4.0 ± 1.0	4.0 ± 1.5	0.445
6–10 mm	9.0 ± 2.0	9.0 ± 2.6	9.0 ± 2.5	0.453
multifocality, n (%)				
presence	20 (48.8%)	25 (61.0%)	45 (54.9%)	0.270
absence	21 (51.2%)	16 (39.0%)	37 (45.1%)	
bilateral unifocality	8 (19.5%)	5 (12.2%)	13 (15.9%)	0.364
bilateral multifocality	9 (22.0%)	9 (22.0%)	18 (22.0%)	1
unilateral unifocality	21 (51.2%)	16 (39.0%)	37 (45.1%)	0.267
unilateral multifocality	3 (7.3%)	11 (26.8%)	14 (17.0%)	**0.019**
TTD (mm)				
median ± IQR	5.0 ± 7.0	9.0 ± 7.2	7.75 ± 6.4	**0.026**
≤10	4.0 ± 5.0	6.0 ± 5.0	5.0 ± 6.0	0.059
>10	12.0 ± 3.9	17.0 ± 12.3	14.0 ± 9.0	**0.036**
number of foci, n (%)				
1	21 (51.2%)	16 (39.0%)	37 (45.1%)	0.267
2	9 (22.0%)	9 (22.0%)	18 (22.0%)	1
3	6 (14.6%)	7 (17.0%)	13 (15.9%)	0.762
≥4	5 (12.2%)	9 (22.0%)	14 (17.0%)	0.240
tumor site, n (%)				
RTL	13 (31.7%)	14 (34.1%)	27 (32.9%)	0.814
LTL	9 (22.0%)	9 (22.0%)	18 (22.0%)	1
RTL + LTL	17 (41.5%)	12 (29.3%)	29 (35.4%)	0.248
isthmus ± other location	2 (4.9%)	6 (14.6%)	8 (9.75%)	0.139

n—data expressed as patients number (%); IQR—interquartile range; TTD—total tumor diameter; RTL—right thyroid lobe; LTL—left thyroid lobe. A statistically significant difference was defined as $p < 0.05$; Bold values are statistically significant.

Multifocality was found in 45 patients (54.9%), with 14 (17.0%) having numerous foci in a single lobe (unilateral multifocality) and 18 patients (22.0%) having multifocality in both lobes (bilateral unifocality). Unifocality was identified in 37 patients (45.1%), with 13 (15.9%) patients having it in both thyroid lobes (bilateral unifocality) and 14 (17.0%) patients having a single focus (unilateral unifocality).

The total tumor diameter (TTD) median was 7.75 mm with a 6.4 IQR, for the group with TTD ≤ 10, the median was 5.0 mm with 6.0 IQR, and for the >10 TTD group the median was 14.0 mm with a 9.0 IQR. There were 37 patients (45.1%) with a single tumoral focus, 18 patients (22.0%) with two tumoral foci, 13 patients (15.9%) with three tumoral foci, and 14 patients (17.0%) with four or more tumoral foci. The largest fraction of patients had tumor localization in both the right and left lobes-29 patients (35.4%), followed by the right thyroid lobe site for 27 patients (32.9%), left lobe for 18 patients (35.4%), and isthmus ± other location for 8 patients (9.7%).

3.2. Comparison between Metastasis and No Metastasis Groups

Gender and age are almost identical characteristics and therefore will not be described comparatively. Naturally, the non-metastatic group is all N0 staged. However, there was one patient in the metastatic group who is classed as N0 (a patient staged M1- with a distant solitary muscle metastasis, in the left gluteus muscle). The patient was operated by total thyroidectomy at the end of 2009. For 8 years, the patient was in complete remission and disease-free. In 2018, thyroglobulin level started to rise, the patient received a dose of radioactive iodine, with a negative post-therapy I-131 whole-body scan. For further evaluation, a F-18 fluorodeoxyglucose (FDG) positron emission tomography/computer tomography (PET/CT) scan was performed, which showed a 39/35/41 mm tumor in the left gluteal muscle with focal pathological uptake SUV lbm max = 16.77, highly suggestive for a metastatic lesion. After surgery and histology exam, the results confirmed papillary thyroid carcinoma metastasis. The patient received another I-131 dose of 5.5 GBq, with negative WBS, and was submitted to external beam therapy; at the moment of writing this paper, the patient was alive and clinically negative [18].

The rest of the patients in the metastatic group were in stages N1a-29 patients (70.7%) and N1b-11 patients (26.8%). All patients in the non-metastatic group were classified as stage I according to AJCC. In the metastatic group, 28 patients (68.3%) were defined as stage I, 12 (29.3%) as stage II, and one (2.4%) as stage IVb (same patient with pN0M1 staging mentioned above). In terms of PTMC subtype, lymphatic, vascular, perineural, and microscopic capsular invasion, no statistically significant differences were identified between the two groups (Table 1).

There was a statistically significant difference between the two groups in terms of multifocality and TTD. The proportion of patients in the metastatic group with unilateral multifocality was significantly higher than in the non-metastatic group (26.8% vs. 7.3%, $p = 0.019$). Based on TTD, the metastatic group had a considerably higher dimension compared to the non-metastatic group (median ± IQR: 9.0 ± 7.2 vs. 5.0 ± 7.0 mm., $p = 0.026$). Furthermore, there was a significant difference between the metastatic group with TTD > 10 mm. compared to the non-metastatic group (median ± IQR: 17.0 ± 12.3 vs. 12.0 ± 3.9 mm., $p = 0.036$).

3.3. Predictors for Metastatic Disease

A multivariate analysis was used to identify which of the statistically significant characteristics may be used as an independent predictor of metastatic disease. The multivariate analysis showed a significant level of $p < 0.0026$, an R2 coefficient of determination of 0.1663, an adjusted R^2 of 0.1342, and a multiple correlation coefficient of 0.4078 (Table 3). TTD and UM were found to be independent predictors of metastatic disease in PTMC, whereas TTD > 10 was not statistically significant. For additional statistical research, a prediction model was created. TTD, UM, and the prediction model were subjected to a ROC analysis (Table 4, Figure 1).

Table 3. Multivariate analysis results showing the characteristics independently associated with metastatic disease in PTMC. Bold values are statistically significant.

Least Squares Multiple Regression						
Sample size			82			
Coefficient of determination R²			0.1663			
R²-adjusted			0.1342			
Multiple correlation coefficient			0.4078			
Residual standard deviation			0.4681			
Regression Equation						
Independent variables	Coefficient	Std. Error	t	p	$r_{partial}$	$r_{semipartial}$
(Constant)	0.2297					
TTD	0.03242	0.01130	2.868	**0.0053**	0.3089	0.2965
UM	0.3312	0.1375	2.409	**0.0183**	0.2632	0.2491
TTD > 10	−0.2383	0.1707	−1.396	0.1566	−0.1561	0.1443
Analysis of Variance						
Source	DF		Sum of Squares		Mean Square	
Regression	3		3.4090		1.1363	
Residual	78		17.0910		0.2191	
F-ratio			5.1861			
Significance level			$p = 0.0026$			

Table 4. The receiver operating characteristic analysis results of the parameters that are independently associated with the presence of PTMC metastatic disease and the prediction model consisting of these parameters. Between the brackets are the values corresponding to the 95%-confidence interval.

Parameter	AUC	Significance Level	J	Cut-Off	Se (%)	Sp (%)
TTD	0.642 (0.529 to 0.745)	0.0197	0.2439	>4.4	78.05 (62.4–89.4)	46.34 (30.7–62.6)
UM	0.598 (0.483 to 0.704)	0.0163	0.1951	>0	26.83 (14.2–42.9)	92.68 (80.1–98.5)
Prediction model	0.734 (0.625 to 0.826)	<0.0001	0.3659	>0.4890	60.98 (44.5–75.8)	75.61 (59.7–87.6)

TTD—total tumor diameter; UM—unilateral multifocality; AUC—area under curve; Se—sensitivity; Sp—specificity.

The cut-off value for TTD of >4.4 mm was found to be an independent predictor of metastatic disease in PTMC ($p = 0.0197$, Se = 78.05%, Sp = 46.34%). The presence of UM was also shown to be an independent predictor ($p = 0.0163$, Se = 26.83%, Sp = 92.68%). The statistical characteristics of TTD and UM were translated by a prediction model with the following statistical values ($p < 0.0001$, Se = 60.98%, Sp = 75.61%).

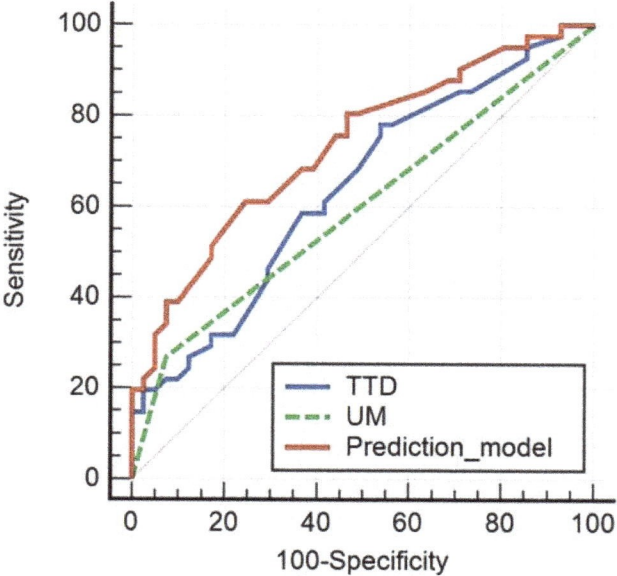

Figure 1. Receiver operating characteristic curve of the two parameters independently associated with the presence of PTMC metastatic disease and the prediction model. TTD-total tumor volume; UM-unilateral multifocality.

4. Discussion

TTD/multifocality in PTMC have been the subject of several recent papers [11–17,19–21]. Most of the research was conducted on a large cohort of patients and provides extremely useful data; nevertheless, European demographic data are scarce, with the majority of studies focusing on Asian populations [11–17,19,20] and one in North America [21]. Furthermore, some of these studies compare risk factors for PTMC and PTC groups, although tumor sizes vary widely and comparative terms can be frequently misunderstood.

In our research, multifocality was found in 54.9% of PTMCs and 48.8% had LNM. There was no statistical difference between the metastatic and non-metastatic groups in terms of multifocality ($p = 0.270$). This result contradicts the findings of most research, which demonstrate a link between multifocality and metastatic disease [4–6,11,12,14]. This contradictory result may be a consequence of the different cohorts (in our study the number of patients in the two groups is equal vs. the other studies that have a much higher number of patients in the non-metastatic group).

Alternatively, a statistically significant difference in unilateral multifocality was observed in our study (26.8% vs. 7.3%, $p = 0.019$). Unilateral multifocality was also shown to be an independent predictor of metastatic disease in our study. Similar to our results, according to Cai et al. [20], patients with unilateral multifocality were more likely than those with bilateral multifocality to develop neck metastases. In contrast, the results published by Yan et al. [19] show that bilateral multifocality, rather than unilateral multifocality, should be considered as an aggressive marker at presentation, and neither is an independent prognostic factor for clinical outcome in PTMC.

When we investigated the TTD, the findings of our research indicated that the metastatic group had a considerably higher dimension compared to the non-metastatic group (median ± IQR: 9.0 ± 7.2 vs. 5.0 ± 7.0 mm, $p = 0.026$). In addition, there was a significant difference between the metastatic group with TTD > 10 mm. compared to the non-metastatic group (median ± IQR: 17.0 ± 12.3 vs. 12.0 ± 3.9 mm., $p = 0.036$). Similar findings were revealed in research published by Feng et al. [11]. The results of his study showed that multifocal PTMC with TTD > 10 mm was more aggressive than unifocal PTMC or multifocal PTMC with TTD ≤ 10 mm. Likewise, the results of Zhao et al. [12] showed that LNM frequency was significantly higher in multifocal PTMCs with TTD > 10 mm than unifocal tumors with a diameter ≤ 10 mm (60.4 vs. 30%, $p < 0.001$).

According to Liu et al. [15]. the risks of LNM, extrathyroidal extension (ETE), infiltration, and the recurrence-free survival were significantly different between PTMCs with a unifocal diameter ≤ 10 mm and multifocal TTD > 10 mm and between multifocal PTMCs with a TTD of ≤1 mm and >10 mm. TTD might be used as a criterion to identify individuals at increased risk of persistence, according to Tam et al. [16], and T1a multifocal PTMCs with TTDs of 1 to 2 cm might be classed as T1b. However, there are also published data that demonstrate that calculating the TTD to assess adverse biological behavior in multifocal PTMC is insufficient and limited [17].

The novel findings of our research showed TTD and UM as independent predictors of metastatic disease in PTMC. The cut-off value of TTD > 4.4 mm independently predicts metastatic disease with a Se of 78.05% and Sp of 46.34%. On the other hand, the presence of UM independently predicts metastatic disease in PTMC (Se = 26.83%, Sp = 92.68%). Integrating TTD and UM statistical characteristics, a prediction model for metastatic disease has been developed (Se = 60.98%, Sp = 75.61%).

The latest consensus statements regarding the strategy for active surveillance of adult low-risk PTMC published by Sugitani et al. [22] on behalf of the Japan Association of Endocrine Surgery Task Force on management for papillary thyroid microcarcinoma consider that no data suggest that tumor multiplicity is associated with tumor enlargement and appearance of LNM; thus, patients with PTMC and multiple lesions can be candidates for active surveillance. Our data and results suggest a special precaution related to multiplicity, the UM being in our cohort an independent factor that predicts metastatic disease.

ATA guidelines [2] do not indicate routinely the Radioactive Iodine Therapy in PTMC, except the association of aggressive histology or other specific individual conditions (ex., discordant thyroglobulin level after surgery, etc.) Considering the abovementioned results, the Radioiodine therapy decision might be better adjusted.

There are several drawbacks to this study. The small number of patients included in the research is one of the limitations. This is since prophylactic lymph node dissection (LND) is not performed routinely in our center, thus the number of patients with a histopathological result of PTMC that includes the status of lymph nodes being very limited. Furthermore, this is a retrospective research based on a single regional center's experience. In light of this, randomized case-control clinical multicenter studies are required.

5. Conclusions

Regardless of how comprehensive the content of the guidelines is, certain therapeutic settings remain insufficiently evaluated. Our data strongly indicate that TTD and UM can be used to predict metastatic disease in PTMC, which may help to better adapt the RAI therapy decision. We believe that TTD and multifocality are tumor features that should be considered in future guidelines.

Author Contributions: Conceptualization, L.H., D.P.; data curation, L.H., P.-A.Ș.; formal analysis, P.-A Ș., L.H.; investigation, L.H., D.P., P.-A.Ș.; methodology, D.P., P.-A.Ș., L.H.; supervision, D.P. All authors have read and agreed to the published version of the manuscript.

Funding: This research received no external funding.

Institutional Review Board Statement: The study was conducted according to the guidelines of the Declaration of Helsinki, and approved by the Institutional Ethics Committee of "Prof. Dr. Ion Chiricuță" Institute of Oncology, Cluj-Napoca (protocol code 178 and date of approval 7 May 2020).

Informed Consent Statement: Informed consent was obtained from all subjects involved in the study.

Conflicts of Interest: The authors declare no conflict of interest.

References

1. Fugazzola, L.; Rossella, E. 2019 European Thyroid Association Guidelines for the Treatment and Follow-Up of Advanced Radioiodine-Refractory Thyroid Cancer. *Eur. Thyroid J.* **2019**, *8*, 227–245. [CrossRef] [PubMed]
2. Haugen, B.; Alexander, E. 2015 American Thyroid Association Management Guidelines for Adult Patients with Thyroid Nodules and Diferentiated Thyroid Cancer. *Thyroid* **2016**, *26*, 1–133. [CrossRef] [PubMed]
3. Bray, F.; Ferlay, J. Global cancer statistics 2018: GLOBOCAN estimates of incidence and mortality worldwide for 36 cancers in 185 countries. *CA Cancer J. Clin.* **2018**, *68*, 394–424. [CrossRef] [PubMed]
4. Wu, X.; Li, B. Risk Factors for Central Lymph Node Metastases in Patients with Papillary Thyroid Microcarcinoma. *Endocr. Pract.* **2018**, *24*, 1057–1062. [CrossRef]
5. Liu, L.; Liang, J. The incidence and risk factors for central lymph node metastasis in cN0 papillary thyroid microcarcinoma: A meta-analysis. *Eur. Arch. Otorhinolaryngol.* **2017**, *274*, 1327–1338. [CrossRef]
6. Kim, S.K.; Park, I. Predictive factors for lymph node metastasis in papillary thyroid microcarcinoma. *Ann. Surg. Oncol.* **2016**, *23*, 2866–2873. [CrossRef]
7. Wang, Y.; Guan, Q. Nomogram for predicting central lymph node metastasis in papillary thyroid microcarcinoma: A retrospective cohort study of 8668 patients. *Int. J. Surg.* **2018**, *55*, 98–102. [CrossRef]
8. Tuttle, R.; Haugen, B. Updated American Joint Committee on Cancer/Tumor-Node-Metastasis Staging System for Differentiated and Anaplastic Thyroid Cancer (Eighth Edition): What Changed and Why? *Thyroid* **2017**, *27*, 751–756. [CrossRef]
9. Haddad, R.; Nasr, C. NCCN Guidelines Insights Thyroid Carcinoma, Version 2.2018. *J. Natl. Compr. Cancer Netw.* **2018**, *16*, 1429–1440. [CrossRef]
10. Filetti, S.; Durante, C.; ESMO Guidelines Committee. Thyroid cancer: ESMO Clinical Practice Guidelines for diagnosis, treatment and follow-UPY. *Ann. Oncol.* **2019**, *30*, 1856–1883. [CrossRef] [PubMed]
11. Feng, J.W.; Pan, H. Total tumor diameter: The neglected value in papillary thyroid microcarcinoma. *J. Endocrinol. Investig.* **2020**, *43*, 601–613. [CrossRef]
12. Zhao, Q.; Ming, J. Multifocality and total tumor diameter predict central neck lymph node metastases in papillary thyroid microcarcinoma. *Ann. Surg. Oncol.* **2013**, *20*, 746–752. [CrossRef] [PubMed]
13. Wu, X.; Li, B. Predicting factors of central lymph node metastases in patients with unilateral multifocal papillary thyroid microcarcinoma. *Gland Surg.* **2020**, *9*, 695–701. [CrossRef] [PubMed]
14. Song, J.; Yan, T. Clinical Analysis of Risk Factors for Cervical Lymph Node Metastasis in Papillary Thyroid Microcarcinoma: A Retrospective Study of 3686 Patients. *Cancer Manag. Res.* **2020**, *12*, 2523–2530. [CrossRef] [PubMed]
15. Liu, C.; Wang, S. Total tumour diameter is superior to unifocal diameter as a predictor of papillary thyroid microcarcinoma prognosis. *Sci. Rep.* **2017**, *7*, 1846. [CrossRef] [PubMed]
16. Tam, A.; Ozdemir, D. Should Multifocal Papillary Thyroid Carcinomas Classified as T1A with a Tumor Diameter Sum of 1 to 2 Centimeters Be Reclassified as T1B? *Endocr. Pract.* **2017**, *23*, 526–535. [CrossRef]
17. Zhou, B.; Wei, L. Does Multifocal Papillary Thyroid Microcarcinoma with a Total Tumor Diameter >1 cm Indicate Poor Biological Behavior? The Evidence is Insufficient. *Endocr. Pract.* **2021**, *27*, 131–136. [CrossRef] [PubMed]
18. Hitu, L.; Cainap, C. Skeletal Muscle Metastasis in Papillary Thyroid Microcarcinoma Evaluated by F18-FDG PET/CT. *Diagnostics* **2020**, *10*, 100. [CrossRef]
19. Yan, T.; Qiu, W. Bilateral multifocality, a marker for aggressive disease, is not an independent prognostic factor for papillary thyroid microcarcinoma: A propensity score matching analysis. *Clin. Endocrinol.* **2021**, *95*, 209–216. [CrossRef]
20. Cai, J.; Fang, F. Unilateral Multifocality and Bilaterality Could Be Two Different Multifocal Entities in Patients with Papillary Thyroid Microcarcinoma. *BioMed Res. Int.* **2020**, *2020*, 9854964. [CrossRef]
21. Pérez-Soto, R.H.; Velázquez-Fernández, D. Preoperative and Postoperative Risk Stratification of Thyroid Papillary Microcarcinoma: A Comparative Study between Kuma Criteria and 2015 American Thyroid Association Guidelines Risk Stratification. *Thyroid* **2020**, *30*, 857–862. [CrossRef] [PubMed]
22. Sugitani, I.; Ito, Y. Indications and Strategy for Active Surveillance of Adult Low-Risk Papillary Thyroid Microcarcinoma: Consensus Statements from the Japan Association of Endocrine Surgery Task Force on Management for Papillary Thyroid Microcarcinoma. *Thyroid* **2021**, *31*, 183–192. [CrossRef] [PubMed]

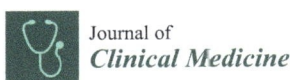

Article

Predictors of Central Compartment Involvement in Patients with Positive Lateral Cervical Lymph Nodes According to Clinical and/or Ultrasound Evaluation

Giuseppa Graceffa [1], Giuseppina Orlando [2,*], Gianfranco Cocorullo [2], Sergio Mazzola [3], Irene Vitale [2], Maria Pia Proclamà [2], Calogera Amato [2], Federica Saputo [1], Enza Maria Rollo [1], Alessandro Corigliano [4], Giuseppina Melfa [2], Calogero Cipolla [1] and Gregorio Scerrino [4]

[1] Unit of Oncological Surgery, Department of Surgical Oncological and Oral Sciences, University of Palermo, Via del Vespro, 129, 90127 Palermo, Italy; giuseppa.graceffa@unipa.it (G.G.); federica.saputo92@gmail.com (F.S.); enzamaria13@gmail.com (E.M.R.); calogero.cipolla@unipa.it (C.C.)

[2] Unit of General and Emergency Surgery, Department of Surgical Oncological and Oral Sciences, Policlinico P. Giaccone, University of Palermo, Via L Giuffré, 5, 90127 Palermo, Italy; gianfranco.cocorullo@unipa.it (G.C.); irenevitale93@gmail.com (I.V.); mariapiaproclama@gmail.com (M.P.P.); calogera.amato92@gmail.com (C.A.); irene_melfa@yahoo.it (G.M.)

[3] Unit of Clinical Epidemiology & Tumor Registry, Department of Laboratory Diagnostics, Policlinico P. Giaccone, University of Palermo, Via L Giuffré, 5, 90127 Palermo, Italy; mazzolasergio@hotmail.it

[4] Unit of Endocrine Surgery, Department of Surgical Oncological and Oral Sciences, Policlinico P. Giaccone, University of Palermo, Via L Giuffré, 5, 90127 Palermo, Italy; alessandro-corigliano@hotmail.it (A.C.); gregorio.scerrino@tiscali.it (G.S.)

* Correspondence: giusi_orlando@hotmail.it

Citation: Graceffa, G.; Orlando, G.; Cocorullo, G.; Mazzola, S.; Vitale, I.; Proclamà, M.P.; Amato, C.; Saputo, F.; Rollo, E.M.; Corigliano, A.; et al. Predictors of Central Compartment Involvement in Patients with Positive Lateral Cervical Lymph Nodes According to Clinical and/or Ultrasound Evaluation. *J. Clin. Med.* **2021**, *10*, 3407. https://doi.org/10.3390/jcm10153407

Academic Editor: Giovanni Conzo

Received: 14 July 2021
Accepted: 29 July 2021
Published: 30 July 2021

Publisher's Note: MDPI stays neutral with regard to jurisdictional claims in published maps and institutional affiliations.

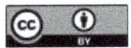

Copyright: © 2021 by the authors. Licensee MDPI, Basel, Switzerland. This article is an open access article distributed under the terms and conditions of the Creative Commons Attribution (CC BY) license (https://creativecommons.org/licenses/by/4.0/).

Abstract: Lymph node neck metastases are frequent in papillary thyroid carcinoma (PTC). Current guidelines state, on a weak level of evidence, that level VI dissection is mandatory in the presence of latero-cervical metastases. The aim of our study is to evaluate predictive factors for the absence of level VI involvement despite the presence of metastases to the lateral cervical stations in PTC. Eighty-eight patients operated for PTC with level II–V metastases were retrospectively enrolled in the study. Demographics, thyroid function, autoimmunity, nodule size and site, cancer variant, multifocality, Bethesda and EU-TIRADS, number of central and lateral lymph nodes removed, number of positive lymph nodes and outcome were recorded. At univariate analysis, PTC location and number of positive lateral lymph nodes were risk criteria for failure to cure. ROC curves demonstrated the association of the number of positive lateral lymph nodes and failure to cure. On multivariate analysis, the protective factors were PTC located in lobe center and number of positive lateral lymph nodes < 4. Kaplan–Meier curves confirmed the absence of central lymph nodes as a positive prognostic factor. In the selected cases, Central Neck Dissection (CND) could be avoided even in the presence of positive Lateralcervical Lymph Nodes (LLN+).

Keywords: papillary thyroid carcinoma; central compartment; lateralcervical lymph nodes; EU-TIRADS; Bethesda; central neck dissection; lateral neck dissection; skip metastasis

1. Introduction

Papillary thyroid carcinoma (PTC) has an extremely strong tendency to metastasize to the neck lymph nodes. This condition can occur in up to 80% of cases [1,2]. There is widespread acceptance of the classification of neck lymph nodes into seven levels, with level VI being the lymph nodes of the central compartment and level VII the lymph nodes of the upper mediastinum. Level I (sub-mental and sub-mandibular lymph nodes) is generally not considered in PTC exeresis, whereas levels II to V are the lymph nodes of the lateral compartment involved in neck dissection [3].

The current ATA guidelines (2015) regarding prophylactic central neck dissection (PCND) limit this indication to stages from T3 (tumor > 4 cm in greatest diameter and/or gross invasion of prethyroid muscles), while therapeutic central neck dissection is indicated in T1 (tumor less than 2 cm) or T2 (tumor size between 2 and 4 cm) only in the clear presence (clinically, ecographically and/or biopsy proven) of central metastases, or in cases of lateral lymphadenopathy [4–6]. Although widely accepted and practiced, this indication, contained in recommendation 36 of the ATA guidelines, is weak, with a low level of evidence [4].

Central neck dissection is not a procedure without complications. Hypoparathyroidism and recurrent laryngeal nerve palsy (both transient or permanent) may occur more frequently than in simple thyroidectomy [7–12].

The realization that central neck dissection is a surgical procedure with additional morbidity may lead to the search for a context in which, even in the presence of metastases to the lateral neck lymph nodes, central neck dissection could be avoided. The occurrence of skip metastasis to the lateral lymph node compartment is well known [13–15]. However, only recently a study appeared in the literature specifically aimed at answering the question of whether prophylactic central compartment dissection is always needed in the presence of lateral neck metastases [16].

The aim of this study is to evaluate predictive factors for the absence of level VI involvement despite the presence of metastases to the lateral cervical stations in PTC, and also to formulate hypotheses on the possible risk of persistence or recurrence directly related to the persistence of level VI lymph nodes.

2. Material and Methods

This retrospective observational cohort study was carried out on patients consecutively that had undergone thyroidectomy from January 2010 to December 2020, with the diagnosis of papillary thyroid carcinoma at two University Surgery Units: the General and Emergency Surgery Unit and the General and Oncology Surgery, both of which are referral centers for endocrine neck surgery in western Sicily. All patients with complete clinical reports regarding preparation for surgery, hospital course and follow-up until 30 June 2021 were included in the study; patients included underwent surgery for PTCs with metastases to the lateral-cervical lymph nodes at the time of surgery and who, therefore, underwent TT + CND + unilateral LND in one step. Surgical procedures were performed by surgeons, belonging to the respective operating units, classifiable as "high volume" according to the unanimous consensus of the international literature [17,18], having all performed over 1000 thyroidectomies with more than 100 procedures/year for a period of activity of 10 or more years.

Exclusion criteria were: surgery for central and/or latero-cervical metastases, which, therefore, underwent Thyroidectomy and/or Central Neck Dissection and/or Lateral Neck Dissection in two or more steps. We also excluded non-papillary thyroid cancers, patients with incomplete clinical documentation, those with malignancy of another site or who had developed an extrathyroid cancer during follow-up, familial thyroid tumors and who had undergone operations performed by operators with a volume of activity of less than 1000 total thyroidectomies or <100 thyroidectomies/year or with a period of "dedicated" activity of less than 10 years.

We considered the following variables (in brackets, the way the variables were assessed): age (continuous), sex (categorical), TSH values detected at the time of preparation for surgery (continuous), autoimmunity (categorical), largest diameter of the nodule measured at ultrasound (continuous), cancer variant (classical, follicular, other, categorical). Based on preoperative ultrasonographic findings, we included the suspicious lesions in the excel sheet classifying them as located in the "upper lobe pole" (=1), "middle lobe" (=2) and "other" (=3), including in this group the isthmic or paraisthmic lesions and the lesions at the lower pole of the thyroid lobe (categorical variable). Moreover, we recorded multifocality (categorical), Bethesda classification (categorical), EU-TIRADS classification (categorical), total number of central lymph nodes removed (continuous), number of positive central lymph nodes (continuous), total number of lateral lymph nodes removed (continuous), number of positive lateral lymph nodes (continuous) and outcome (unfavorable, yes/no, categorical). The categories that we considered as "unfavorable" outcomes fell into two different patterns: patients with "persistence", in whom there was proven locoregional disease before six months after postoperative radioiodine ablation, and patients with "recurrence", in whom new disease occurred after this cut-off time. The presence of locoregional disease (persistence or recurrence) was assessed by integrating the results of laboratory tests (thyroglobulin [Tg] > 10 ng/mL after appropriate discontinuation of L-Tyroxine treatment in the absence of anti-Tg antibodies), ultrasound (presence of suspected locoregional tissue) and fine-needle aspiration biopsy of tissue detected on ultrasound, which in turn was evaluated by cytology and Tg assay on the eluate. In two cases, there was persistence of elevated Tg values in the absence of locoregional recurrence on instrumental exams: these patients were excluded from the study because of the uncertainty of considering them as loco-regional recurrence, systemic recurrence or false positive result.

For the purpose of the Kaplan–Meier curves, the date on which the recurrence was detected was reported. Disease-free patients were conventionally verified as of 30 June 2021.

Among the variables included in the statistical evaluation, location within the thyroid lobe was documented in the literature as a risk factor for skip metastasis [13–15], while variables such as the threshold value of metastatic lateral lymph nodes and the total number of central lymph nodes removed were derived from the study results. TIRADS and cytology (classified according to Bethesda) were included in order to evaluate whether these two simple datapoints from the preoperative diagnostic procedure could be used as indicators and guide the choice of surgery.

2.1. Surgery

The surgical procedure has always been performed as a 'formally' total thyroidectomy. In the patients undergoing Intraoperative Nerve Monitoring, if the surgical protocol required to suspend the operation at lobectomy with removal of the central hemicompartment ipsilateral to the cancer (two-staged thyroidectomy), we excluded these patients (two in the whole cohort) from the study. Central neck dissection was always bilateral, with excision of both periricurrential and paratracheal chains, and lateral neck dissection extended at least to IIa-III-IV levels, while IIb and V levels were removed in the presence of gross and/or multiple latero-cervical metastases detected by ultrasound or in the presence of involvement of these stations.

2.2. Radioiodine Ablation and Endocrinological Treatment

All patients with metastatic lateral lymph node (LLN+) underwent radioiodine ablation, at a dosage of about 100–150 mCi, after suspension of L-thyroxine treatment until TSH values > 30 microIU/mL were reached. This treatment was performed 4–8 weeks after surgery and, after post-treatment whole-body scan, suppressive therapy with L-thyroxine was reimposed with the aim of bringing TSH to about 0.5 microIU/mL.

2.3. Statistical Analysis

In a first step, a univariate analysis was carried out in which Fisher's exact test for categorical variables and Mann–Whitney's test for continuous variables were applied.

ROC curves were then realized in order to evaluate the accuracy of the variables "number of central lymph node (CLN)", "number of lateral lymph node (LLN)" and "number of LLN+" as predictors of the occurrence of metastatic central lymph node (CLN+ $\geq$ 1).

Moreover, a multivariate logistic analysis was performed in which the following variables were included: Age, Sex, TIRADS, Location, CLN and LLN+. From the various models, the best fit was chosen. Akaike's Information Criterion (AIC) was used as an indicator of the quality of the fit of the multiple logistic regression function to the needs of the study.

Finally, Kaplan–Meier curves were created in the following three groups: CLN+ = 0, All cases and CLN+ $\geq$ 1. The statistical significance of the differences between the Kaplan–Meier curves was checked with the Log Rank test.

Statistical elaborations were carried out with the software RStudio (version 3.4.1 of 30 June 2017) for R (version 2.1) The ROC Curves and Kaplan–Meier were made using the application packages "pROC" and "Survival".

3. Results

Eighty-eight patients in follow-up from 6 months to 10 years (mean 4.6 years) with a mean age of 46 years (range: 14–82) met the inclusion criteria.

3.1. Univariate Analysis

From the univariate analysis (Table 1) the variables with p-value < 0.05 were: Location, TIRADS, CLN and LLN+. The location, TIRADS and LLN+ seem to be a moderately accurate predictor of CLN+. Comparing the ROC curves, in which the specificity/sensitivity relationship was calculated using CLN+ as a reference we note that the number of LLN is a poor predictor of CLN+ (Figure 1). In fact, the Area Under the Curve (AUC) values were = 0.57 and 95% confidence interval (CI) (0.44–0.68), with a threshold value of 28.5. Specificity, therefore, was 1% CI (1–1) and sensitivity = 0.18 with 95% CI (0.09–0.29). The numbers of CLN and LLN+ were found to be a moderately accurate predictor of CLN+ with AUC = 0.73 and 95% CI (0.61–0.82) with a cutoff value = 7.5, specificity = 0.84% CI (0.72–0.97) and sensitivity = 0.46 with 95% CI (0.34–0.59) and AUC = 0.83 and 95% CI (0.73–0.92) with a cutoff value of 2.5, specificity = 0.81% CI (0.66–0.94) and sensitivity = 0.77 with 95% CI (0.66–0.88), respectively.

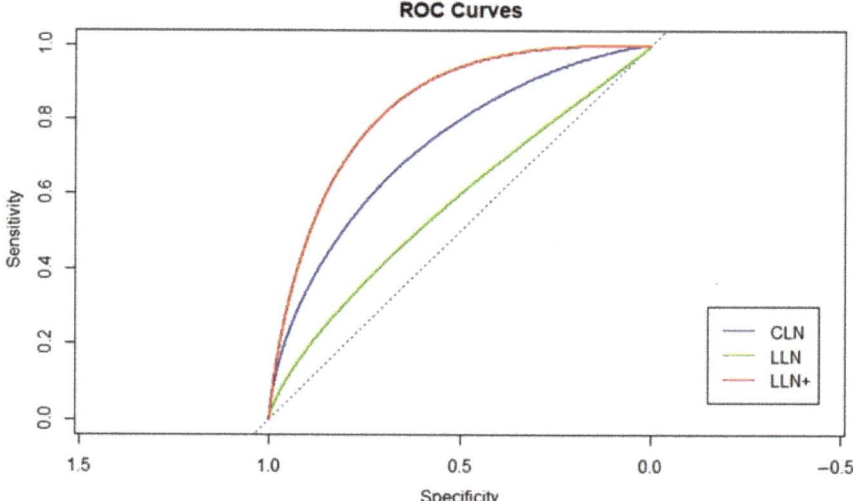

Figure 1. The number of LLN is a poor predictor of CLN+ $\geq$ 1.

3.2. Multivariate Analysis

The multivariate analysis (Table 2) revealed that the best-fitting model according to AIC (=67.98) included the following variables: Age, Sex, Localization, CLN > 7 and LLN+ < 4. The model shows that center-lobar cancer localization and LLN+ < 4 appear to be protective values (CLN+ = 0 and no recurrence) with ORs of 0.005 95%IC (8.12×10^{-5}–8.21×10^{-2}) (p-value < 0.05) and 0.020 95%IC (7.81×10^{-4}–0.164) (p-value < 0.05), respectively.

Table 1. The number of CLN and LLN+ were found to be a moderately accurate predictor of CLN+ ≥ 1. TIRADS Classification: TIRADS I: Normal thyroid US; TIRADS II: Benign Aspects; TIRADS III: Probably Benign Aspects, TIRADS IV A Low Suspicious Aspect; TIRADS IVB 1 or 2 signs of High suspicious aspects and no Adenopathy; TIRADS 5: ≥3 of High Suspicious aspects and/or Adenopathy. The Bethesda System for Reporting Thyroid Cytopathology: Bethesda I: Nondiagnostic or Unsatisfactory; Bethesda II: Benign; Bethesda III: Atypia of undetermined significance or follicular lesion of undetermined significance; Bethesda IV: Follicular neoplasm or suspicious for a follicular neoplasm; Bethesda V: Suspicious for malignancy; Bethesda VI: Malignant. Nodule location: Site 1: upper lobe pole; Site 2: middle lobe; Site 3: isthmic, paraisthmic or lower pole [19,20].

Variable	CLN+ 0_Recovery	CLN+ ≥ 1	Total	OR (95%CI)	p-Value
Age	47	46			0.677
Sex M	6	22	28	2.77	0.05849
Sex F	26	34	60	(0.92–9.60)	
Total	32	56	88		
TSH	2.19	2.15			0.5318
Autoimmunity YES	7	12	19	0.97	0.9999
Autoimmunity NO	25	44	69	(0.31–3.32)	
Total	32	56	88		
Size 1	27	44	71		
Size 2	2	6	8		0.8454
Size 3	3	6	9		
Total	32	56	88		
Site 1	12	31	43		
Site 2	13	1	14		8.141×10^{-6}
Site 3	7	24	31		
Total	32	56	88		
Multifocality NO	40	9	49	0.37	0.2136
Multifocality YES	36	3	39	(0.06–1.65)	
Total	32	56	88		
Bethesda 1	1	1	2		
Bethesda 2	3	4	7		
Bethesda 3	9	11	20		
Bethesda 4	15	22	37		0.3606
Bethesda 5	4	13	17		
Bethesda 6	0	5	5		
Total	32	56	88		
TIRADS 3	2	1	3		
TIRADS 4	14	10	24		0.008372
TIRADS 5	16	45	61		
Total	32	56	88		
CLN	4.4	7.5			0.0008543
LLN	17.31	19.57			0.3917
LLN+	1.81	4.36			5.741×10^{-7}

ROC Curves. Bold format of data mean p-Values < 0.05.

From the analysis of Kaplan–Meier curves (Figure 2), it can be seen that the difference in disease-free survival between the group of patients in which no central lymph nodes were found and the group with metastatic central lymph nodes was significant ($p < 0.05$).

Finally, we found it interesting to note that patients with CLN = 0 had a small number of metastatic LLN (4 or less) and none of them experienced persistence or disease recurrence.

Variables found to be non-significant in the univariate analysis (age, sex, TSH levels, autoimmunity, multifocality, Bethesda category, TIRADS category) were not considered in the multivariate analysis.

Variables found.

Table 2. The model shows that center-lobar cancer localization and LLN+ < 4 appear to be protective values.

Variable	OR	IC (Inf) 95%	IC (Sup) 95%	p-Value
Age	0.959	0.907	1.007	0.10725
Sex	0.564	0.073	3.448	0.54998
Site 2	0.005	$8.12e^{-5}$	$8.21e^{-2}$	0.00210 **
Site 3	1.224	0.275	5.491	0.78752
CLN > 7	1.587	1.231	2.195	0.00149 **
LLN+ < 4	0.020	$7.81e^{-4}$	0.164	0.00238 **

** mean p-values lower than 0.05.

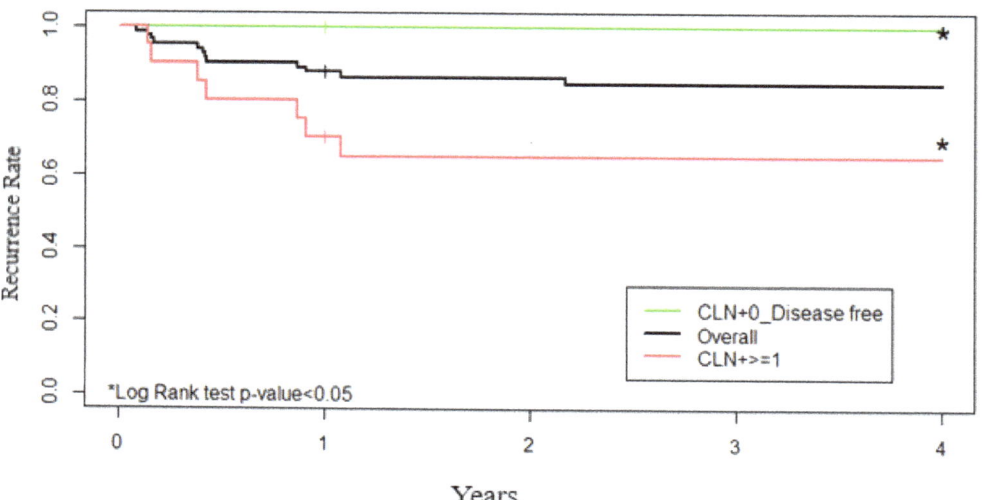

Figure 2. The group of patients with no central lymph nodes involvement has longer disease-free survival than the group with metastatic central lymph nodes ($p < 0.05$). Kaplan–Meier Curves.

4. Discussion

Nowadays, the role of PCND in PTC is still debated, with studies proposing to avoid this procedure for early stages and limit CND to cases of clinically positive central lymph nodes [21,22] and others showing benefits even for stages below T3 [23–25]. Given the advantages, especially from the point of view of postoperative radiometabolic treatment, and possible complications such as hypoparathyroidism and recurrent nerve palsy, careful case selection and consensus in the context of the multidisciplinary team has been proposed by others [26]. In any case, the position that PCND does not change the overall survival rate of PTC seems to be prevalent [27–29].

Currently, the ATA, CCN and ESES guidelines consider the presence of lateral neck metastases as an indication for CND [4,6,30]. This is also supported by the order of the lymphatic diffusion pathways, which, however, may vary for portions of thyroid tissue located near the upper poles of the gland, as stated in several studies [13,14,31–33]. This was also confirmed in a detailed anatomical study [34].

Central lymph node metastases in PTC are extremely frequent (up to 80%), but most of them are microscopic, detected after careful histopathological evaluation and have no clinical significance [2,16,35]. On the other hand, in studies considering prophylactic lateral cervical dissection, the occurrence of metastases in levels II–V was well above 50% [36], although there is very little support for such a choice and not much data available on the subject. These data have to be compared with those related to the risk of PTC recurrence, which is very low in the most common variants of PTC and, in any case, ranging from

1% to 40% [16,37], and, in an even clearer perspective, in the 5-year disease-free survival, which reaches 98% [4]. This debate could be concluded by stating that, obviously within certain limits, there is no correlation between central or lateral lymph node metastases, rate of locoregional recurrence and in general the prognosis of PTC [4,16,21,38]. These limits may be constituted by the real numerical and especially volumetric consistency of the affected lymph nodes [16], as well as by the prognostic factors of cancer, which, however, most likely act independently from lymph node metastases [39].

The attitude taken at our institution with regard to PCND has gone from a gradual enthusiasm that had extended its indications also to early stages of PTC (T2 and sometimes T1), which culminated in the middle of the last decade [9,24], to a gradual alignment with the actual indications of the main scientific societies mentioned above, so that, in fact, we now perform PCND only in T3 and in N1b with any T.

In this study, we found a relapse rate of 13.7% (12), similar to percentage described in several other studies [40,41].

The number of patients with positive LLN but without central compartment involvement was very high (32 = 36.4%). This high prevalence of LLN+ without CLN+ would be sufficient to justify further investigation, which led to our results.

An aspect that we found interesting in our study was the finding that the presence of few positive LLNs (<4) seems to be protective compared to the presence of CLN metastases; therefore, in such circumstances, the presence of a sporadic metastasis in the lateral site might be predictive of skip metastasis. A finding that could be investigated in the future is the association of more advanced TIRADS with the increased likelihood of central metastases in the presence of known LLN metastases. Although we are not able to give a definite interpretation to this statistical finding, we believe we can explain this effect by a probably greater aggressiveness of the tumor that could tend to be associated with more advanced morphological aspects. A similar association was not found when evaluating cytological features with the Bethesda system, whose degree of alterations do not correlate in any way (indeed we did not expect it) with a more extensive metastatic spread of the tumor.

The first interesting result of our study is evidenced by the multivariate analysis, which confirms the importance of the apical location in the thyroid lobe as a risk factor for the presence of possible skip metastases and, conversely, a certain "protective" role of cancer locations other than this one in the context of the thyroid lobe.

Another attractive finding arising from the results of the Kaplan–Meier curves is the better disease-free survival reported in the group of patients without involvement of CLN, even with LLN+, demonstrating a role of the CLN− as a positive prognostic factor in terms of persistence or recurrence. Conversely, the simultaneous presence of CLN+ and LLN+ entails in a worse prognosis. All these results could constitute a further justification to limit prophylactic CND in the presence of isolated skip metastases, provided that these do not hide central metastases [40].

We are aware of several biases in our study: firstly, its retrospective nature; secondly, the expertise-dependence of lymph node clearing during lymph node dissections; and thirdly, we consider the study to be very large, with follow-up ranging from 6 months to 10 years. Furthermore, the empiricism with which recurrence was established and with which, in turn, it is distanced from persistence. Furthermore, the enrolment of laterocervical dissections less extensive than II–V may constitute a bias but this type of surgical choice is justified and validated in the literature [41–43].

Another bias is the lack of evaluation of some prognostic factors, such as angioinvasiveness, extracapsular or extranodal extension, but usually, such evaluations are not reliably answered during the preoperative workup and, on the other hand, our intention was to find reliable answers to the question "what to do if a certain condition is found" in a real scenario. Finally, we did not compare a population of patients who underwent CLND plus LLND versus only LLND. In this perspective, the comparison between the two groups should be considered virtual.

5. Conclusions

At present, we cannot consider the data obtained from this study sufficient to lead to the adoption of new treatment protocols.

Far from providing definitive data on the existence of a category of PTC patients in whom level VI dissection can be avoided even in the presence of lateral cervical metastases, this study aims to provide further food for thought and add data to achieve the goal of avoiding central compartment dissection, albeit in a restricted category of patients, and thus limiting risks and sequelae of this not entirely harmless procedure.

Author Contributions: Conceptualization, G.G., C.C. and G.S.; Data curation, S.M., I.V., M.P.P., C.A., F.S., E.M.R. and A.C.; Formal analysis, S.M.; Investigation, G.O., G.C. and G.M.; Methodology, G.G., G.O., G.C., G.M., C.C. and G.S.; Software, A.C.; Supervision, G.S.; Validation, C.C. and G.S.; Writing–original draft, G.G.; Writing–review & editing, G.S. All authors have read and agreed to the published version of the manuscript.

Funding: This research received no external funding.

Institutional Review Board Statement: The study was conducted according to the guidelines of the Declaration of Helsinki and Ethics review and approval for this study was waived because of our institution's nonrequirement for retrospective studies.

Informed Consent Statement: Informed consent was obtained from all subjects involved in the study. This retrospective study analyzes anonymized data already in institutional database.

Data Availability Statement: Digital and paper archives of the Department of Surgical Oncological and Oral Sciences, Policlinico P. Giaccone, University of Palermo, Via L Giuffré, 5, 90127 Palermo, Italy.

Conflicts of Interest: The authors declare no conflict of interest.

References

1. Eltelety, A.M.; Terris, D.J. Neck Dissection in the Surgical Treatment of Thyroid Cancer. *Endocrinol. Metab. Clin. N. Am.* **2019**, *48*, 143–151. [CrossRef] [PubMed]
2. Thompson, A.M.; Turner, R.M.; Hayen, A.; Aniss, A.; Jalaty, S.; Learoyd, D.L.; Sidhu, S.; Delbridge, L.; Yeh, M.W.; Clifton-Bligh, R.; et al. A preoperative nomogram for the prediction of ipsilateral central compartment lymph node metastases in papillary thyroid cancer. *Thyroid* **2014**, *24*, 675–682. [CrossRef]
3. Sakorafas, G.H.; Koureas, A.; Mpampali, I.; Balalis, D.; Nasikas, D.; Ganztzoulas, S. Patterns of Lymph Node Metastasis in Differentiated Thyroid Cancer; Clinical Implications with Particular Emphasis on the Emerging Role of Compartment-Oriented Lymph Node Dissection. *Oncol. Res. Treat.* **2019**, *42*, 143–147. [CrossRef] [PubMed]
4. Haugen, B.R.; Alexander, E.K.; Bible, K.C.; Doherty, G.M.; Mandel, S.J.; Nikiforov, Y.E.; Pacini, F.; Randolph, G.W.; Sawka, A.M.; Schlumberger, M.; et al. 2015 American Thyroid Association Management Guidelines for Adult Patients with Thyroid Nodules and Differentiated Thyroid Cancer: The American Thyroid Association Guidelines Task Force on Thyroid Nodules and Differentiated Thyroid Cancer. *Thyroid* **2016**, *26*, 1–133. [CrossRef] [PubMed]
5. Doubleday, A.; Sippel, R.S. Surgical options for thyroid cancer and post-surgical management. *Expert Rev. Endocrinol. Metab.* **2018**, *13*, 137–148. [CrossRef] [PubMed]
6. Sancho, J.J.; Lennard, T.W.J.; Paunovic, I.; Triponez, F.; Sitges-Serra, A. Prophylactic central neck disection in papillary thyroid cancer: A consensus report of the European Society of Endocrine Surgeons (ESES). *Langenbeck's Arch. Surg.* **2014**, *399*, 155–163. [CrossRef] [PubMed]
7. Palestini, N.; Borasi, A.; Cestino, L.; Freddi, M.; Odasso, C.; Robecchi, A. Is central neck dissection a safe procedure in the treatment of papillary thyroid cancer? Our experience. *Langenbeck's Arch. Surg.* **2008**, *393*, 693–698. [CrossRef] [PubMed]
8. Mazzaferri, E.L.; Doherty, G.M.; Steward, D.L. The pros and cons of prophylactic central compartment lymph node dissection for papillary thyroid carcinoma. *Thyroid* **2009**, *19*, 683–689. [CrossRef] [PubMed]
9. Scerrino, G.; Di Giovanni, S.; Salamone, G.; Melfa, G.I.; Inviati, A.; Raspanti, C.; Gulotta, G. Surgical complications in prophylactic central neck dissection: Preliminary findings from a retrospective cohort study. *Minerva Chir.* **2014**, *69* (Suppl. S1), 131–134.
10. Lombardi, D.; Accorona, R.; Paderno, A.; Cappelli, C.; Nicolai, P. Morbidity of central neck dissection for papillary thyroid cancer. *Gland. Surg.* **2017**, *6*, 492–500. [CrossRef]
11. Calò, P.; Conzo, G.; Raffaelli, M.; Medas, F.; Gambardella, C.; De Crea, C.; Gordini, L.; Patrone, R.; Sessa, L.; Erdas, E.; et al. Total thyroidectomy alone versus ipsilateral versus bilateral prophylactic central neck dissection in clinically node-negative differentiated thyroid carcinoma. A retrospective multicenter study. *Eur. J. Surg. Oncol. EJSO* **2017**, *43*, 126–132. [CrossRef]
12. Liu, X.; Zhang, D.; Zhang, G.; Zhao, L.; Zhou, L.; Fu, Y.; Li, S.; Zhao, Y.; Li, C.; Wu, C.-W.; et al. Laryngeal nerve morbidity in 1.273 central node dissections for thyroid cancer. *Surg. Oncol.* **2018**, *27*, A21–A25. [CrossRef] [PubMed]

13. Lee, Y.S.; Shin, S.-C.; Lim, Y.-S.; Lee, J.-C.; Wang, S.-G.; Son, S.-M.; Kim, I.-J.; Lee, B.-J. Tumor location-dependent skip lateral cervical lymph node metastasis in papillary thyroid cancer. *Head Neck* **2014**, *36*, 887–891. [CrossRef] [PubMed]
14. Attard, A.; Paladino, N.C.; Monte, A.I.L.; Falco, N.; Melfa, G.; Rotolo, G.; Rizzuto, S.; Gulotta, E.; Salamone, C.; Bonventre, S.; et al. Skip metastases to lateral cervical lymph nodes in differentiated thyroid cancer: A systematic review. *BMC Surg.* **2019**, *18* (Suppl. S1), 112. [CrossRef] [PubMed]
15. Hu, D.; Lin, H.; Zeng, X.; Wang, T.; Deng, J.; Su, X. Risk Factors for and Prediction Model of Skip Metastasis to Lateral Lymph Nodes in Papillary Thyroid Carcinoma. *World J. Surg.* **2019**, *44*, 1498–1505. [CrossRef]
16. Harries, V.; BS, M.M.; Wang, L.Y.; Tuttle, R.M.; Wong, R.J.; Shaha, A.R.; Shah, J.P.; Patel, S.G.; Ganly, I. Is a Prophylactic Central Compartment Neck Dissection Required in Papillary Thyroid Carcinoma Patients with Clinically Involved Lateral Compartment Lymph Nodes? *Ann. Surg. Oncol.* **2021**, *28*, 512–518. [CrossRef] [PubMed]
17. Melfa, G.; Porrello, C.; Cocorullo, G.; Raspanti, C.; Rotolo, G.; Attard, A.; Gullo, R.; Bonventre, S.; Gulotta, G.; Scerrino, G. Surgeon volume and hospital volume in endocrine neck surgery: How many procedures are needed for reaching a safety level and acceptable costs? A systematic narrative review. *Il G. Di Chir.* **2018**, *39*, 5–11. [CrossRef] [PubMed]
18. Lorenz, K.; Raffaeli, M.; Barczyński, M.; Lorente-Poch, L.; Sancho, J. Volume, outcomes, and quality standards in thyroid surgery: An evidence-based analysis—European Society of Endocrine Surgeons (ESES) positional statement. *Langenbeck's Arch. Surg.* **2020**, *405*, 401–425. [CrossRef]
19. Cibas, E.S.; Ali, S.Z. The 2017 Bethesda System for Reporting Thyroid Cytopathology. *Thyroid* **2017**, *27*, 1341–1346. [CrossRef]
20. Grant, E.G.; Tessler, F.N.; Hoang, J.K.; Langer, J.E.; Beland, M.D.; Berland, L.L.; Cronan, J.J.; Desser, T.S.; Frates, M.C.; Hamper, U.M.; et al. Thyroid Ultrasound Reporting Lexicon: White Paper of the ACR Thyroid Imaging, Reporting and Data System (TIRADS) Committee. *J. Am. Col. Radiol.* **2015**, *12*, 1272–1279. [CrossRef]
21. Sippel, R.S.; Robbins, S.E.; Poehls, J.L.; Pitt, S.C.; Chen, H.; Leverson, G.; Long, K.L.; Schneider, D.F.; Connor, N.P. A randomized controlled clinical trial.: No clear benefit to prophylactic central neck dissection in patients with clinically node negative papillary thyroid cancer. *Ann. Surg.* **2020**, *272*, 496–503. [CrossRef] [PubMed]
22. Gambardella, C.; Tartaglia, E.; Nunziata, A.; Izzo, G.; Siciliano, G.; Cavallo, F.; Mauriello, C.; Napolitano, S.; Thomas, G.; Testa, D.; et al. Clinical significance of prophylactic central compartment neck dissection in the treatment of clinically node-negative papillary thyroid cancer patients. *World J. Surg. Oncol.* **2016**, *14*, 1–5. [CrossRef] [PubMed]
23. Barczyński, M.; Konturek, A.; Stopa, M.; Nowak, W. Prophylactic central neck dissection for papillary thyroid cancer. *BJS* **2013**, *100*, 410–418. [CrossRef] [PubMed]
24. Scerrino, G.; Attard, A.; Melfa, G.; Raspanti, C.; Di Giovanni, S.; Attard, M.; Inviati, A.; Mazzola, S.; Modica, G.; Gulotta, G.; et al. Role of prophylactic central neck dissection in cN0-papillary thyroid carcinoma: Results from a high-prevalence area. *Minerva Chir.* **2015**, *71*, 159–167.
25. Yazıcı, D.; Çolakoğlu, B.; Sağlam, B.; Sezer, H.; Kapran, Y.; Aydın, Ö.; Demirkol, M.O.; Alagöl, F.; Terzioğlu. T. Effect of prophylactic central neck dissection on the surgical outcomes in papillary thyroid cancer: Experience in a single center. *Eur. Arch. Oto-Rhino-Laryngol.* **2020**, *277*, 1491–1497. [CrossRef]
26. Chen, L.; Wu, Y.-H.; Lee, C.-H.; Chen, H.-A.; Loh, E.-W.; Tam, K.-W. Prophylactic Central Neck Dissection for Papillary Thyroid Carcinoma with Clinically Uninvolved Central Neck Lymph Nodes: A Systematic Review and Meta-analysis. *World J. Surg.* **2018**, *42*, 2846–2857. [CrossRef]
27. Leboulleux, S.; Rubino, C.; Baudin, E.; Caillou, B.; Hartl, D.M.; Bidart, J.M.; Travagli, J.P.; Schlumberger, M. Prognostic factors for persistent or recurrent disease of papillary thyroid carcinoma with neck lymph node metastases and/or tumor extension beyond the thyroid capsule at initial diagnosis. *J. Clin. Endocrinol. Metab.* **2005**, *90*, 5723–5729. [CrossRef]
28. Toniato, A.; Boschin, I.M.; Casara, D.; Mazzarotto, R.; Rubello, D.; Pelizzo, M. Papillary Thyroid Carcinoma: Factors Influencing Recurrence and Survival. *Ann. Surg. Oncol.* **2008**, *15*, 1518–1522. [CrossRef]
29. Bardet, S.; Malville, E.; Rame, J.P.; Babin, E.; Samama, G.; De Raucourt, D.; Michels, J.J.; Reznik, Y.; Henry-Amar, M. Macroscopic lymph-node involvement and neck dissection predict lymph-node recurrence in papillary thyroid carcinoma. *Eur. J. Endocrinol.* **2008**, *158*, 551–560. [CrossRef]
30. National Comprehensive Cancer Network. NCCN Clinical Practice Guidelines in Oncology-Thyroid Carcinoma. Available online: https://www.nccn.org/ (accessed on 20 April 2019).
31. Zhang, L.; Wei, W.-J.; Ji, Q.-H.; Zhu, Y.-X.; Wang, Z.-Y.; Wang, Y.; Huang, C.-P.; Shen, Q.; Li, D.-S.; Wu, Y. Risk Factors for Neck Nodal Metastasis in Papillary Thyroid Microcarcinoma: A Study of 1056 Patients. *J. Clin. Endocrinol. Metab.* **2012**, *97*, 1250–1257. [CrossRef]
32. Xiang, D.; Xie, L.; Xu, Y.; Li, Z.; Hong, Y.; Wang, P. Papillary thyroid microcarcinomas located at the middle part of the middle third of the thyroid gland correlates with the presence of neck metastasis. *Surgery* **2015**, *157*, 526–533. [CrossRef]
33. Zhan, X.; Xue, S.; Yin, Y.; Chen, G. Related factors for skip metastasis of neck lymph node in papillary thyroid carcinoma. *Zhonghua Wai Ke Za Zhi Chin. J. Surg.* **2017**, *55*, 599–602. [PubMed]
34. Likhterov, I.; Dos Reis, L.L.; Urken, M.L. Central compartment management in patients with papillary thyroid cancer presenting with metastatic disease to the lateral neck: Anatomic pathways of lymphatic spread. *Head Neck* **2017**, *39*, 853–859. [CrossRef] [PubMed]

35. Randolph, G.W.; Duh, Q.Y.; Heller, K.S.; LiVolsi, V.A.; Mandel, S.J.; Steward, D.L.; Tufano, R.P.; Tuttle, R.M. The prognostic significance of nodal metastases from papillary thyroid carcinoma can be stratified based on the size and number of metastatic lymph nodes, as well as the presence of extranodal extension. *Thyroid* **2012**, *22*, 1144–1152. [CrossRef] [PubMed]
36. Mulla, M.G.; Knoefel, W.T.; Gilbert, J.; McGregor, A.; Schulte, K.M. Lateral cervical lymph node metastases in papillary thyroid cancer: A systematic review of imaging-guided and prophylactic removal of the lateral compartment. *Clin. Endocrinol.* **2012**, *77*, 126–131. [CrossRef]
37. National Cancer Institute. Surveillance, Epidemiology, and End Results Program (SEER): Thyroid Cancer. Available online: https://seer.cancer.gov/statfacts/html/thyro.html (accessed on 30 June 2021).
38. Viola, D.; Materazzi, G.; Valerio, L.; Molinaro, E.; Agate, L.; Faviana, P.; Seccia, V.; Sensi, E.; Romei, C.; Piaggi, P.; et al. Prophylactic central compartment lymph node dissection in papillary thyroid carci-noma: Clinical implications derived from the first prospective randomized controlled single institution study. *J. Clin. Endocrinol. Metab.* **2015**, *100*, 1316–1324. [CrossRef]
39. Cipriani, N.A. Prognostic Parameters in Differentiated Thyroid Carcinomas. *Surg. Pathol. Clin.* **2019**, *12*, 883–900. [CrossRef]
40. Lee, D.Y.; Oh, K.H.; Cho, J.-G.; Kwon, S.-Y.; Woo, J.-S.; Baek, S.-K.; Jung, K.-Y. The Benefits and Risks of Prophylactic Central Neck Dissection for Papillary Thyroid Carcinoma: Prospective Cohort Study. *Int. J. Endocrinol.* **2015**, *2015*, 571480. [CrossRef]
41. Chéreau, N.; Buffet, C.; Trésallet, C.; Tissier, F.; Leenhardt, L.; Menegaux, F. Recurrence of papillary thyroid carcinoma with lateral cervical node metastases: Predictive factors and operative management. *Surgery* **2016**, *159*, 755–762. [CrossRef]
42. Chinn, S.; Zafereo, M.; Waguespack, S.G.; Edeiken, B.S.; Roberts, D.B.; Clayman, G.L. Long-Term Outcomes of Lateral Neck Dissection in Patients with Recurrent or Persistent Well-Differentiated Thyroid Cancer. *Thyroid* **2017**, *27*, 1291–1299. [CrossRef]
43. Hartl, D.M.; Al Ghuzlan, A.; Borget, I.; Leboulleux, S.; Mirghani, H.; Schlumberger, M. Prophylactic Level II Neck Dissection Guided by Frozen Section for Clinically Node-Negative Papillary Thyroid Carcinoma: Is It Useful? *World J. Surg.* **2013**, *38*, 667–672. [CrossRef] [PubMed]

Article

Tall Cell Variant versus Conventional Papillary Thyroid Carcinoma: A Retrospective Analysis in 351 Consecutive Patients

Alessandro Longheu *, Gian Luigi Canu, Federico Cappellacci, Enrico Erdas, Fabio Medas and Pietro Giorgio Calò

Department of Surgical Sciences, University of Cagliari, S. S. 554, Bivio Sestu, 09042 Monserrato, Italy; gianlu_5@hotmail.it (G.L.C.); fedcapp94@gmail.com (F.C.); erdasenrico@libero.it (E.E.); fabiomedas@gmail.com (F.M.); pgcalo@unica.it (P.G.C.)
* Correspondence: alex1283@tiscali.it; Tel.: +39-393473779728

Abstract: Background: The aim of this retrospective study was to investigate clinical and pathological characteristics of the tall cell variant of papillary thyroid carcinoma compared to conventional variants. Methods: The clinical records of patients who underwent surgical treatment between 2009 and 2015 were analyzed. The patients were divided into two groups: those with a histopathological diagnosis of tall cell papillary carcinoma were included in Group A, and those with a diagnosis of conventional variants in Group B. Results: A total of 35 patients were included in Group A and 316 in Group B. All patients underwent total thyroidectomy. Central compartment and lateral cervical lymph node dissection were performed more frequently in Group A (42.8% vs. 18%, $p = 0.001$, and 17.1% vs. 6.9%, $p = 0.04$). Angiolymphatic invasion, parenchymal invasion, extrathyroidal extension, and lymph node metastases were more frequent in Group A, and the data reached statistical significance. Local recurrence was more frequent in Group A (17.1% vs. 6.3%, $p = 0.02$), with two patients (5.7%) in Group A showing visceral metastases, whereas no patient in Group B developed metastatic cancer ($p = 0.009$). Conclusions: Tall cell papillary carcinoma is the most frequent aggressive variant of papillary thyroid cancer. Tall cell histology represents an independent poor prognostic factor compared to conventional variants.

Keywords: tall cell variant of papillary thyroid carcinoma; conventional papillary thyroid carcinoma; thyroid surgery

1. Introduction

Papillary thyroid carcinoma (PTC) is the most common malignant endocrine tumor. The prognosis for patients with PTC is almost the same as that of individuals who never had cancer, and only a few patients with PTC are affected by a biologically aggressive tumor [1,2]. The most common of PTC aggressive subtypes is the tall cell variant (TCV). TCV was first described by Hawk and Hazard in 1976 [3] and represents from 4% to 19% of all PTCs [4,5]. Several studies have demonstrated that this variant is generally underdiagnosed [6–9]. The definition of TCV includes the presence of a tumor whose cells are two to three times as tall as they are wide, eosinophilic cytoplasm, basilar-oriented nuclei, and the nuclear features of PTC [3,10,11]. TCV is generally considered a more aggressive variant of PTC and frequently has lymph node metastases and/or distant metastases, with a poorer prognosis [12–14] compared to conventional PTC (cPTC). The aim of this retrospective study was to investigate the clinical and pathological characteristics of TCV-PTC compared to conventional variants.

2. Materials and Methods

2.1. Study Design

This is a retrospective cohort study on patients who underwent thyroidectomy in our Unit of General and Endocrine Surgery (University of Cagliari, Cagliari, Italy) after the histopathological diagnosis of cPTC or TCV-PTC between January 2009 and December 2015. We identified cPTC with a classical variant, a follicular variant, and an oncocytic variant. Other biologically aggressive variants of PTC, papillary thyroid microcarcinoma, follicular carcinoma, medullary carcinoma, anaplastic carcinoma, secondary tumors, and tumors with a tall cell component < 50% were excluded. The patients were identified from a prospectively maintained institutional database, and those with incomplete or lost data at follow-up were excluded from the study. The patients were divided into 2 groups: those with a histopathological diagnosis of TCV-PTC were included in Group A, while those with a histopathological diagnosis of cPTC were included in Group B. Demographic data (sex and age), preoperative findings (cytological diagnosis and echographic features), surgical treatment (total thyroidectomy ± central compartment neck dissection ± modified lateral neck dissection), surgical outcomes (operative time and postoperative stay), histopathological findings, complications (hypoparathyroidism, recurrent laryngeal nerve injury, postsurgical cervical hematoma, wound infection, and chylous fistula), and follow-up data (local recurrence and distant metastases) were recorded.

2.2. Preoperative Evaluation

For each patient, preoperative assessment consisted of free triiodothyronine (FT3), free thyroxine (FT4), and thyroid-stimulating hormone (TSH) blood measurements; high-resolution ultrasound (US) of the neck; and fibrolaryngoscopy for assessment of vocal fold mobility. In the case of suspicious nodules, US-guided fine-needle aspiration cytology was performed.

2.3. Surgical Procedure

All operations were performed under general anesthesia by the three most skilled endocrine surgeons of our unit. Recurrent laryngeal nerves and parathyroid glands were systematically searched and identified. Intraoperative nerve monitoring (IONM) was routinely used to facilitate nerve identification and to confirm its functional integrity. Hemostasis was mainly achieved using energy-based devices. One or two closed-suction drains were placed below the strap muscles. The cervical linea alba and platysma were sutured with absorbable sutures, and the skin was closed by a continuous intradermal suture. The duration of the surgical procedure, from skin incision to skin closure, was estimated in minutes.

2.4. Postoperative Management and Follow-Up

The serum calcium and PTH levels were assayed pre- and postoperatively. Postsurgical hypoparathyroidism was defined as PTH < 10 pg/mL following the operation (normal range = 10–65 pg/mL). Permanent hypoparathyroidism was defined as PTH concentrations below the normal range for more than 12 months. In case of suspected recurrent laryngeal nerve injury, a fibrolaryngoscopy was performed to assess vocal cord mobility. Postoperative radioactive iodine therapy (RAI) was administered, according to the 2009 American Thyroid Association guidelines, in case of gross extrathyroidal extension, primary tumor size greater than 4 cm, distant metastases, or selected patients with a primary tumor, ranging from 1 to 4 cm, confined to the thyroid gland but with a significant risk of recurrence. Follow-up consisted of neck US examination and dosage of thyroglobulin (Tg) and thyroglobulin antibodies (TgAb) levels every six months during suppressive L-thyroxine treatment (a serum Tg level of 0.2 ng/mL was considered as undetectable). In patients with suspicious recurrence, a whole-body ^{131}I scanning after recombinant human thyrotropin (rhTSH) was performed. The diagnosis of disease recurrence in the cervical lymph nodes was based on serum Tg level monitoring, US-guided fine-needle aspiration cytology (FNAC), and Tg washing of FNAC aspirates.

2.5. Statistical Analysis

Statistical analyses were performed with MedCalc® (Ostend, Belgium) 19.1.3. The Fisher exact test or chi-squared test was used for categorical variables, and the t-test for continuous variables. The Kaplan–Meier method was used to analyze disease-free survival curves. p-values < 0.05 were considered statistically significant.

3. Results

As reported in Table 1, 351 patients were included in this study: 35 (9.97%) in Group A and 316 (90.03%) in Group B. Women were more numerous than men in both groups. The mean age was 49.3 ± 18.2 years in Group A and 50.6 ± 14.9 in Group B ($p = 0.6$). An indeterminate or suspicious nodule was identified in 8 (22.8%) cases in Group A and 131 (41.4%) in Group B ($p = 0.04$), whereas a carcinoma was diagnosed in 14 (40%) patients in Group A and 24 (7.5%) in Group B ($p < 0.0001$). Suspicious echographic features were found in 14 (40%) patients in Group A and 119 (37.6%) in Group B ($p = 0.8$). Benign thyroid disease (multinodular goiter and hyperthyroidism) was associated with thyroid cancer in 10 (28.5%) patients in Group A and 87 (27.5%) in Group B ($p = 0.8$).

Table 1. Demographic and preoperative data.

	Group A ($n = 35$)	Group B ($n = 316$)	p-Value
Sex Male Female	 14 (40%) 21 (60%)	 80 (25.31%) 236 (74.68%)	0.07
Age (years, mean ± SD)	49.34 ± 18.22	50.62 ± 14.9	0.6
Indeterminate or suspicious nodule on cytology	8 (22.85%)	131 (41.45%)	0.04
Diagnosis of carcinoma on cytology	14 (40%)	24 (7.59%)	<0.0001
Suspicious nodule on US	14 (40%)	119 (37.65%)	0.8
Benign disease (multinodular goiter and hyperthyroidism)	10 (28.57%)	87 (27.53%)	0.8

All patients underwent total thyroidectomy; central neck compartment lymphadenectomy was associated with thyroidectomy in 15 (42.8%) patients in Group A and 57 (18.03%) in Group B ($p < 0.001$), whereas modified lateral neck dissection was performed in 6 (17.1%) patients in Group A and 22 (6.9%) in Group B ($p = 0.04$). The mean surgical time was 121 ± 29.01 min in Group A and 100 ± 28.91 min in Group B ($p = 0.0004$). The mean postoperative stay was 2.74 ± 0.97 days in Group A and 2.68 ± 0.93 in Group B ($p = 0.7$) (Table 2).

Table 2. Surgical procedure and postoperative stay.

	Group A ($n = 35$)	Group B ($n = 316$)	p-Value
Total thyroidectomy and central compartment dissection	15 (42.85%)	57 (18.03%)	<0.001
Total thyroidectomy and modified lateral neck dissection	6 (17.14%)	22 (6.96%)	0.04
Surgical time (min, mean ± SD)	121 ± 29.01	100 ± 28.91	0.0004
Postoperative stay (days, mean ± SD)	2.74 ± 0.97	2.68 ± 0.93	0.7

The mean tumor size was 2.39 ± 1.27 cm in Group A and 2.22 ± 1.25 cm in Group B ($p = 0.03$); thyroid weight was 31.9 ± 42.99 g in Group A and 33.91 ± 42.37 g in Group B ($p = 0.7$). Multicentric cancer was found in 11 (31.42%) patients in Group A and in 110 (31.64%) in Group B ($p = 1$), angiolymphatic invasion in 6 (17.14%) patients in Group A and in 16 (5.06%) in Group B ($p = 0.01$), parenchymal invasion in 13 (37.14%) patients in Group A and in 56 (17.72%) in Group B ($p = 0.004$), and extrathyroidal extension in 11

(31.42%) patients in Group A and in 16 (5.06%) in Group B ($p < 0.0001$). Cervical lymph node metastases were found in 16 (45.71%) patients in Group A and in 42 (13.29%) in Group B ($p < 0.0001$) (Table 3).

Table 3. Histopathological diagnosis.

	Group A (n = 35)	Group B (n = 316)	p-Value
Tumor size (cm, mean ± SD)	2.69 ± 1.27	2.22 ± 1.25	0.03
Thyroid weight (grams, mean ± SD)	31.9 ± 42.99	33.91 ± 42.37	0.7
Multicentric carcinoma	11 (31.42%)	100 (31.64%)	1
Angiolymphatic invasion	6 (17.14%)	16 (5.06%)	0.01
Carcinoma infiltrating the glandular parenchyma	13 (37.14%)	56 (17.72%)	0.004
Extrathyroidal extension	11 (31.42%)	16 (5.06%)	<0.0001
Node metastases	16 (45.71%)	42 (13.29%)	<0.0001

In Group A, postoperative hematoma occurred in one (2.85%) patient, transient recurrent laryngeal nerve palsy in one (2.85%), transient hypoparathyroidism in 11 (31.42%), and permanent hypoparathyroidism in three (8.5%), whereas wound infection, permanent recurrent laryngeal nerve palsy, and chylous fistula did not occur. In Group B, postoperative hematoma occurred in four (1.26%) patients, transient recurrent laryngeal nerve palsy in four (1.26%), transient hypoparathyroidism in 87 (27.53%), and permanent hypoparathyroidism in 20 (6.3%), whereas wound infection, permanent recurrent laryngeal nerve palsy, and chylous fistula did not occur (Table 4).

Table 4. Postoperative complications.

	Group A (n = 35)	Group B (n = 316)	p Value
Postoperative hematoma	1 (2.85%)	4 (1.26%)	0.4
Wound infection	0	0	
Transient recurrent laryngeal nerve palsy	1 (2.85%)	4 (1.26%)	0.4
Permanent recurrent laryngeal nerve palsy	0	0	
Transient hypoparathyroidism	11 (31.42%)	87 (27.53%)	0.6
Permanent hypoparathyroidism	3 (8.5%)	20 (6.3%)	0.6
Chylous fistula	0	0	

The mean follow-up was 79.4 ± 25.9 months in Group A and 98.4 ± 26.5 in Group B ($p = 0.09$). Local recurrence affected 6 (17.1%) patients in Group A and 20 (6.3%) in Group B ($p = 0.02$); 2 (5.71%) patients in Group A developed distant metastases, whereas distant metastases did not occur in Group B ($p = 0.009$) (Table 5).

Table 5. Local recurrence and distant metastases.

	Group A (n = 35)	Group B (n = 316)	p-Value
Local recurrence	6 (17.1%)	20 (6.3%)	0.02
Distant metastases	2 (5.71%)	0	0.009
Follow-up (months, mean ± SD)	79.4 ± 25.9	98.4 ± 26.5	0.09

Five-year disease-free survival was 82.3% in Group A and 92.8% in Group B ($p = 0.0018$) (Figure 1).

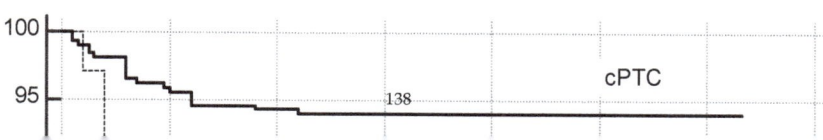

4. Discussion

Only a few patients with PTC are affected by a clinically aggressive tumor, and the most common of these subtypes is TCV-PTC, which was first described by Hawk and Hazard in 1976 [3]. The definition accepted widely by pathologists includes the presence of a papillary tumor whose cells are at least twice as long as they are wide [3,11]. Currently, this variant is underdiagnosed: several studies have demonstrated that when cases diagnosed as cPTC were reviewed by endocrine pathologists, 1–13% of the tumors were identified as TCV-PTC [6,15,16]. One of the obstacles to the correct diagnosis of TCV-PTC is the lack of consensus as to how much of the tumor must be composed of tall cells to make a diagnosis. The cutoff varies from one institution to another, from 30% to 70% [10,17,18], and any tumor that contains a smaller percentage of tall cells than the institutional cutoff is classified as PTC with tall cell features [18]. In our institute, tumors with less than 50% tall cells are excluded by the diagnosis of TCV-PTC, and they were excluded from this study because the implications of the presence of a small number of tall cells in a thyroid tumor are currently debated [6–9]. However, some authors found an association between PTC with tall cell features and a poorer prognosis than cPTC [19–22]. FNAC is the most useful tool in the preoperative diagnosis of papillary carcinoma. The accuracy of FNAC can reach more than 95% in adequate specimens [23].

The cytological features of TCV-PTC have been well described [24]. Nevertheless, preoperative diagnosis of TCV-PTC on FNAC is difficult, and it is more common for patients to be diagnosed postoperatively after histopathological examination [25]. Use of molecular testing and immunochemistry may aid in the preoperative diagnosis of TCV-PTC and other more aggressive variants of PTC: the BRAF V600E mutation is highly prevalent in TCV-PTC, with reports ranging from 66% to 100% [26–31]. The conventional smear is the standard diagnostic method for detecting thyroid lesions. Liquid-based cytology can improve detection of tall cells, because the cytoplasm of the cells is not well preserved in the conventional smear. Liquid-based cytology allows distinguishing TCV-PTC from PTC with tall cell features, and the residual material in fixative solution allows further studies to be carried out, such as immunostaining or molecular testing [32]. In 1976, Hawk and Hazard retrospectively reviewed 197 cases of PTC from 1921 to 1960. Four patients with a diagnosis of TCV-PTC died of the disease, and the mean follow-up was 7.8 years. The authors were the first to describe an association of TC cytology with larger tumors and older age [3]. In 2004, Sywak et al. reviewed 209 cases of TCV-PTC. The authors of this study found high rates of extracapsular spread of tumors (67%) and cervical adenopathy (57%); 25% of the patients showed locoregional recurrence and 22% developed distant metastases [33]. In the same year, Machens et al. found the association between TC cytology and distant metastases (50% in the TCV-PTC cohort vs. 31% in PTC) [34]. In 2007, Ghossein et al. reported that TCV-PTC without extrathyroidal extension has a more aggressive behavior than conventional intrathyroidal PTC, with a significantly higher nodal metastatic rate independent of tumor diameter, sex, and age [16]. In 2010, Jalisi et al. published a systematic literature review to evaluate the prognosis of TCV compared to cPTC. The TCV patients showed a higher rate of extrathyroidal extension (cumulative average of 60.3%), a higher rate of distant metastases at diagnosis (cumulative average of 15%), and nodal metastases (cumulative average of 58.1%). The cumulative average recurrence and the cumulative average disease-related mortality were higher in the TCV group versus cPTC group (42.5% vs. 9.8% and 23.6% vs. 1.5%, respectively) [35]. In a large multicenter study, Shi et al. confirmed the association between PTC-TCV and high-risk parameters, including extrathyroidal invasion, lymph node metastasis, stage III/IV, disease recurrence, mortality, and the use of radioiodine treatment [36].

In our study, the histopathological and prognostic data of patients with a diagnosis of TCV-PTC agreed with the data reported in previous studies. TCV-PTC showed a greater diameter than cPTC (2.69 vs. 2.22 cm), and angiolymphatic invasion, thyroid parenchymal invasion, extrathyroidal extension, and lymph node metastases were greater in TCV-PTC than cPTC (17.14% vs. 5.06%, 37.14% vs. 17.72%, 31.42% vs. 5.06%, and 45.71% vs. 13.29%, respectively). TCV-PTC also showed higher rates of local recurrence (17.1% vs. 6.3%) and distant metastases (5.71% vs. 0%). Five-year disease-free survival in patients with a diagnosis of PTC-TCV was 82.3% in the TCV-PTC group, whereas it was 92.3% in the cPTC group. All these findings reached statistical significance. Local recurrences in TCV-PTC patients were identified early in the follow-up. They all occurred within 16 months of surgery, while the few distant metastases occurred within 24 months. Similarly, local recurrences in the cPTC group were early, all occurring within 25 months of surgery. Clinical aggressiveness of TCV-PTC seems to be related to certain factors elaborated by the tumor. The high expression of Muc1 and type IV collagenase in TCV-PTC may allow for degradation of stroma, and this can be responsible for the greater invasiveness compared to usual and follicular variants of PTC [37,38]. The clinical behavior of TCV-PTC may also be related to the higher prevalence of activating point mutations of the BRAF compared to cPTC [38]. Indeed, tumors characterized by BRAF mutations in their molecular profile have a higher rate of extrathyroidal extension and nodal metastases and show a higher stage than BRAF-negative tumors [28]. The impact of TC cytology on prognosis requires a more aggressive therapeutic approach than typically followed in other PTC variants. However, the main problem is that TCV-PTC is diagnosed on histopathological examination after the initial thyroid surgery has been performed. If a patient is diagnosed with TCV-PTC and has undergone partial thyroidectomy, the patient should return to the operating room to perform a completion thyroidectomy associated with central neck dissection followed by RAI. If a total thyroidectomy is performed, the therapeutic choices to consider are the execution of central neck dissection followed by RAI versus RAI alone, and if the tumor is not iodocaptant, external beam radiation can be a therapeutic option [35]. Sywak et al. described that the treatment of choice of TCV-PTC is represented by total thyroidectomy associated with cervical lymph node dissection in the case of lymph node involvement, and en bloc resection of the perithyroidal tissues is necessary if their involvement is detected before or during surgery [33]. Prendiville et al. found that all patients with TCV-PTC require aggressive surgical treatment in association with RAI, levothyroxine suppressive therapy, and close follow-up [15].

In agreement with these findings, all patients enrolled in this study underwent total thyroidectomy, while more conservative surgery was not performed. Central compartment lymph node dissection and modified lateral neck dissection were performed more frequently in TCV-PTC patients than in cPTC patients (42.85% vs. 18.03% $p = 0.001$ and 17.14% vs. 6.96% $p = 0.04$, respectively). Consequently, the mean operative time increased in TCV-PTC patients (121 ± 29.01 min vs. 100 ± 28.91 min $p = 0.0004$), with no differences in postoperative stay between the two groups. In this study, the problem of difficult preoperative diagnosis of TCV-PTC emerged. In the case of postoperative diagnosis of TCV-PTC, no patient underwent rescue central compartment lymph node dissection because, in our clinical practice, total thyroidectomy was always associated with a central or modified lateral neck dissection in the case of clinical or ultrasound findings suggestive of lymph node involvement [39,40]. Total thyroidectomy is a safe procedure and showed a similar low complication rate in the two study groups. TCV-PTC patients should always be considered at intermediate risk of recurrence. Among the factors known to confer an intermediate risk of recurrence are extrathyroidal extension, lymph node metastases at the time of surgical treatment or I^{131} uptake outside the thyroid lodge on a post-therapy whole-body scan (Rx-WBS) performed after initial radioablative therapy [41,42], aggressive tumor histology, and vascular invasion [15,43,44]. All patients enrolled in this study underwent at least one course of RAI because it is always indicated when individual histology confers an intermediate risk of recurrence [45].

Our study has a main limitation. It is based on a retrospective analysis from a single institution. However, as ours is a high-volume center in a region where thyroid disease is endemic, our results are in line with those reported in the literature.

5. Conclusions

TCV is the most frequent aggressive histopathological variant of PTC. Our patients with a diagnosis of TCV-PTC showed larger tumor diameter and higher frequency of angiolymphatic invasion, extrathyroidal invasion, and lymph node metastases at the time of surgery than cPTC patients, and this resulted in a higher rate of local recurrence and distant metastases and in a less favorable clinical outcome. In this study, TC histology was therefore confirmed as an independent negative prognostic factor. Among the authors, there is the general consensus that the surgical treatment of TCV-PTC should be aggressive, with the execution of total thyroidectomy associated with central neck dissection followed by RAI. This good practice of therapeutic conduct is contrasted by TCV-PTC being largely underdiagnosed, being usually identified on definitive histopathological examination in patients with a generic preoperative diagnosis of suspicious or indeterminate nodule or PTC. We think that a good therapeutic option is to combine total thyroidectomy with the execution of central and/or modified lateral compartment lymph node dissection in the case of clinical or ultrasound findings suggestive of lymph node involvement, associated with RAI. Surgery is safe, and the complication rate is similar to that of cPTC patients. Further studies are needed to increase the chances of preoperative diagnosis of aggressive variants of PTC and to perform a tailored surgical treatment based on precise preoperative findings.

Author Contributions: Conceptualization, A.L. and P.G.C.; methodology, A.L., G.L.C., F.M., E.E., and F.C.; formal analysis, A.L., G.L.C., and F.M.; investigation, F.M., E.E., and P.G.C.; data curation, E.E. and F.C.; writing—original draft preparation, A.L. and G.L.C.; writing—review and editing, A.L. and F.C.; visualization, F.M.; supervision, F.M. and P.G.C. All authors have read and agreed to the published version of the manuscript.

Funding: This research received no external funding.

Institutional Review Board Statement: The study was conducted in accordance with the Declaration of Helsinki, and the protocol was approved by the Ethics Committee of A.O.U. Cagliari (Project identification code: NP/2019/3369).

Informed Consent Statement: Informed consent was administered to every participant included in the study.

Data Availability Statement: Data will be made available under reasonable request.

Conflicts of Interest: The authors declare no conflict of interest.

References

1. LiVolsi, V.A. Papillary carcinoma tall cell variant (TCV): A review. *Endocr. Pathol.* **2010**, *21*, 12–15. [CrossRef] [PubMed]
2. Calò, P.G.; Medas, F.; Loi, G.; Erdas, E.; Pisano, G.; Nicolosi, A. Differentiated thyroid cancer in the elderly: Our experience. *Int. J. Surg.* **2014**, *12*, 140–143. [CrossRef] [PubMed]
3. Hawk, W.A.; Hazard, J.B. The many appearances of papillary carcinoma of the thyroid. *Clevel. Clin. Q.* **1976**, *43*, 207–215. [CrossRef] [PubMed]
4. Muzaffar, M.; Nigar, E.; Mushtaq, S.; Mamoon, N. The morphological variants of papillary carcinoma of the thyroid: A clinicopathological study-AFIP experience. *J. Pak. Med. Assoc.* **1998**, *48*, 133–137.
5. Pilotti, S.; Collini, P.; Manzari, A.; Marubini, E.; Rilke, F. Poorly differentiated forms of papillary thyroid carcinoma: Distinctive entities or morphological patterns? *Semin. Diagn. Pathol.* **1995**, *12*, 249–255.
6. Therry, J.H.; St John, S.A.; Karkowski, F.J.; Suarez, J.R.; Yassa, N.H.; Platica, C.D.; Marti, J.R. Tall cell papillary thyroid cancer: Incidence and prognosis. *Am. J. Surg.* **1994**, *168*, 459–461. [CrossRef]
7. Leung, A.K.; Chow, S.M.; Law, S.C. Clinical features and outcome of the tall cell variant of papillary thyroid carcinoma. *Laryngoscope* **2008**, *118*, 32–38. [CrossRef]
8. Ito, Y.; Hirokawa, M.; Fukushima, M.; Inoue, H.; Yabuta, T.; Uruno, T.; Kihara, M.; Higashiyama, T.; Takamura, Y.; Miya, A.; et al. Prevalence and prognostic significance of poor differentiation and tall cell variant in papillary carcinoma in Japan. *World J. Surg.* **2008**, *32*, 1535–1543. [CrossRef]
9. Ruter, A.; Nishiyama, R.; Lennquist, S. Tall-cell variant of papillary thyroid cancer: Disregarded entity? *World J. Surg.* **1997**, *21*, 15–20. [CrossRef]
10. Jonhson, T.L.; Lloyd, R.V.; Thompson, N.W.; Beierwaltes, W.H.; Sisson, J.C. Prognostic implications of the tall cell variant of papillary thyroid carcinoma. *Am. J. Surg. Pathol.* **1988**, *12*, 22–27. [CrossRef]
11. DeLellis, R.A. *Pathology and Genetics of Tumours of Endocrine Organs*; IARC Press: Lyon, France, 2004.

12. Angeles-Angeles, A.; Chable-Montero, F.; Martinez-Benitez, B.; Albores-Saavedra, J. Unusual metastases of papillary thyroid carcinoma: Report of 2 cases. *Ann. Diagn. Pathol.* **2009**, *13*, 189–196. [CrossRef]
13. Tosi, A.L.; Ragazzi, M.; Asioli, S.; Del Vecchio, M.; Cavalieri, M.; Eusebi, L.H.; Foschini, M.P. Breast tumor resembling the tall cell variant of papillary thyroid carcinoma: Report of 4 cases with evidence of malignant potential. *Int. J. Surg. Pathol.* **2007**, *15*, 14–19. [CrossRef]
14. Longheu, A.; Medas, F.; Pisano, G.; Gordini, L.; Nicolosi, A.; Sorrenti, S.; Erdas, E.; Calò, P.G. Differentiated thyroid cancer in patients ≥75 years: Histopathological features and results of surgical treatment. *Int. J. Surg.* **2016**, *33*, 159–163. [CrossRef] [PubMed]
15. Prendiville, S.; Burman, K.D.; Ringel, M.D.; Shmookler, B.M.; Deeb, Z.E.; Wolfe, K.; Azumi, N.; Wartofsky, L.; Sessions, R.B. Tall cell variant: An aggressive form of papillary thyroid carcinoma. *Otolaryngol. Head Neck Surg.* **2000**, *122*, 352–357. [CrossRef] [PubMed]
16. Ghossein, R.A.; Leboeuf, R.; Patel, K.N.; Rivera, M.; Katabi, N.; Carlson, D.L.; Tallini, G.; Shaha, A.; Singh, B.; Tuttle, R.M. Tall cell variant of papillary thyroid carcinoma without extrathyroid extension: Biologic behavior and clinical implications. *Thyroid* **2007**, *17*, 655–661. [CrossRef] [PubMed]
17. Ghossein, R.; LiVolsi, V.A. Papillary thyroid carcinoma tall cell variant. *Thyroid* **2008**, *18*, 1179–1181. [CrossRef] [PubMed]
18. Akslen, L.A. Prognostic importance of histologic grading in papillary thyroid carcinoma. *Cancer* **1993**, *72*, 2680–2685. [CrossRef]
19. Ganly, I.; Ibrahimpasic, T.; Rivera, M.; Nixon, I.; Palmer, F.; Patel, S.G.; Tuttle, R.M.; Shah, J.P.; Ghossein, R. Prognostic implications of papillary thyroid carcinoma with tall-cell features. *Thyroid* **2014**, *24*, 662–670. [CrossRef]
20. Vuong, H.G.; Long, N.P.; Anh, N.H.; Nghi, T.D.; Hieu, M.V.; Hung, L.P.; Nakazawa, T.; Katoh, R.; Kondo, T. Papillary thyroid carcinoma with tall cell features i sas aggressive as tall cell variant: A meta-analysis. *Endocr. Connect.* **2018**, *7*, 286–293. [CrossRef]
21. Bongers, P.J.; Kluijfhout, W.P.; Verzijl, R.; Lustgarten, M.; Vermeer, M.; Goldstein, D.P.; Devon, K.; Rotstein, L.E.; Asa, S.L.; Brierley, J.D.; et al. Papillary thyroid cancers with focal tall cell change are as aggressive as tall cell variants and should not be considered a slow-risk disease. *Ann. Surg. Oncol.* **2019**, *26*, 2533–2539. [CrossRef]
22. Beninato, T.; Scognamiglio, T.; Kleiman, D.A.; Uccelli, A.; Vaca, D.; Fahey, T.J.; Zarnegar, R. Ten percent tall cells confer the aggressive feaures of the tall cell variant of papillary thyroid carcinoma. *Surgery* **2013**, *154*, 1331–1336. [CrossRef] [PubMed]
23. Baloch, Z.W.; LiVolsi, V.A. Fine-needle aspiration on thyroid nodules: Past, present, and future. *Endocr. Pract.* **2004**, *10*, 234–241. [CrossRef] [PubMed]
24. Guan, H.; VandenBussche, C.J.; Erozan, Y.S.; Rosenthal, D.L.; Tatsas, A.D.; Olson, M.T.; Zheng, R.; Auger, M.; Ali, S.Z. Can the tall cell variant of papillary thyroid carcinoma be distinguished from the conventional type in fine needle aspirates? A cytomorphologic study with assessment of diagnostic accuracy. *Acta Cytol.* **2013**, *57*, 534–542. [CrossRef] [PubMed]
25. Kuo, E.J.; Goffredo, P.; Sosa, J.A.; Roman, S.A. Aggressive variants of papillary thyroid microcarcinoma are associated with extrathyroidal spread and lymph-node metastases: A population-level analysis. *Thyroid* **2013**, *23*, 1305–1311. [CrossRef] [PubMed]
26. Lee, X.; Gao, M.; Ji, Y.; Yu, Y.; Feng, Y.; Li, Y.; Zhang, Y.; Cheng, W.; Zao, W. Analysis of differential BRAF(V600E) mutational status in high aggressive papillary thyroid microcarcinoma. *Ann. Surg. Oncol.* **2009**, *16*, 240–245. [CrossRef] [PubMed]
27. Virk, R.K.; Van Dyke, A.L.; Finkelstein, A.; Prasad, A.; Gibson, J.; Hui, P.; Theoharis, C.G.; Carling, T.; Roman, S.A.; Sosa, J.A.; et al. BRAF(V600E) mutation in papillary thyroid microcarcinoma: A genotype-phenotype correlation. *Mod. Pathol.* **2013**, *26*, 62–70. [CrossRef]
28. Adeniran, A.J.; Zhu, Z.; Gandhi, M.; Steward, D.L.; Fidler, J.P.; Giordano, T.J.; Biddinger, P.W.; Nikiforov, Y.E. Correlation between genetic alterations and microscopic features, clinical manifestations, and prognostic characteristics of thyroid papillary carcinomas. *Am. J. Surg. Pathol.* **2006**, *30*, 216–222. [CrossRef]
29. Sheu, S.Y.; Grabellus, F.; Schwertheim, S.; Handke, S.; Worm, K.; Schmis, K.W. Lack of correlaion Between BRAF V600E mutational status and and the expression profile of a distinct set of miRNAs in papillary thyroid carcinoma. *Horm. Metab. Res.* **2009**, *41*, 482–487. [CrossRef]
30. Basolo, F.; Torregrossa, L.; Giannini, L.; Miccoli, M.; Lupi, C.; Sensi, E.; Berti, P.; Elisei, R.; Vitti, P.; Baggiani, A.; et al. Correlation between the BRAF V600E mutaton and tumor invasiveness in papillary thyroid carcinomas smaller than 20 millimeters: Analysis of 1060 cases. *J. Clin. Endocrinol. Metab.* **2010**, *95*, 4197–4205. [CrossRef]
31. Finkelstein, A.; Levy, G.H.; Hui, P.; Prasad, A.; Virk, R.; Chieng, D.C.; Carling, T.; Roman, S.A.; Sosa, J.A.; Udelsman, R.; et al. Papillary thyroid carcinomas with and without BRAF V600E mutations are morphologically distinct. *Histopathology* **2012**, *60*, 1052–1059. [CrossRef]
32. Lee, S.H.; Jung, C.K.; Bae, J.S.; Jung, S.L.; Choi, Y.J.; Kang, C.S. Liquid-based citology improves preoperative diagnostic accuracy of the tall cell variant of papillary thyroid carcinoma. *Diagn. Cytopathol.* **2013**, *42*, 11–17. [CrossRef] [PubMed]
33. Sywak, M.; Pasieka, J.L.; Ogilvie, T. A review of thyroid cancer with intermediate differentiation. *J. Surg. Oncol.* **2004**, *86*, 44–54. [CrossRef] [PubMed]
34. Machens, A.; Holzhausen, H.; Lautenschlager, C.; Dralle, H. The tall-cell variant of papillary thyroid carcinoma: A multivariate analysis of clinical risk factors. *Langenbeck Arch. Surg.* **2004**, *389*, 278–282. [CrossRef] [PubMed]
35. Jalisi, S.; Ainsworth, T.; LaValley, M. Prognostic outcomes of tall cell variant papillary thyroid cancer: A meta-analysis. *J. Thyroid Res.* **2010**. [CrossRef]

36. Shi, X.; Liu, R.; Basolo, F.; Giannini, R.; Shen, X.; Teng, D.; Guan, H.; Shan, Z.; Teng, W.; Musholt, T.; et al. Differential clinicopathological risk and prognosis of major papillary thyroid cancer variants. *J. Clin. Endocrinol. Metab.* **2016**, *101*, 264–274. [CrossRef]
37. Nishida, T.; Katayama, S.; Tsujimoto, M.; Nakamura, J.; Matsuda, H. Clinicopathological significance of poorly differentiated thyroid carcinoma. *Am. J. Surg. Pathol.* **1999**, *23*, 205–211. [CrossRef]
38. Campo, E.; Merino, M.J.; Liotta, L.; Neumann, R.; Stetler-Stevenson, W. Distribution of the 72-kd type IV collagenase in non neoplastic and neoplastic thyroid tissue. *Hum. Pathol.* **1992**, *23*, 1395–1401. [CrossRef]
39. Calò, P.G.; Medas, F.; Pisano, G.; Boi, F.; Baghino, G.; Mariotti, S.; Nicolosi, A. Differentiated thyroid cancer: Indications and extent of central neck dissection-our experience. *Int. J. Surg. Oncol.* **2013**. [CrossRef]
40. Medas, F.; Canu, G.L.; Cappellacci, F.; Boi, F.; Lai, M.L.; Erdas, E.; Calò, P.G. Predictive factors of lymph node metastasis in patients with papillary microcarcinoma of the thyroid: Retrospective analysis on 293 cases. *Front. Endocrinol.* **2020**, *11*, 551. [CrossRef]
41. Cailleux, A.F.; Baudin, E.; Travagli, J.P.; Ricard, M.; Schlumberger, M. Is diagnostic iodine-131 scanning useful after total thyroid ablation for differentiatd thyroid cancer? *J. Clin. Endocrinol. Metab.* **2000**, *85*, 175–178. [CrossRef]
42. Bachelot, A.; Cailleux, A.F.; Klain, M.; Baudin, E.; Ricard, M.; Bellon, N.; Caillou, B.; Travagli, J.P.; Schlumberger, M. Relationship between tumor burden and serum thyroglobulin level in patients with papillary and follicular thyroid carcinoma. *Thyroid* **2002**, *12*, 707–711. [CrossRef] [PubMed]
43. Akslen, L.A.; LiVolsi, V.A. Prognostic significance of histologic grading compared with subclassification of papillary thyroid carcinoma. *Cancer* **2000**, *88*, 1902–1908. [CrossRef]
44. Wenig, B.M.; Thompson, L.D.; Adair, C.F.; Shmookler, B.; Heffess, C.S. Thyroid papillary carcinoma of columnar cell type: A clinicopathologic study of 16 cases. *Cancer* **1998**, *82*, 740–753. [CrossRef]
45. Cooper, D.S.; Doherty, G.M.; Haugen, B.R.; Kloos, R.T.; Lee, S.L.; Mandel, S.J.; Mazzaferri, E.L.; McIver, B.; Pacini, F.; Schlumberger, M.; et al. Revised American Thyroid Association management guidelines for patients with thyroid nodules and differentiated thyroid cancer. *Thyroid* **2009**, *19*, 1167–1214. [CrossRef]

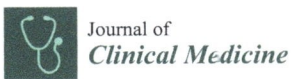

Review

Poorly Differentiated Thyroid Carcinoma: Single Centre Experience and Review of the Literature

Maria Irene Bellini [1,2,*], Marco Biffoni [2,†], Renato Patrone [3,†], Maria Carola Borcea [2], Maria Ludovica Costanzo [2], Tiziana Garritano [2], Rossella Melcarne [2], Rosa Menditto [2], Alessio Metere [4], Chiara Scorziello [2], Marco Summa [2], Luca Ventrone [2], Vito D'Andrea [2] and Laura Giacomelli [2]

1. Azienda Ospedaliera San Camillo Forlanini, 00152 Rome, Italy
2. Department of Surgical Sciences, Sapienza University of Rome, 00161 Rome, Italy
3. ICTUS, University of Naples Federico II, Via Pansini 5, 80131 Naples, Italy
4. General Surgery Department, Ospedale dei Castelli (O.D.C.), Via Nettunense Km 11,5, 00040 Rome, Italy
* Correspondence: m.irene.bellini@gmail.com
† Marco Biffoni and Renato Patrone contributed equally to this research.

Abstract: There is controversy in the literature regarding a distinct subset of thyroid carcinoma whose histologically classification falls between well-differentiated and anaplastic carcinomas, previously identified as 'poorly differentiated thyroid carcinoma' (PDTC), or 'insular carcinoma', in view of the peculiar morphological characteristics of the cell groupings. The correct diagnosis and treatment of this entity have important prognostic and therapeutic significance. In this review, we describe the epidemiology, diagnosis, and management of PDTC and report our single centre experience to add to the limited evidence existing in the literature.

Keywords: poorly differentiated thyroid cancer; total thyroidectomy; fine-needle aspiration cytology

1. Epidemiology

Poorly differentiated thyroid carcinoma (PDTC) is a rare disease, with an intermediate biological behaviour between well-differentiated (papillary and follicular) and undifferentiated (anaplastic) carcinoma; it can arise de novo in the gland or represent the evolution of an unknown differentiated carcinoma [1]. According to published studies, only 27% of cases are diagnosed correctly before surgical intervention; about 80% of PDTC have a poorly differentiated component of ≥50%, and only 20% a lower percentage [2].

PDTC-reported incidence varies according to the geographic area considered: less than 1% of the whole thyroid cancers diagnosed in Japan [3], 2–3% in North American [4], and 15% of those diagnosed in northern Italy [5]. The frequency is higher in older age and more prevalent in women (2.1:1 female to male ratio), particularly in areas of endemic goitre [6].

In PDTC, regional lymph nodal or distant metastases are common at diagnosis, with about 70% of patients presenting with locally advanced disease and a median 5 years-survival of 50–60% [7].

2. Ultrasonographic Features

Ultrasound (US) scan of the neck is an essential imaging technique for the evaluation of thyroid disease [8], and it is used to guide fine-needle aspiration cytologic (FNAC) and core-needle biopsy procedures [9]. PDTC should be suspected when a circumscribed margin and an oval-to-round shape nodule of around 3–3.5 cm [7,10] are visualised, particularly if there is a concomitant irregular rich blood flow [11,12]. Notably, the so-called 'sword sign' is of particular importance, and it is observed only in poorly or undifferentiated thyroid carcinomas, with Colour Doppler US [13,14]. The reason for these appearances is supposed to be in relation to the abnormal circumscribed proliferation driven by genetic mutations

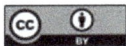

and following atypical hyperplasia of thyroid follicular epithelial cells. This is commonly observed in immune diseases, as for example, in Hashimoto thyroiditis [15], and other goitre diseases where the abnormal lymphocytes stimulation might occur with higher frequency. Since only poorly differentiated or anaplastic carcinomas display external or internal jugular vein central invasion, Doppler US, preferable during Valsalva manoeuvre, is vital to correctly plan the surgical strategy [16]. Microcalcifications presence could also be considered as a sign of malignancy in suspicious nodules, as they mostly represent psammoma bodies and might raise awareness of an occult ipsilateral or contralateral disease [17].

3. Histological Examination

Since its original description in 1983 by Japanese authors [18], the controversy surrounding the intrinsic nature of PDTC has been debated. Dr. Juan Rosai, who contributed significantly to this debate, observed that the main growth pattern was insular, therefore proposed the name of 'insular carcinoma' [19]. He also highlighted that this feature was already been described earlier on as a 'proliferating goitre' by Dr. Langhans, although such entity did not overlap with the solid, trabecular, and/or scirrhous patterns above identified by the Japanese authors. Thus, the controversy in the histological diagnosis, in addition to possible different geographical and ethnic factors are the main drivers of the ongoing debate.

From 2004, the WHO classified PDTC as a non-follicular non-papillary, thyroglobulin-producing thyroid carcinoma [20] with an intermediated behaviour between well-differentiated and anaplastic carcinoma, whose distinctive hallmarks of adverse prognosis are high mitotic index and the presence of necrosis.

In 2006, a proposed diagnostic algorithm, known as the 'Turin proposal' defined the following diagnostic criteria [21]: (1) presence of a solid/trabecular/insular pattern of growth in a malignant (invasive) thyroid lesion of follicular derivation in the majority of the tumour; (2) lack of the conventional papillary carcinoma nuclear features; (3) presence of mitotic activity $>3 \times 10$ HPF or tumour necrosis or convoluted nuclei. Albeit simplifying the diagnosis, limitations inherent criteria reproducibility have been highlighted [22]—namely, what percentage of poorly differentiated tissue was needed in a tumour to allow for such a diagnosis and to affect patient prognosis, specifically considering the fact that the 2004 WHO classification did not offer a cut-off value.

Finally, the Memorial Sloan Kettering Cancer Centre (MSKCC) criteria for PDTC are less restrictive and only consider an elevated mitotic index (>5/10 HPFs) and/or tumour necrosis regardless of tumour growth patterns and nuclear aspects [23].

4. Histological Variants of Poorly Differentiated Carcinoma

The oncocytic variant of PDTC is even more controversial, and although it is recognised as an independent entity by the WHO [20], it was not originally included in the Turin proposal. The presence of necrosis in this tumour variant is the main characteristic, which is common to oncocytic lesions in general, where spontaneous or FNA-initiated infarction and focal necrosis often occur. It is important, however, to identify oncocytic PDTC early, as it is associated with worse outcomes in comparison with conventional PDTC [24].

5. Cytology: The Bethesda System for Reporting Thyroid Cytopathology (TBSRTC)

The needle aspiration under ultrasound guidance is the most frequently used examination for diagnostic purposes [25]; however, the amount of material may be low or inadequate for diagnosis. In these cases, with high suspicion of malignancy, a core biopsy is recommended rather than FNAC repetition to increase the accuracy of percutaneous needle diagnostics, as a first-line tool in selected cases [26].

The Bethesda System for Reporting Thyroid Cytopathology (TBSRTC) regulates the management of patients after FNAC [27], as summarised in Table 1.

Table 1. The Bethesda System for Reporting Thyroid Cytopathology (TBSRTC) classification.

Diagnostic Category	Risk of Malignancy (%)	Recommendation
I. Non-diagnostic or unsatisfactory	1–4	Repeat FNAC with Ultrasound guidance
II. Benign	0–3	Clinical Follow-up
III. AUS or FLUS	5–15	Repeat FNAC
IV. Suspected follicular neoplasm/Follicular neoplasm	15–30	Hemithyroidectomy
V. Suspected Malignancy	60–75	Near total thyroidectomy or hemithyroidectomy
VI. Malignancy	97–99	Total thyroidectomy

AUS: Atypia of undetermined significance; FLUS: follicular lesion of undetermined significance; FNAC: fine-needle aspiration cytology.

A difference exists for category IV (follicular neoplasm) cases which undergo hemithyroidectomy and category V (suspected malignancy) which undergo total thyroidectomy. Single cases of PDTC might be placed in either of these categories because of morphological overlapping, as previously mentioned, but surgical intervention is always recommended, given the malignant nature of PDTC. Furthermore, it has been reported that only 32.5% of PDTC cases are correctly diagnosed by FNAC, whose main feature appears to be the architectural pattern of cellular nests and three-dimensional clusters, along with loosely cohesive singly dispersed cells in the background. This latter feature represents a highly distinctive tract of PDTC.

In view of the controversy related to the interpretation of the cytological appearance, an integration with ultrasound findings might be useful in the intermediate (IV) Bethesda category, where completion of the thyroidectomy would be the safest approach if an initial lobectomy was performed. However, in cases where morphological features are indicative of TBSRTC category V or VI, a preoperative histological diagnosis before surgery is not necessary, as the treatment will not be affected.

6. Immunohistochemistry

In addition to the cytohistological tracts, the diagnosis is based on a panel of immunohistochemical stains, summarised in Table 2. Although PDTC loses the component of well-differentiated thyroid carcinoma, it produces thyroglobulin, contains colloids, and retains the ability to respond to radioactive iodine [28]. Furthermore, since it originates from a gland, it is derived from epithelial cells, thus maintaining the immunophenotypic characteristic of expressing cytokeratins, as reported by Dettmer et al. [29].

Table 2. Common immunohistochemical staining used in poorly differentiated thyroid carcinoma (PDTC).

Immunohistochemical Staining	PDTC
Calcitonin	−
Chromogranin A	no data
Synaptophysin	no data
Thyroglobulin	+
Galectin-3	−/+
HBME-1	−/+
PanCK	+
TTF1	−/−

Table 2. Cont.

Immunohistochemical Staining	PDTC
CK7	−/+
CK19	−/+
PAX8	−/+

7. Molecular Biology

BRAF and RAS mutations remain the principal genes involved in aggressive thyroid carcinomas, occurring in 33% and 45% of the PDTCs, respectively [30,31]. Notably, there is a correlation between the genes involved and the phenotype displayed, with 42% of RAS mutations in identifiable PDTCs according to both Turin proposal and MSKCC criteria, and with BRAF mutation only accounting for 78% of the MSKCC-diagnosed PDTCs. Additionally, BRAF-mutated PDTCs are more frequently responsible for a loco-regional disease, while on the contrary, RAS-mutated follicular carcinomas tend to present with distant metastases.

It has also been demonstrated that the co-existence of BRAF/RAS and TERT genetic alterations has a detrimental impact on the aggressiveness of thyroid carcinoma. More specifically, TERT promoter and TP53 mutations, as well as PIK3CA–PTEN–AKT–mTOR pathway, SWI–SNG complex synergistically concur to worse outcomes in PDTC [32].

The median mutation burden detected in PDTC is 2, and an above-median number of somatic mutations is associated with a larger tumour size of >4 cm, a higher frequency of distant metastasis, and shorter overall survival [30].

8. TNM Classification

In October 2016, the American Joint Committee on Cancer (AJCC) published the 8th edition of the AJCC/TNM cancer staging system, and it has been introduced in clinical practice since 1 January 2018 [33,34] (Table 3).

Table 3. TNM classification.

Primary tumour (pT):
TX: Primary tumour cannot be assessed
T0: No evidence of primary tumour
T1: Tumour ≤2 cm in greatest dimension limited to the thyroid
T1a: Tumour ≤1 cm in greatest dimension limited to the thyroid
T1b: Tumour >1 cm but ≤2 cm in greatest dimension limited to the thyroid
T2: Tumour >2 cm but ≤4 cm in greatest dimension limited to the thyroid
T3: Tumour >4 cm limited to the thyroid or gross extrathyroidal extension invading only strap muscles
T3a: Tumour >4 cm limited to the thyroid
T3b: Gross extrathyroidal extension invading only strap muscles (sternohyoid, sternothyroid, thyrohyoid, or omohyoid muscles) from a tumour of any size
T4: Includes gross extrathyroidal extension into major neck structures
T4a: Gross extrathyroidal extension invading subcutaneous soft tissues, larynx, trachea, oesophagus, or recurrent laryngeal nerve from a tumour of any size
T4b: Gross extrathyroidal extension invading prevertebral fascia or encasing carotid artery or mediastinal vessels from a tumour of any size

Table 3. Cont.

Regional lymph node (pN):
NX: Regional lymph nodes cannot be assessed
N0: No evidence of regional lymph node metastasis
N0a: One or more cytologic or histologically confirmed benign lymph nodes
N0b: No radiologic or clinical evidence of locoregional lymph node metastasis
N1: Metastasis to regional nodes
N1a: Metastasis to level VI or VII (pretracheal, paratracheal, prelaryngeal/Delphian or upper mediastinal) lymph nodes; this can be unilateral or bilateral disease
N1b: Metastasis to unilateral, bilateral, or contralateral lateral neck lymph nodes (levels I, II, III, IV, or V) or retropharyngeal lymph nodes
Distant metastasis (M):
M0: No distant metastasis
M1: Distant metastasis

9. Management

As for well-differentiated thyroid cancers, the initial phase is managed by the endocrinologist and the surgeon, with an adequate staging of the disease in a short time, the main requirement to correctly plan the treatment and achieve the best recurrence-free survival outcomes [7,10]. The initial diagnosis is clinical and cytohistological. The presence of rapidly growing thyroid nodule with a tendency to involve loco-regional structures (nodes), but also to eventually metastasise, is already clinically suggestive of an aggressive carcinoma. It is recommended to consider the clinical, US, and cytological major features including the rapid growth of a well-defined mass, as well as its heterogeneity and hypoechogenicity, trying to target the strong hypoechoic area when performing the FNAC. The same alert should rise for fast-growing suspicious lymph nodes, mainly at the subcortical area (where the metastatic cell nests develop; in fact, necrosis is often acellular and located centrally within the metastatic node), to give rise to the diagnosis of PDTC

Yet, as previously mentioned, cytological diagnosis of PDTC based on FNAC is challenging, in view of the rarity of the disease, the nonspecific cytological features, the overlap with cytological characteristics of follicular neoplasms, and the frequent presence of the poorly differentiated component within the well-differentiated tumour.

Elimination of PDTC can be achieved by complete surgical removal and treatment of a limited loco-regional disease, with a high remission (94.3%) [35], very close to that of well-differentiated carcinoma and superior to that of anaplastic carcinoma [36]. The increase in survival is associated with the young age (<60 years), the limited size of the tumour, the absence of distant metastases, the co-existence of a well-differentiated thyroid tumour, and a greater extension of neck surgery, as indicated in Table 4, our single centre experience. Surgical intervention in operable cases involves total thyroidectomy associated with complete recurrent and lateral cervical lymphadenectomy.

Table 4. Our single centre experience.

Pt	Sex	Age (Years)	FU (Months)	FNAC	AP (mm)	T (mm)	L (mm)	Surgery	Histology	Lymphadenectomy	pT	pN
1	M	58	60	-	-	-	-	TT	PDTC	Radical lymphadenectomy + laryngectomy	4a	0/8
2	F	85	24	4	-	-	-	TT	PDTC	Periglandular nodes	4a	1a 1/2
3	M	64	24	4	24	13	27	TT	PDTC	2 loco-regional nodes	4a	0/2
4	F	54	24	recurrence	7.5; 18.9	4.6; 8.8	11.6; 20	Nodule removal	PDTC	-	-	-
4	F	55	12	recurrence x2	0.08	0.05	0.05	Nodule removal	PDTC	-	-	-
5	M	56	12	3	46	38	41	TT	PDTC	N	3a	-
6	F	55	12	3	50.8	37.7	61.2	TT	Oncocytic	Latero-cervical II-IV	3b	1b (10/43)
7	F	80	12	-	-	-	-	TT	PDTC	Latero-cervical III-IV-VI-VIII	4	1b 6/44

AP: anteroposterior diameter; FNAC: fine-needle aspiration cytology; FU: follow-up; L: lateral diameter; pN: primary nodes; pT: primary tumour; Pt: patient; T: transversal diameter; TT: total thyroidectomy.

Our previous experience also showed that the presence of lateral cervical lymph nodes at the time of diagnosis is higher for patients older than 71 years [37], confirming the significance of age as a prognostic factor, especially in thyroid cancers.

Finally, in terms of follow-up, given the differentiation of the thyroid cell, the use of thyroglobulin dosage in the follow-up is an indicator for relapse of the disease, and for the same reason, there is support for the use of a suppressive hormone replacement therapy or for the use of radioactive iodine (even in the presence of mixed forms). This is particularly relevant in the radioiodine-resistant forms, and even though chemotherapy is currently not standard of care, emerging positive effects have been reported into two large trials [38,39], in which monoclonal antibodies, sorafenib and lenvatinib, were administered.

10. Conclusions

Poorly differentiated thyroid carcinoma diagnosis is challenging; thus, this disease might remain underdiagnosed. The Turin proposal—namely, a high mitotic index and a solid/trabecular or insular pattern, are the most broadly in use diagnostic algorithm, and it is important to determine the percentage of poorly differentiated disease to correctly estimate recurrence-free survival and plan treatment accordingly. The genetic landscape of PDTC is in continuous evolution and surgical radical treatment offers excellent survival.

Author Contributions: Conceptualization: M.I.B., M.B., L.G., V.D., R.P.; methodology: M.I.B., L.G., V.D.; validation: M.B., V.D., L.G.; formal analysis: T.G., R.M. (Rosa Menditto), A.M., M.S., L.V.; investigation: M.B., L.G.; resources: M.I.B., M.B., R.P., L.G., M.C.B., M.L.C., R.M. (Rossella Melcarne), C.S., V.D.; data curation: M.I.B., M.B., L.G., V.D.; writing: M.I.B., writing—review and editing, L.G., V.D., R.P.; supervision: L.G., V.D. All authors have read and agreed to the published version of the manuscript.

Funding: No external source funded this study.

Institutional Review Board Statement: The study, performed in accordance to the Declaration of Helsinki principles, is a retrospective analysis. The data used were anonymised; the study did not require patient or public involvement nor affected patient care. The study fell under the category of research through the use of anonymised data of existing databases which, based on the Health Research Authority criteria, does not require proportional or full ethics review and approval.

Informed Consent Statement: As a retrospective chart analysis, no informed consent was required.

Data Availability Statement: The data used to support the findings of this study are included within the article and are available on request from the corresponding author.

Conflicts of Interest: The authors declare no conflict of interest.

Abbreviations

FNAC	Fine-needle aspiration cytology
PDTC	Poorly differentiated thyroid carcinoma
TBSRTC	Bethesda System for Reporting Thyroid Cytopathology
US	Ultrasound

References

1. Kim, M.-H.; Lee, T.H.; Lee, J.S.; Lim, D.-J.; Lee, P.C.-W. Hif-1α Inhibitors Could Successfully Inhibit the Progression of Differentiated Thyroid Cancer in Vitro *Pharmaceuticals* **2020**, *13*, 208. [CrossRef]
2. Dettmer, M.; Schmitt, A.; Steinert, H.; Haldemann, A.; Meili, A.; Moch, H.; Komminoth, P.; Perren, A. Poorly differentiated thyroid carcinomas: How much poorly differentiated is needed? *Am. J. Surg. Pathol.* **2011**, *35*, 1866–1872. [CrossRef]
3. Kakudo, K.; Bai, Y.; Katayama, S.; Hirokawa, M.; Ito, Y.; Miyauchi, A.; Kuma, K. Classification of follicular cell tumors of the thyroid gland: Analysis involving Japanese patients from one institute. *Pathol. Int.* **2009**, *59*, 359–367. [CrossRef]
4. Sanders, E.M., Jr.; LiVolsi, V.A.; Brierley, J.; Shin, J.; Randolph, G.W. An evidence-based review of poorly differentiated thyroid cancer. *World J. Surg.* **2007**, *31*, 934–945.
5. Asioli, S.; Erickson, L.A.; Righi, A.; Jin, L.; Volante, M.; Jenkins, S.; Papotti, M.; Bussolati, G.; Lloyd, R.V. Poorly differentiated carcinoma of the thyroid: Validation of the Turin proposal and analysis of IMP3 expression. *Mod. Pathol.* **2010**, *23*, 1269–1278. [CrossRef] [PubMed]
6. Ibrahimpasic, T.; Ghossein, R.; Shah, J.P.; Ganly, I. Poorly Differentiated Carcinoma of the Thyroid Gland: Current Status and Future Prospects. *Thyroid* **2019**, *29*, 311–321. [CrossRef] [PubMed]
7. Lee, D.Y.; Won, J.-K.; Lee, S.-H.; Park, D.J.; Jung, K.C.; Sung, M.-W.; Wu, H.-G.; Kim, K.H.; Park, Y.J.; Hah, J.H. Changes of Clinicopathologic Characteristics and Survival Outcomes of Anaplastic and Poorly Differentiated Thyroid Carcinoma. *Thyroid* **2016**, *26*, 404–413. [CrossRef]
8. Grani, G.; Ramundo, V.; Falcone, R.; Lamartina, L.; Montesano, T.; Biffoni, M.; Giacomelli, L.; Sponziello, M.; Verrienti, A.; Schlumberger, M.; et al. Thyroid Cancer Patients with No Evidence of Disease: The Need for Repeat Neck Ultrasound. *J. Clin. Endocrinol. Metab.* **2019**, *104*, 4981–4989. [CrossRef] [PubMed]
9. Fresilli, D.; David, E.; Pacini, P.; Del Gaudio, G.; Dolcetti, V.; Lucarelli, G.; Di Leo, N.; Bellini, M.; D'Andrea, V.; Sorrenti, S.; et al. Thyroid Nodule Characterization: How to Assess the Malignancy Risk. Update of the Literature. *Diagnostics* **2021**, *11*, 1374. [CrossRef]
10. Lee, D.Y.; Won, J.-K.; Choi, H.S.; Park, D.J.; Jung, K.C.; Sung, M.-W.; Kim, K.H.; Hah, J.H.; Park, Y.J. Recurrence and Survival after Gross Total Removal of Resectable Undifferentiated or Poorly Differentiated Thyroid Carcinoma. *Thyroid* **2016**, *26*, 1259–1268. [CrossRef]
11. Hahn, S.Y.; Shin, J.H. Description and Comparison of the Sonographic Characteristics of Poorly Differentiated Thyroid Carcinoma and Anaplastic Thyroid Carcinoma. *J. Ultrasound Med.* **2016**, *35*, 1873–1879. [CrossRef] [PubMed]
12. Lacout, A.; Marcy, P.-Y. Highlights on power Doppler US of thyroid malignancy. *Radiology* **2010**, *257*, 586–587. [CrossRef]
13. Marcy, P.-Y.R.; Thariat, J.; Bozec, A.; Poissonnet, G.; Benisvy, D.; Dassonville, O. Venous obstruction of thyroid malignancy origin: The Antoine Lacassagne Institute experience. *World J. Surg. Oncol.* **2009**, *7*, 40. [CrossRef]
14. Lacout, A.; Marcy, P.Y.; Thariat, J. RE: Role of Duplex Doppler US for Thyroid Nodules: Looking for the "Sword" Sign. *Korean J. Radiol.* **2011**, *12*, 400–401. [CrossRef]
15. Dailey, M.E.; Lindsay, S.; Skahen, R. Relation of thyroid neoplasms to Hashimoto disease of the thyroid gland. *Arch. Surg.* **1955**, *70*, 291–297. [CrossRef] [PubMed]
16. Hyer, S.L.; Dandekar, P.; Newbold, K.; Haq, M.; Wechalakar, K.; Harmer, C. Thyroid cancer causing obstruction of the great veins in the neck. *World J. Surg. Oncol.* **2008**, *6*, 36. [CrossRef]
17. Ferreira, L.B.; Gimba, E.; Vinagre, J.; Sobrinho-Simões, M.; Soares, P. Molecular Aspects of Thyroid Calcification. *Int. J. Mol. Sci.* **2020**, *21*, 7718. [CrossRef]
18. Sakamoto, A.; Kasai, N.; Sugano, H. Poorly differentiated carcinoma of the thyroid. A clinicopathologic entity for a high-risk group of papillary and follicular carcinomas. *Cancer* **1983**, *52*, 1849–1855. [CrossRef]
19. Carcangiu, M.L.; Zampi, G.; Rosai, J. Poorly differentiated ("insular") thyroid carcinoma. A reinterpretation of Langhans' "wuchernde Struma". *Am. J. Surg. Pathol.* **1984**, *8*, 655–668. [CrossRef]
20. DeLellis, R.A.; Lloyd, R.V.; Heitz, P.U.; Eng, C. (Eds.) *Pathology and Genetics of Tumours of Endocrine Organs*; IARC Press: Lyon, France, 2004.
21. Volante, M.; Collini, P.; Nikiforov, Y.E.; Sakamoto, A.; Kakudo, K.; Katoh, R.; Lloyd, R.V.; LiVolsi, V.A.; Papotti, M.; Sobrinho-Simoes, M.; et al. Poorly Differentiated Thyroid Carcinoma: The Turin Proposal for the Use of Uniform Diagnostic Criteria and an Algorithmic Diagnostic Approach. *Am. J. Surg. Pathol.* **2007**, *31*, 1256–1264. [CrossRef] [PubMed]
22. Volante, M.; Bussolati, G.; Papotti, M. The story of poorly differentiated thyroid carcinoma: From Langhans' description to the Turin proposal via Juan Rosai. *Semin. Diagn. Pathol.* **2016**, *33*, 277–283. [CrossRef]

23. Hiltzik, D.; Carlson, D.L.; Tuttle, R.M.; Chuai, S.; Ishill, N.; Shaha, A.; Shah, J.P.; Singh, B.; Ghossein, R.A. Poorly differentiated thyroid carcinomas defined on the basis of mitosis and necrosis: A clinicopathologic study of 58 patients. *Cancer* **2006**, *106*, 1286–1295. [CrossRef] [PubMed]
24. Önenerk, M.; Canberk, S.; Güneş, P.; Erkan, M.; Kilicoglu, G.Z. Oncocytic variant of poorly differentiated thyroid carcinoma: "Is diagnosis possible by fine-needle aspiration?". *CytoJournal* **2016**, *13*, 23. [CrossRef] [PubMed]
25. Bellevicine, C.; Vigliar, E.; Malapelle, U.; Pisapia, P.; Conzo, G.; Biondi, B.; Vetrani, A.; Troncone, G. Cytopathologists can reliably perform ultrasound-guided thyroid fine needle aspiration: A 1-year audit on 3715 consecutive cases. *Cytopathology* **2015**, *27*, 115–121. [CrossRef]
26. Jung, C.K.; Baek, J.H. Recent Advances in Core Needle Biopsy for Thyroid Nodules. *Endocrinol. Metab.* **2017**, *32*, 407–412. [CrossRef]
27. Melo-Uribe, M.A.; Sanabria, Á.; Romero-Rojas, A.; Pérez, G.; Vargas, E.J.; Gutiérrez, V.; Abaúnza, M. The Bethesda system for reporting thyroid cytopathology in Colombia: Correlation with histopathological diagnoses in oncology and non-oncology institutions. *J. Cytol.* **2015**, *32*, 12–16. [CrossRef] [PubMed]
28. Dettmer, M.S.; Schmitt, A.; Komminoth, P.; Perren, A. Poorly differentiated thyroid carcinoma: An underdiagnosed entity. *Pathologe* **2020**, *40*, 227–234. [CrossRef]
29. Durante, C.; Tallini, G.; Puxeddu, E.; Sponziello, M.; Moretti, S.; Ligorio, C.; Cavaliere, A.; Rhoden, K.J.; Verrienti, A.; Maranghi, M.; et al. BRAF(V600E) mutation and expression of proangiogenic molecular markers in papillary thyroid carcinomas. *Eur. J. Endocrinol.* **2011**, *165*, 455–463. [CrossRef]
30. Landa, I.; Ibrahimpasic, T.; Boucai, L.; Sinha, R.; Knauf, J.A.; Shah, R.; Dogan, S.; Ricarte-Filho, J.C.; Krishnamoorthy, G.P.; Xu, B.; et al. Genomic and transcriptomic hallmarks of poorly differentiated and anaplastic thyroid cancers. *J. Clin. Investig.* **2016**, *126*, 1052–1066. [CrossRef]
31. Sykorova, V.; Dvorakova, S.; Vcelak, J.; Vaclavikova, E.; Halkova, T.; Kodetova, D.; Lastuvka, P.; Betka, J.; Vlcek, P.; Reboun, M.; et al. Search for new genetic biomarkers in poorly differentiated and anaplastic thyroid carcinomas using next generation sequencing. *Anticancer Res.* **2015**, *35*, 2029–2036.
32. Xu, B.; Ghossein, R. Genomic Landscape of poorly Differentiated and Anaplastic Thyroid Carcinoma. *Endocr. Pathol.* **2016**, *27*, 205–212. [CrossRef]
33. Amin, M.B.; Greene, F.L.; Edge, S.B.; Compton, C.C.; Gershenwald, J.E.; Brookland, R.K.; Meyer, L.; Gress, D.M.; Byrd, D.R.; Winchester, D.P. The Eighth Edition AJCC Cancer Staging Manual: Continuing to build a bridge from a population-based to a more "personalized" approach to cancer staging. *CA Cancer J. Clin.* **2017**, *67*, 93–99. [CrossRef]
34. Tuttle, R.M.; Haugen, B.; Perrier, N.D. Updated American Joint Committee on Cancer/Tumor-Node-Metastasis Staging System for Differentiated and Anaplastic Thyroid Cancer (Eighth Edition): What Changed and Why? *Thyroid* **2017**, *27*, 751–756. [CrossRef] [PubMed]
35. Ibrahimpasic, T.; Ghossein, R.; Carlson, D.L.; Chernichenko, N.; Nixon, I.; Palmer, F.L.; Lee, N.Y.; Shaha, A.R.; Patel, S.G.; Tuttle, R.M.; et al. Poorly Differentiated Thyroid Carcinoma Presenting with Gross Extrathyroidal Extension: 1986–2009 Memorial Sloan-Kettering Cancer Center Experience. *Thyroid* **2013**, *23*, 997–1002. [CrossRef] [PubMed]
36. Conzo, G.; Polistena, A.; Calò, P.G.; Bononi, P.; Gambardella, C.; Mauriello, C.; Tartaglia, E.; Avenia, S.; Sanguinetti, A.; Medas, F.; et al. Efficacy of combined treatment for anaplastic thyroid carcinoma: Results of a multinstitutional retrospective analysis. *Int. J. Surg.* **2014**, *12*, S178–S182. [CrossRef]
37. Falvo, L.; Catania, A.; Sorrenti, S.; D'Andrea, V.; Berni, A.; De Stefano, M.; De Antoni, E. Prognostic significance of the age factor in the thyroid cancer: Statistical analysis. *J. Surg. Oncol.* **2004**, *88*, 217–222. [CrossRef] [PubMed]
38. Brose, M.S.; Nutting, C.M.; Jarzab, B.; Elisei, R.; Siena, S.; Bastholt, L.; de la Fouchardiere, C.; Pacini, F.; Paschke, R.; Shong, Y.K.; et al. Sorafenib in radioactive iodine-refractory, locally advanced or metastatic differentiated thyroid cancer: A randomised, double-blind, phase 3 trial. *Lancet* **2014**, *384*, 319–328. [CrossRef]
39. Schlumberger, M.; Tahara, M.; Wirth, L.J.; Robinson, B.; Brose, M.S.; Elisei, R.; Habra, M.A.; Newbold, K.; Shah, M.H.; Hoff, A.O.; et al. Lenvatinib versus Placebo in Radioiodine-Refractory Thyroid Cancer. *N. Engl. J. Med.* **2015**, *372*, 621–630. [CrossRef]

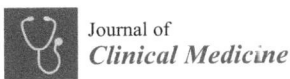

Review

The Role of CEUS in the Evaluation of Thyroid Cancer: From Diagnosis to Local Staging

Salvatore Sorrenti [1], Vincenzo Dolcetti [2], Daniele Fresilli [2], Giovanni Del Gaudio [2], Patrizia Pacini [2], Pintong Huang [3,4], Chiara Camponovo [5], Andrea Leoncini [6], Vito D'Andrea [1], Daniele Pironi [1], Fabrizio Frattaroli [7], Pierpaolo Trimboli [5,8], Maija Radzina [9,10] and Vito Cantisani [2,*]

1. Department of Surgical Sciences, Faculty of Medicine, Sapienza University of Rome, Piazzale Aldo Moro 5, 00185 Rome, Italy; salvatore.sorrenti@uniroma1.it (S.S.); vito.dandrea@uniroma1.it (V.D.); daniele.pironi@uniroma1.it (D.P.)
2. Department of Radiological, Oncological, and Pathological Sciences, Faculty of Medicine, Sapienza University of Rome, Piazzale Aldo Moro 5, 00185 Rome, Italy; vincenzodolcetti@gmail.com (V.D.); daniele.fresilli@hotmail.it (D.F.); g.d.gaudio@gmail.com (G.D.G.); patry.shepsut91@gmail.com (P.P.)
3. Department of Ultrasound in Medicine, The Second Affiliated Hospital of Zhejiang University, School of Medicine, Zhejiang University, Hangzhou 310009, China; huangpintong@zju.edu.cn
4. Research Center of Ultrasound in Medicine and Biomedical Engineering, The Second Affiliated Hospital of Zhejiang University School of Medicine, Zhejiang University, Hangzhou 310009, China
5. Clinic for Endocrinology and Diabetology, Lugano Regional Hospital, Ente Ospedaliero Cantonale (EOC), 6900 Lugano, Switzerland; Chiara.Camponovo@eoc.ch (C.C.); Pierpaolo.Trimboli@eoc.ch (P.T.)
6. Servizio di Radiologia e Radiologia Interventistica, Istituto di Imaging della Svizzera Italiana (IIMSI), Ente Ospedaliero Cantonale (EOC), 6900 Lugano, Switzerland; andrea.leoncini@eoc.ch
7. Department of Surgery "P. Stefanini", Faculty of Medicine, Sapienza University of Rome, Piazzale Aldo Moro 5, 00185 Rome, Italy; fabrizio.frattaroli@uniroma1.it
8. Faculty of Biomedical Sciences, Università della Svizzera Italiana (USI), 6900 Lugano, Switzerland
9. Radiology Research Laboratory, Riga Stradins University, LV-1007 Riga, Latvia; mradzina@gmail.com
10. Medical Faculty, University of Latvia; Diagnostic Radiology Institute, Paula Stradina Clinical University Hospital, LV-1007 Riga, Latvia
* Correspondence: vito.cantisani@uniroma1.it

Abstract: Ultrasound often represents the first diagnostic step for thyroid nodule evaluation in clinical practice, but baseline US alone is not always effective enough to achieve thyroid nodule characterization. In the last decades new ultrasound techniques, such as CEUS, have been introduced to evaluate thyroid parenchyma as recommended by EFSUMB guidelines, for use in clinical research field, although its role is not yet clear. Several papers show the potential utility of CEUS in the differential diagnosis of benign and malignant thyroid nodules and in the analysis of lymph node involvement in neoplastic pathology. Therefore, we carried out an evaluation of the literature concerning the role of CEUS in three specific areas: the characterization of the thyroid nodule, the evaluation of minimally invasive treatment and loco-regional staging of the lymph node in proven thyroid cancer. According to evidence reported, CEUS can also play an operative role in nodular thyroid pathology as it is able to guide ablation procedures on thyroid nodule and metastatic lymph nodes, to assess the radicality of surgery, to evaluate disease relapse at the level of the margins of ablated regions and to monitor the clinical evolution of necrotic areas in immediate post-treatment setting.

Keywords: thyroid nodule; CEUS; RF Ablation; thyroid nodule diagnosis; lymph node

1. Introduction

Ultrasound often represents the first diagnostic step for thyroid nodule evaluation in clinical practice. The thyroid nodule is one of the most common endocrinological disease and its incidental finding is very frequent during diagnostic neck examinations. In fact it is reported in about 10% of CT and MRI and 40–50% of ultrasound neck examinations [1,2].

It is noteworthy that the incidence of the thyroid nodule increases significantly as well as that of the malignant rate. [3]. However, baseline US alone is not always effective to achieve thyroid nodule characterization; that is why, especially in recent years, the support of other imaging modalities have become increasingly necessary to limit as much as possible the use of Fine Needle Aspiration Biopsy/Cytology, Core biopsy or even the diagnostic thyroidectomy.

CT and MRI (DWI, DCE-MRI and hybrid PET/MRI techniques) play a primary role, especially, in the visualization of deep metastatic lesions and in the evaluation of the response to treatment in non-differentiated thyroid cancer histological types [4], in the localized disease, whereas the use of Contrast-Enhanced-Ultrasonography for a second level evaluation is extensively preferable. Currently, the latest guidelines for the use of CEUS propose its employment in the evaluation of organs such as liver, kidney, testis and lymph nodes [5–8], and in the context of diagnostic procedures such as monitoring stent-graft status and in ultrasound-guided biopsies [9]. Conversely, the role of CEUS in the evaluation of nodular and diffuse thyroid pathology is not universally accepted and standardized, as it is not recommended by EFSUMB in its latest Guidelines as routine clinical practice, although it enjoys a significantly active research field [5].

The main diagnostic application of the methodology in this area of interest is represented by the characterization of the different microvascular patterns, with diagnostic accuracy superior to Color-Doppler alone [10]. Through the analysis of qualitative and quantitative parameters, CEUS is in fact able to identify pathological changes in the vascularity of both the thyroid nodule and the lymph nodes of the central and lateral compartments of the neck. CEUS is, therefore, a potentially useful tool in the differential diagnosis of benign and malignant pathologies. This is so even in the cases of nodules with indeterminate cytology, and in the analysis of lymph node involvement in neoplastic pathology. Indeed, it has been reported that increases in ultrasonographic diagnostic accuracy, especially if associated with factor BRAF V600E [11,12] or integrated with superb microvascular imaging (SMI) [13], ultrasound elastography and shear wave elastography [14].

CEUS can also play an operative role as well as a diagnostic one in nodular thyroid pathology: in fact, it can be used to guide ablation procedures on thyroid nodule and metastatic lymph nodes, to study the radicality of surgery, to evaluate the disease relapse at the level of the margins of ablated regions and to monitor the clinical evolution of necrotic areas in the immediate post-operative setting. [15,16].

Therefore, the purpose of this work was to carry out a narrative literature review on the role of CEUS regarding three specific areas: (1) characterization of the thyroid nodule; (2) evaluation of minimally invasive treatment (above all in percutaneous laser, microwave and radiofrequency ablation); (3) loco-regional staging of the lymph node in proven thyroid cancer patients.

2. Materials and Methods

The study was conducted mainly focusing on papers published over the last decade, as these are based on stronger scientific evidence and larger samples on which to perform retrospective studies with greater statistical significance. Research on online databases such as PubMed and Google Scholar was performed:

- to evaluate the role of CEUS in discriminating benign from malignant thyroid nodules using "CEUS or Contrast-Enhanced Ultrasonography" and "thyroid nodule or thyroid cancer" as MESH terms;
- to investigate the role of CEUS in evaluating the efficacy of treatment performed on thyroid nodules and nodal involvement the MESH terms "CEUS or Contrast-Enhanced Ultrasonography" and "thyroid nodule or thyroid cancer" and "after treatment" were used. Additionally, to evaluate the actual effectiveness of CEUS in detecting nodal metastatic involvement "CEUS or Contrast-Enhanced Ultrasonography" and "thyroid cancer lymph nodes or thyroid metastatic lymph nodes or thyroid cancer lymphatic nodes" were used as MESH terms. In this case, 118 studies were

identified from January 2010, but only 80 of them were retrieved because of their true adherence to the topic.

3. Results and Discussion
3.1. CEUS r in the Diagnosis of Thyroid Nodule

Even if conventional US is recognized as the pivotal diagnostic tool to characterize thyroid nodules, some limitations, such as low reproducibility and operator-dependent performance, may reduce its diagnostic value. Furthermore, several additional US applications, including CEUS, have been reported recently in order to improve US performance in the diagnosis of thyroid nodule. In fact, CEUS actually allows us to enhance the microvascular blood flow of the nodule and then assess perfusion and vascular distribution in real time during the US examination [17]. Unfortunately, the technique has not as yet been fully standardized, there are no fixed references for quantitative or qualitative assessment and, importantly, no single CEUS parameter seems to be sensitive and specific enough for a diagnosis of malignancy. However, while the thyroid gland is rich in microvessels and after the injection of contrast agent, the parenchyma of normal thyroid exhibits rapid uniform enhancement, the vascular structures of nodules reveal enhancement in contrast with that of normal tissue [18]. These characteristics can enable the use of CEUS in the diagnosis of thyroid cancer.

Several studies showed that malignant nodules have specific CEUS enhancement patterns (i.e., heterogeneous or low enhancement) [19,20] and some relevant meta-analyses found a good level of performance for CEUS when discriminating thyroid cancer from benign lesions. One systematic review with meta-analysis [21] included articles reporting data regarding 1515 thyroid nodules with histological diagnoses only and their pre-operative CEUS evaluations. This study recorded a pooled sensitivity, specificity, positive predictive value and negative predictive value for CEUS of 85%, 82%, 83% and 85%, respectively, without inconsistency of sensitivity and with mild inconsistency of specificity [21]. A second meta-analysis, including further preliminary studies and comprehensive heterogeneity analyses carried out to assess the performance of CEUS in identifying benign and malignant thyroid nodules, confirmed that CEUS yielded high pooled sensitivity and specificity (87% and 83%) with an AUC of 0.92, indicating that it might be a tool of considerable value in the diagnosis of thyroid nodules [22]. However, there also existed a considerable heterogeneity between the studies included, which might compromise the reliability of the results [22]. This meta-analysis concluded that CEUS might provide high accuracy for the identification of thyroid nodules, but that there is still insufficient evidence that the features of CEUS can improve the diagnostic accuracy of US imaging reporting systems (such as TIRADS) at present [22]. In addition to these evidence-based data, the diagnostic value of CEUS regarding specific clusters of nodules, such as thyroid lesions with calcification, has been said to score high when selecting those in which biopsy is indicated [23]. Anyway, these results have been confirmed by all the studies [24]. It is important to note that the features of CEUS were closely related to nodule size in several studies; Yuan et al. indicated that patterns of real-time CEUS are significantly different when it comes to discerning between benign and malignant thyroid nodules, and have important clinical value [25]. Ma et al. showed that heterogeneous enhancement was an independent predictor of papillary thyroid microcarcinoma [26]. Xu et al. reported that TIRADS classification plus CEUS may be more accurate than TIRADS classification alone [27].

In addition to the above findings in literature regarding clinical applications of CEUS, some general considerations should be taken into account about its use to discriminate between thyroid cancer and benign thyroid nodules. It is well acknowledged that CEUS is associated with a rate of adverse events close to zero (1:10,000 vs. 1–12:100 of iodinated contrast agents) [5]. CEUS has a reasonable cost in many countries but is expensive in others. Only one nodule can be evaluated for each injection of contrast agent. To date, no established criterion for the patterns of enhancement and classification of thyroid nodules exists, so that it cannot be widely used worldwide [18]. Finally, CEUS is not included in any TIRADS, making it controversial in clinical practice [28].

3.2. The Role of CEUS in the Evaluation of Thyroid Nodules after Thermal Ablation and Radioactive Iodine Therapy

Traditionally surgery has been the main option for the treatment of thyroid nodules, however it presents several drawbacks, such as general anesthesia, scarring and the risk of induced hypothyroidism [29]. Thermal ablation has been increasingly applied in recent years to reduce the invasiveness of treatment in patients with benign thyroid nodules, recurrent thyroid cancer and metastatic cervical lymph nodes. Among the image-guided thermal ablation techniques available for solid- and mixed-structure nodules, the most commonly used are the following-laser (LA) and radiofrequency ablation (RFA) [30,31], microwave ablation [15,32,33], and the latest one introduced-high-frequency ultrasound (HIFU) [34,35]. Ultrasound (US) guided non-thermal ethanol ablation is performed in predominantly cystic nodules [36]. Some guidelines and documents expressing consensus suggest the use of image-guided thermal ablation as an alternative to surgery in patients with symptomatic thyroid nodules, more recently as first-line treatment [29,37,38]. At present, many studies have indicated a role for thermal ablation in primary thyroid microcarcinoma (PTMC) with low recurrence rate [39]. All diseases and their treatment require proper follow-up period selection, clinically relevant history data and knowledge about expected outcomes. Ultrasound is one of the most accessible methods for this purpose with all its multiparametric-spectrum advantages.

3.2.1. Benign Nodules

One should be aware of the strict criteria regarding the use of thermal ablation procedures when seeking expected findings during follow-up examinations. Thyroid nodules should be symptomatic or cause mass effect and need to be confirmed as benign with at least two US-guided fine-needle aspirations (FNA) or core-needle biopsy (CNB) before treatment. A single benign diagnosis on FNA or CNB is sufficient when the nodule presents US features highly specific for benignity (isoechoic spongiform nodules or partially cystic nodules) or in the case of an autonomously functioning thyroid nodule (AFTN) at very low risk of malignancy (less than 1%) [40]. The most important indicator of the efficacy of treatment is reduction of the thyroid nodule's volume after treatment. Reported mean data for thermal ablation varies from 50.7 to 93.5% of volume reduction [41].

Percutaneous ethanol injection (PEI) has been used for decades in thyroid nodule treatment [36] since it presents shorter procedure time and less periprocedural pain than thermal ablative procedures [42]. PEI efficacy is mainly related to proportion of solid and cystic component and is reported to be effective in the treatment of cystic nodules, especially with cystic components of >90% [43]. Reported volume reduction has been observed in 82.4–96.9% cases of cystic nodules and 65.8–86.2% in predominantly cystic nodules. This can be explained by the fact that solid components are thought to be more resistant to ethanol and that increased vascularity of nodules increases the drainage of ethanol [44].

Nevertheless, the best treatment modality for predominantly cystic thyroid nodules is still under debate because the reported recurrence rate after PEI is 26–38.3% [45], therefore, a combination of both methods may be advised for benign thyroid nodules.

Even though thermal ablation is a safe and effective procedure in predominantly solid nodules, the pattern of regrowth from margins can occur during follow-up, with a rate of 5.5% and 9% for RFA and laser ablation, respectively [46,47]. Rarely, nodules disappear completely, generally leaving scar tissue–which appears predominantly hypoechoic or has hyperechoic areas in the center of the area treated. Follow-up periods can affect study results concerning volume reduction [48]. As the size of thyroid nodules reduces gradually-mostly rapidly at the end of the first month and continues further up until at least 6–36 months. In the literature examined the primary outcome of image-guided thermal ablations was associated with a volume reduction ratio (VRR) of 60%, 66%, 62% and 53%

at months 6, 12, 24 and 36. On the whole, RFA was associated with a VRR of 68%, 75% and 87%, respectively. Laser ablation was associated with a VRR of 48%, 52%, 45% and 44%, respectively. [21], suggestive of clinically significant and long-lasting volume reduction of benign thyroid nodules with some risk of regrowth (20% in the RFA and 38% in the LA) and needing lower retreatment after RFA over a 5-year follow-up period associated with a young age, large baseline volume and treatment with low-energy delivery [30]. Further promising results are also shown in the use of HIFU in a study by Trimboli et al., a reduction of at least 50% was observed at months 6, 12 and 24 in 6.4%, 16.1% and 22.5% nodules, respectively [34], while reduction of volume of 31.5% and 31.9% at 12 and 36 months, respectively, was observed in a European multicenter study [35].

US is the most widely used imaging modality for the assessment of early signs of a potential future regrowth of a nodule. Usually, the efficacy of an ablation technique is defined in terms of volume reduction >50% of the initial volume and is evaluated at one year after treatment [31,47]. Recently, some authors introduced the initial ablation ratio (IAR) as a quantitative early indicator correlated with the reduction ratio of volume during follow-up [31]. In their paper, Sim et al. evaluated the IAR identifying the ablated area on standard B-mode ultrasound images [47]. According to this study, IAR is the ratio of the ablated volume to the total volume of the nodule. If the IAR after RFA is <70%, the nodule is likely to regrow [47]. However, some limitations of US, such as low reproducibility and operator-depending performance and measuring, might reduce its accuracy in the evaluation of the ablated volume of the thyroid nodule. In particular, the ablated area can be difficult to demarcate clearly with B-mode, as it can appear as an isoechoic area compared with nonablated surrounding thyroid tissue. In these cases, a contrast-enhanced ultrasound (CEUS) is advocated after ablation to better identify the necrotic area, showing reduction in the variation of measurements and may impact on IAR definition in thyroid ablations [5].

CEUS is applied in some centers to precisely delineate the ablated area in thyroid nodules treated with image-guided thermal ablation (Figure 1a–d) [49,50]. In addition, US contrast agents can be directly administered to complete a standard US examination. They are safe, requires no preliminary blood testing and are well tolerated by patients. [50]. Ma et al. [51] evaluated the single-session complete ablation rate of US-guided percutaneous laser ablations for benign thyroid nodules and found that all decreased from the original size within 1 day after ablation and suggested CEUS as the main method for the evaluation of treatment efficacy. During the procedure, if CEUS shows nodules with a small amount of residual tissue at the edge, the patient requires further ablation treatment until the remnants of the lesion disappear completely. CEUS helps to clarify boundaries between viable and nonviable tissue. This might prove helpful when seeking a more precise and reproducible measure of the ablated area right after the ablation procedure and e during follow up imaging-early (3 months) and intermediate term (6 and 12 months) are the intervals suggested for follow-up with subsequent monitoring for up to 1–2 years, in order to reveal regrowth [38]. Follow-up periods can be discontinued if treated nodules disappear completely or remain as small scarring tissue [48].

3.2.2. Malignant Nodules and Lymph Nodes

In cases of PTMC the retrospective studies have reported minor recurrence rates, e.g., from Yan et al. with the largest sample sizes (414 cases), the overall incidence of local tumor progression rate after RFA was only 3.62% including LNM (0.97%) and recurrence PTMC (2.42%) [39]. In addition, the patients who received additional RFA achieved good therapeutic results during follow-up. However, in a recent study, compared with PTMC, PTC (diameter > 10 mm, T1bN0M0) patients who were enrolled to undergo the TA had a relatively higher residual lesion and LNM ratio (3.03%, two in 66 cases 1.52%, one in 66 cases, respectively) [52].

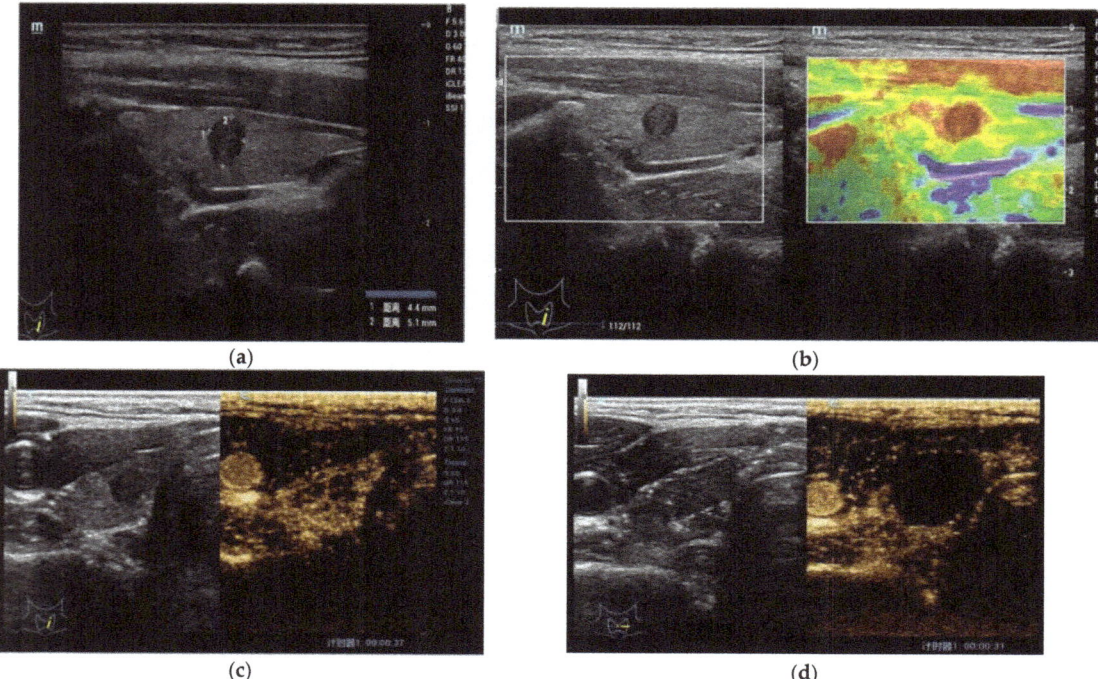

Figure 1. (**a**) At B-mode US, the shape of the lesion appeared taller-than-wide, hypoechoic with regular margins without internal microcalcifications (EU-TIRADS 5); (**b**) At qualitative USE evaluation, the lesion appeared stiff (completely red in the color box); (**c**) At CEUS evaluation, the lesion appeared richly vascularized similar to surrounding thyroid parenchyma without strong wash-out. At FNAC the lesion was classified as Tir 5. (**d**) After Radiofrequency Ablation, the lesion and surrounding parenchyma does not show enhancement in the CEUS mode.

In cases of Primary Thyroid Microcarcinoma (PTMC) Zhang et al. suggested that the characteristics of high specificity, sensitivity and accuracy of CEUS might also be applied to the postoperative evaluation of PTMC and at the same time, used to access the exact ablation zone and detect the residual enhancement of suspicious lesions [53]. Even though, the postoperative pathology reports confirmed the presence of incomplete ablation in all cases where 66.7% of them presented LNM. Therefore, the authors concluded that thermal ablation should be recommended with caution as a treatment for operable patients with PTC. Of the thermal treatment methods, RFA yielded a relatively lower complete ablation rate compared with MWA and LA in recently published research. This phenomenon might be explained as follows: first, a part of the macro-calcification might not have been totally ablated, secondly, MWA is rarely affected by the heat-sink effect (local cooling of the thermal process by adjacent blood flow) that is thought to contribute to incomplete ablation and local recurrence after RFA [54]. The use of US and contrast-enhanced ultrasound (CEUS) examinations before ablation, in a study by Zhang et al. of 92 cases, confirmed by core biopsy before and after treatment, revealed that RFA can effectively eliminate low-risk PTMC with no signs of recurrence or residual tumor during follow-up periods of up to 12–18 months [55]. In a critical view of the satisfactory results of residual volume, there were great differences in the absorption rate, ranging from 10.2% to 100%, after thermal ablation in different trials [52]. PTMC is a slowly progressing disease and requires a longer and more active follow-up period to verify the efficacy of treatment [33]. Two main criteria are mandatory to evaluate ablated tissue vascularity and serum thyroglobulin (Tg) levels. Vascularity may be assessed by imaging: computed tomography [56], magnetic resonance imaging within staging protocol [57] and Color Doppler ultrasound or CEUS-loss of color signal or absence of contrast uptake within a treated lesion that was previously vascularized is adequate evidence of appropriate thermal coagulation.

The main features to be assessed in ultrasonography are: changes in nodule size, echogenicity and vascularity. Ablation areas are hypoechoic and tend to reduce in sizes. The presence of intra-nodal vascularity after RFA is an important indicator of the need to repeat the RFA procedure [58] because it should disappear in fully ablated regions. In a study a of the prognostic value of CEUS, patterns and tumor size, a comparison was made between extrathyroid extension (ETE) and non-ETE groups showing that the time from peak to one-half tumor size and wash-in slope were significantly different between the ETE and non-ETE groups [44]. Xiang et al. [59] evaluated the CEUS in the detection of neck lymph node metastasis for papillary thyroid carcinoma. The results approved heterogeneous enhancement, perfusion defects, microcalcification and centripetal/hybrid enhancement as specific criteria for malignant lymph nodes.

Hypo-enhancement and absent enhancement are considered major CEUS patterns characteristic of malignant thyroid nodules [23,60–62], and absent enhancement especially for thyroid tumors of 10 mm or less in diameter. The main reason that malignant thyroid tumors show a lack of blood supply is related to their complex neovascularization-once the growth becomes greater than neovascularization, tumor necrosis and embolus formation leads to hypo-enhancement on CEUS. Moreover, Zhou et al. [63] found that instead of hypo-enhancement, the nodule-to-perinodule peak intensity ratio showed the best diagnostic efficiency, with an optimal cut-off value of 0.9 [15].

In conclusion, CEUS is a precise tool before and after thyroid treatment, to use to assess the margins of recent ablation or recurrence but overlapping data between CEUS qualitative and quantitative evaluation parameters and criteria of benign and malignant features indicate a limitation in the interpretation of the nodules after treatment and create difficulties when interpreting tumor microvascularity interpretation. No single indicator is sufficiently sensitive or specific [5]. Therefore, the results should be interpreted in conjunction with clinical and case-history data, conventional US and the findings of other imaging examinations if one is to improve diagnostic accuracy in the assessment of thyroid nodules after treatment.

3.2.3. Radioactive Iodine Therapy (RAI)

In patients operated for papillary thyroid carcinoma (PTC), US should be used a few months later in all patients as part of the investigation defining the response to adjuvant therapy with radioactive iodine (RAI) therapy [64–66]. After this first assessment, the American Thyroid Association (ATA) [65] and the European Thyroid Association (ETA) [64] only exclude the need for repeat US in patients (1) with low-risk rates, (2) with excellent response to therapy and (3) with persistently negative unstimulated Tg (u-Tg) and anti-Tg antibodies (TgAb). Even in these cases, the recommendation of repeating a US at least every 12–24 months within the first 5 years has recently been reiterated [66]. However, US frequently reveals false positive lesions that raise patient concern and required fine-needle aspiration (FNA) [67]. Most patients with PTC (except high-risk ones) will not develop disease after treatment with RAI [65]. Consequently, the detection of a neck recurrence requires that a US be performed in many patients as well as several examinations per patient [67], sometimes followed by FNA, resulting in unnecessary expenditure. These cases might be the subject of possible CEUS evaluation pre and post RAI.

In patients with macroscopically complete tumor resection who have recently received RAI, a postoperative US (before RAI) has been shown to be a valuable procedure [64–66,68,69] and CEUS may bring an added value. The indication of a US could be selective in the first years after RAI when postoperative US has ruled out persistent neck disease after total thyroidectomy, e.g., Rosario et al. [70] suggests that low- or intermediate-risk patients with papillary thyroid carcinoma without persistent disease after total thyroidectomy (including postoperative US and whole-body scanning) do not require repeated US examinations during the first two years after treatment with RAI. In the following years and up until the fifth year, this imaging method can be restricted to patients with u-Tg $\geq$ 1 ng/mL [67] and seems to be unnecessary in patients with undetectable Tg and TgAb.

3.3. Evaluation of Lymph-Node Local Staging Using CEUS

A correct locoregional staging of thyroid cancer through the identification of metastatic lymph nodes (LN) is essential for proper clinical and surgical management, for the treatment plan and the prognostic evaluation. Metastases from thyroid carcinoma, especially in papillary thyroid cancer (PTC) which is the most common thyroid cancer, are found in 20–50% of all cases, even in small or occult neoplastic nodules [71]. Patients with cervical lymph node metastasis (CLNM) increase the recurrence risk of PTC, and associated PTC-related death [72]. A key role in detecting pathological lymph nodes is played by ultrasound, which is more effective than mere physical examination through the palpation of the neck. At the same time, it is very effective from a cost-benefit point of view due to its widespread diffusion and accessibility. Compared to the other techniques used for the evaluation of the lymph nodes (CT, MRI techniques and PET), it turns out to be the cheapest and least invasive. This is true also during the follow-up phase [73]. Moreover, ultrasound contrast agents can be used in patients with impaired renal function and have a lower incidence of severe allergic reactions than CT and MRI contrast agents [74].

The main B-mode sonographic features of neoplastic lymph nodes are a long-axis diameter to short-axis diameter ratio (L/S ratio) of lesser than 2, a round shape, fatty hilum loss, hyper-echogenicity and the presence of calcifications and cystic components. However, all these signs can coexist both in healthy and pathological lymph nodes or have low specificity for malignancy [74]. Furthermore, there is a large discrepancy of results among the studies that analyze the effectiveness of preoperative ultrasound in the diagnosis of CLNM. As shown in the Zhao et al. and Li et al. meta-analysis, preoperative ultrasound demonstrates an intermediate sensitivity and a good but not excellent diagnostic efficacy in the diagnosis of central and lateral CLNM of PTC [75].

Thus, nowadays, CEUS might improve ultrasound diagnostic accuracy for cervical lymph node staging after PTC diagnosis. In fact, CEUS can be useful for the characterization of focal US alterations in patients with suspicious LN metastatic involvement. Specifically, CEUS emphasizes the micro-vascularization of the lymph node, where perfusion defects are a sign of metastatic involvement: poor or absent vascularization can be identified in widespread metastatic infiltration, corresponding to large areas of necrosis [8]. CEUS might also be useful for characterizing focal cortical thickening identified on grey-scale ultrasonography. Metastatic deposits are less vascularized than the adjacent nodal parenchyma, which is more evident during the parenchymal phase due to earlier contrast washout. On the contrary, more often focal thickening in benign LN displays the same enhancement features as the adjacent nodal tissue [8]. Furthermore, to improve differentiation between benign and metastatic LN perfusion kinetics has been examined too. Benign LN shows a centrifugal progression of enhancement, while a prominent centripetal enhancement is more often observed in a metastatic LN. By analysing signal time-intensity curves and the parametric images obtained through the perfusion parameters, it has also been noted that in metastatic LN compared to non-pathological LN, the difference between peak signal intensity in hyper enhancing and hypo enhancing regions is emphasized more [76].

In most of these studies the conventional US and CEUS combination is compared to histological examinations (by dissection, gun biopsy) or FNA cytology as gold standard. Hong et al. found some US and CEUS parameters useful in differential diagnosis between benign vs. metastatic LN with high specificity and statistical significance. In particular: L/S ratio < 2, ill-defined margins, hyper-echogenicity, cystic necrosis, calcification and peripheral vascularity are found at baseline US; meanwhile, centripetal or asynchronous perfusion (Figure 2a,b), non- or hyper-enhancement, perfusion defects and ring enhancing margins are found using CEUS; lymph nodes with one or more of the previous features are considered metastatic [77].

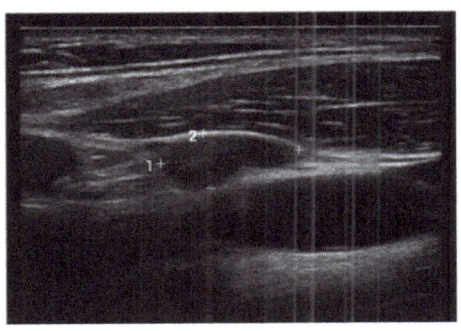 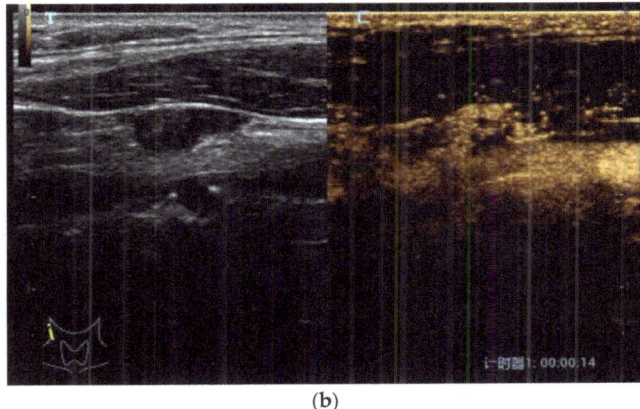

(a) (b)

Figure 2. (a) At B-mode US in Patient with papillary thyroid carcinoma, a laterocervical node showed irregular shape, hypoechoic aspect and regular margins with no internal microcalcifications or cystic changes (low metastatic risk); (b) At CEUS, the laterocervical node presented rich heterogeneous and centripetal vascularization (high metastatic risk). The histological examination confirmed that it was a metastatic node of a papillary thyroid cancer.

The six largest studies regarding differentiation between benign and metastatic cervical lymp nodes, conducted between 2014 and 2019, show that CEUS has a good diagnostic accuracy superior to standard US and Color-Doppler grayscale alone [59,74,77–79] (Table 1).

Table 1. Comparison of the papers based on the number of patients included in each single study and on the number of patients with at least one malignant nodule detected using CEUS; the values for sensitivity, specificity, PPV and NPV were obtained though comparison with the histological examination.

Authors of the Studies	Total Patients	Patients ± Total Patients	Sensitivity (%)	Specificity (%)	PPV [1]	NPV [2]	Accuracy
Xiang et al. [59]	82	65/82	82%	65%	90%	48%	79%
Zhan et al. [74]	56	33/56	65%	100%	100%	63%	78%
Hong et al. [77]	573	253/573	85%	94%	94%	86%	89%
Wang et al. [78]	285	102/285	67%	64–85% [3]	-	-	-
Chen et al. [79]	206	46/206	90%	89%	90%	86%	89%
Tao et al. [4] [80]	275	127/275	72%	74%	70%	75%	73%

[1] Positive Predictive Value; [2] Negative Predictive Value; [3] The study divides patients into two groups, PTC (>10 mm), PTMC (<10 mm); [4] The evaluation is based on a prediction model combining both the parameters obtained from the CEUS and clinical parameters.

Furthermore, both Hong et al. and Chen et al. demonstrate how a combination of US and CEUS is more accurate on the whole than any of these two techniques used individually: the Hong et al. paper reported a detected a B mode US + CEUS accuracy of 92.2% (vs. 89.3% of CEUS and 84.6% of grayscale US alone) [77]; the Chen et al. paper reported a B mode US + CEUS accuracy of 92.7% (vs. 89.1% of CEUS and 80.0% of grayscale US alone) [79].

In addition, Zhan et al. proved that homogeneity, cystic change or calcification and above, all peak-time intensity, were the three strongest independent predictors for CLNM using CEUS [74]. However, only one previous study showed that no single conventional ultrasonography or CEUS characteristics were conclusive enough to distinguish metastatic thyroid nodules from indolent ones; anyway iso- or hypo-enhancements at peak time, especially in combination with several other parameters, might still be good predictors for CLNM prognoses in PTC patients [81].

In conclusion, although the studies published to date are still too few, besides being based on limited sample populations and the sensitivity and specificity values reported are quite inhomogeneous, it is possible to state that CEUS could play a role in loco-regional lymph-node evaluation in patients with malignant thyroid nodule.

Author Contributions: Conceptualization, S.S., V.C. and V.D. (Vito D'Andrea); methodology, V.C.; software, P.H.; validation, S.S., V.C. and D.F.; formal analysis, V.C., M.R., P.T. and V.D. (Vincenzo Dolcetti); investigation, C.C.; data curation, C.C., V.D., G.D.G. and P.P.; writing—original draft preparation, M.R., P.T. and V.D. (Vincenzo Dolcetti); writing—review and editing, S.S., D.P., F.F., A.L., V.D. (Vito D'Andrea), V.C. and D.F.; supervision, S.S. and V.C.; project administration, V.C. All authors have read and agreed to the published version of the manuscript.

Funding: This research received no external funding.

Informed Consent Statement: Not applicable.

Acknowledgments: Renzo Mocini for English Editing.

Conflicts of Interest: Vito Cantisani declares to have lectured for Bracco, Samsung and Canon; the other authors declare no conflict of interest.

References

1. Nachiappan, A.C.; Metwalli, Z.A.; Hailey, B.S.; Patel, R.A.; Ostrowski, M.L.; Wynne, D.M. The Thyroid: Review of Imaging Features and Biopsy Techniques with Radiologic-Pathologic Correlation. *RadioGraphics* **2014**, *34*, 276–293. [CrossRef]
2. Xie, C.; Cox, P.; Taylor, N.; LaPorte, S. Ultrasonography of thyroid nodules: A pictorial review. *Insights Imaging* **2016**, *7*, 77–86. [CrossRef]
3. Mohorea, I.S.; Socea, B.; Șerban, D.; Ceausu, Z.; Tulin, A.; Melinte, V.; Ceausu, M. Incidence of thyroid carcinomas in an extended retrospective study of 526 autopsies. *Exp. Ther. Med.* **2021**, *21*, 607. [CrossRef]
4. Kushchayev, S.V.; Kushchayeva, Y.S.; Tella, S.H.; Glushko, T.; Pacak, K.; Teytelboym, O.M. Medullary Thyroid Carcinoma: An Update on Imaging. *J. Thyroid Res.* **2019**, *2019*, 1893047. [CrossRef]
5. Sidhu, P.S.; Cantisani, V.; Dietrich, C.F.; Gilja, O.H.; Saftoiu, A.; Bartels, E.; Bertolotto, M.; Calliada, F.; Clevert, D.A.; Cosgrove, D.; et al. The EFSUMB Guidelines and Recommendations for the Clinical Practice of Contrast-Enhanced Ultrasound (CEUS) in Non-Hepatic Applications: Update 2017 (Long Version). *Ultraschall Med.* **2018**, *39*, e2–e44, English. [CrossRef]
6. Dietrich, C.F.; Nolsøe, C.P.; Barr, R.G.; Berzigotti, A.; Burns, P.N.; Cantisani, V.; Chammas, M.C.; Chaubal, N.; Choi, B.I.; Clevert, D.A.; et al. Guidelines and Good Clinical Practice Recommendations for Contrast-Enhanced Ultrasound (CEUS) in the Liver-Update 2020 WFUMB in Cooperation with EFSUMB, AFSUMB, AIUM, and FLAUS. *Ultrasound Med. Biol.* **2020**, *46*, 2579–2604. [CrossRef]
7. Ricci, P.; Laghi, A.; Cantisani, V.; Paolantonio, P.; Pacella, S.; Pagliara, E.; Arduini, F.; Pasqualini, V.; Trippa, F.; Filpo, M.; et al. Contrast-enhanced sonography with SonoVue: Enhancement patterns of benign focal liver lesions and correlation with dynamic gadobenate dimeglumine-enhanced MRI. *AJR Am. J. Roentgenol.* **2005**, *184*, 821–827. [CrossRef]
8. Cantisani, V.; Bertolotto, M.; Weskott, H.P.; Romanini, L.; Grazhdani, H.; Passamonti, M.; Drudi, F.M.; Malpassini, F.; Isidori, A.; Meloni, F.M.; et al. Growing indications for CEUS: The kidney, testis, lymph nodes, thyroid, prostate, and small bowel. *Eur. J. Radiol.* **2015**, *84*, 1675–1684. [CrossRef]
9. Cantisani, V.; Grazhdani, H.; Clevert, D.A.; Iezzi, R.; Aiani, L.; Martegani, A.; Fanelli, F.; Di Marzo, L.; Wlderk, A.; Cirelli, C.; et al. EVAR: Benefits of CEUS for monitoring stent-graft status. *Eur. J. Radiol.* **2015**, *84*, 1658–1665. [CrossRef]
10. Cantisani, V.; Consorti, F.; Guerrisi, A.; Guerrisi, I.; Ricci, P.; Di Segni, M.; Mancuso, E.; Scardella, L.; Milazzo, F.; D'Ambrosio, F.; et al. Prospective comparative evaluation of quantitative-elastosonography (Q-elastography) and contrast-enhanced ultrasound for the evaluation of thyroid nodules: Preliminary experience. *Eur. J. Radiol.* **2013**, *82*, 1892–1898. [CrossRef]
11. Zhan, J.; Zhang, L.H.; Yu, Q.; Li, C.L.; Chen, Y.; Wang, W.P.; Ding, H. Prediction of cervical lymph node metastasis with contrast-enhanced ultrasound and association between presence of BRAFV600E and extrathyroidal extension in papillary thyroid carcinoma. *Ther. Adv. Med. Oncol.* **2020**, *12*. [CrossRef] [PubMed]
12. Zhu, X.; Peng, X.; Zhu, L.; Xie, L.; Cheng, F.; Zhou, B. Evaluation of the diagnostic performance of contrast-enhanced ultrasound combined with BRAF V600E gene detection in nodules of unclear significance by thyroid fine-needle aspiration. *Gland Surg.* **2021**, *10*, 328–335. [CrossRef] [PubMed]
13. Lu, R.; Meng, Y.; Zhang, Y.; Zhao, W.; Wang, X.; Jin, M.; Guo, R. Superb microvascular imaging (SMI) compared with conventional ultrasound for evaluating thyroid nodules. *BMC Med. Imaging* **2017**, *17*, 65. [CrossRef]

14. Gay, S.; Schiaffino, S.; Santamorena, G.; Massa, B.; Ansaldo, G.; Turtulici, G.; Giusti, M. Thyroid Team at the Policlinico San Martino, Genoa. Role of Strain Elastography and Shear-Wave Elastography in a Multiparametric Clinical Approach to Indeterminate Cytology Thyroid Nodules. *Med. Sci. Monit.* **2018**, *24*, 6273–6279. [CrossRef]
15. Zhang, L.; Zhou, W.; Zhan, W.; Peng, Y.; Jiang, S.; Xu, S. Percutaneous Laser Ablation of Unifocal Papillary Thyroid Microcarcinoma: Utility of Conventional Ultrasound and Contrast-Enhanced Ultrasound in Assessing Local Therapeutic Response. *World J. Surg.* **2018**, *42*, 2476–2484. [CrossRef] [PubMed]
16. Zhang, L.; Zhou, W.; Zhan, W. Role of ultrasound in the assessment of percutaneous laser ablation of cervical metastatic lymph nodes from thyroid carcinoma. *Acta Radiol.* **2018**, *59*, 434–440. [CrossRef]
17. Greis, C. Quantitative evaluation of microvascular blood flow by contrast-enhanced ultrasound (CEUS). *Clin. Hemorheol. Microcirc.* **2011**, *49*, 137–149. [CrossRef]
18. Giusti, M.; Orlandi, D.; Melle, G.; Massa, B.; Silvestri, E.; Miruto, F.; Turtulici, G. Is there a real diagnostic impact of elastosonography and contrast-enhanced ultrasonography in the management of thyroid nodules? *J. Zhejiang Univ. Sci. B* **2013**, *14*, 195–206. [CrossRef]
19. Zhang, Y.; Zhou, P.; Tian, S.M.; Zhao, Y.F.; Li, J.L.; Li, L. Usefulness of combined use of contrast-enhanced ultrasound and TI-RADS classification for the differentiation of benign from malignant lesions of thyroid nodules. *Eur. Radiol.* **2017**, *27*, 1527–1536. [CrossRef] [PubMed]
20. Wang, Y.; Nie, F.; Liu, T.; Yang, D.; Li, Q.; Li, J.; Song, A. Revised Value of Contrast-Enhanced Ultrasound for Solid Hypo-Echoic Thyroid Nodules Graded with the Thyroid Imaging Reporting and Data System. *Ultrasound Med. Biol.* **2018**, *44*, 930–940. [CrossRef]
21. Trimboli, P.; Castellana, M.; Virili, C.; Havre, R.F.; Bini, F.; Marinozzi, F.; D'Ambrosio, F.; Giorgino, F.; Giovanella, L.; Prosch, H.; et al. Performance of contrast-enhanced ultrasound (CEUS) in assessing thyroid nodules: A systematic review and meta-analysis using histological standard of reference. *Radiol. Med.* **2020**, *125*, 406–415. [CrossRef]
22. Zhang, J.; Zhang, X.; Meng, Y.; Chen, Y. Contrast-enhanced ultrasound for the differential diagnosis of thyroid nodules: An updated meta-analysis with comprehensive heterogeneity analysis. *PLoS ONE* **2020**, *15*, e0231775. [CrossRef]
23. Jiang, J.; Shang, X.; Wang, H.; Xu, Y.B.; Gao, Y.; Zhou, Q. Diagnostic value of contrast-enhanced ultrasound in thyroid nodules with calcification. *Kaohsiung J. Med. Sci.* **2015**, *31*, 138–144. [CrossRef]
24. Friedrich-Rust, M.; Sperber, A.; Holzer, K.; Diener, J.; Grünwald, F.; Badenhoop, K.; Weber, S.; Kriener, S.; Herrmann, E.; Bechstein, W.O.; et al. Real-time elastography and contrast-enhanced ultrasound for the assessment of thyroid nodules. *Exp. Clin. Endocrinol. Diabetes* **2010**, *118*, 602–609. [CrossRef]
25. Yuan, Z.; Quan, J.; Yunxiao, Z.; Jian, C.; Zhu, H. Contrast-enhanced ultrasound in the diagnosis of solitary thyroid nodules. *J. Cancer Res. Ther.* **2015**, *11*, 41–45. [CrossRef]
26. Ma, H.J.; Yang, J.C.; Leng, Z.P.; Chang, Y.; Kang, H.; Teng, L.H. Preoperative prediction of papillary thyroid microcarcinoma via multiparameter ultrasound. *Acta Radiol.* **2017**, *58*, 1303–1311. [CrossRef]
27. Xu, Y.; Qi, X.; Zhao, X.; Ren, W.; Ding, W. Clinical diagnostic value of contrast-enhanced ultrasound and TI-RADS classification for benign and malignant thyroid tumors: One comparative cohort study. *Medicine* **2019**, *98*, e14051. [CrossRef]
28. Durante, C.; Grani, G.; Lamartina, L.; Filetti, S.; Mandel, S.J.; Cooper, D.S. The Diagnosis and Management of Thyroid Nodules: A Review. *JAMA* **2018**, *319*, 914–924. [CrossRef]
29. Kim, J.; Baek, J.H.; Lim, H.K.; Ahn, H.S.; Baek, S.M.; Choi, Y.J.; Choi, Y.J.; Chung, S.R.; Ha, E.J.; Hahn, S.Y.; et al. 2017 Thyroid Radiofrequency Ablation Guideline: Korean Society of Thyroid Radiology. *Korean J. Radiol.* **2018**, *19*. [CrossRef]
30. Bernardi, S.; Giudici, F.; Cesareo, R.; Antonelli, G.; Cavallaro, M.; Deandrea, M.; Giusti, M.; Mormile, A.; Negro, R.; Palermo, A.; et al. Five-Year Results of Radiofrequency and Laser Ablation of Benign Thyroid Nodules: A Multicenter Study from the Italian Minimally Invasive Treatments of the Thyroid Group. *Thyroid* **2020**, *30*, 1759–1770. [CrossRef]
31. Mauri, G.; Gennaro, N.; Lee, M.K.; Baek, J.H. Laser and Radiofrequency Ablations for Benign and Malignant Thyroid Tumors. *Int. J. Hyperth.* **2019**, *36*, 13–20. [CrossRef]
32. Yan, J.; Qiu, T.; Lu, J.; Wu, Y.; Yang, Y. Microwave ablation induces a lower systemic stress response in patients than open surgery for treatment of benign thyroid nodules. *Int. J. Hyperth.* **2018**, *34*, 606–610. [CrossRef]
33. Teng, D.K.; Li, W.H.; Du, J.R.; Wang, H.; Yang, D.Y.; Wu, X.L. Effects of Microwave Ablation on Papillary Thyroid Microcarcinoma: A Five-Year Follow-Up Report. *Thyroid* **2020**, *30*, 1752–1758. [CrossRef]
34. Trimboli, P.; Pelloni, F.; Bini, F.; Marinozzi, F.; Giovanella, L. High-intensity focused ultrasound (HIFU) for benign thyroid nodules: 2-year follow-up results. *Endocrine* **2019**, *65*, 312–317. [CrossRef]
35. Monpeyssen, H.; Ben Hamou, A.; Hegedüs, L.; Ghanassia, É.; Juttet, P.; Persichetti, A.; Bizzarri, G.; Bianchini, A.; Guglielmi, R.; Raggiunti, B.; et al. High-intensity focused ultrasound (HIFU) therapy for benign thyroid nodules: A 3-year retrospective multicenter follow-up study. *Int. J. Hyperth.* **2020**, *37*, 1301–1309. [CrossRef]
36. Bernardi, S.; Stacul, F.; Zecchin, M.; Dobrinja, C.; Zanconati, F.; Fabris, B. Radiofrequency ablation for benign thyroid nodules. *J. Endocrinol. Investig.* **2016**, *39*, 1003–1013. [CrossRef]
37. Dietrich, C.F.; Müller, T.; Bojunga, J.; Dong, Y.; Mauri, G.; Radzina, M.; Dighe, M.; Cui, X.W.; Grünwald, F.; Schuler, A.; et al. Statement and Recommendations on Interventional Ultrasound as a Thyroid Diagnostic and Treatment Procedure. *Ultrasound Med. Biol.* **2018**, *44*, 14–36. [CrossRef]

38. Papini, E.; Monpeyssen, H.; Frasoldati, A.; Hegedüs, L. European Thyroid Association Clinical Practice Guideline for the Use of Image-Guided Ablation in Benign Thyroid Nodules. *Eur. Thyroid J.* **2020**, *9*, 172–185. [CrossRef]
39. Yan, L.; Lan, Y.; Xiao, J.; Lin, L.; Jiang, B.; Luo, Y. Long-term outcomes of radiofrequency ablation for unifocal low-risk papillary thyroid microcarcinoma: A large cohort study of 414 patients. *Eur. Radiol.* **2021**, *31*, 685–694. [CrossRef]
40. Park, H.S.; Baek, J.H.; Park, A.W.; Chung, S.R.; Choi, Y.J.; Lee, J.H. Thyroid Radiofrequency Ablation: Updates on Innovative Devices and Techniques. *Korean J. Radiol.* **2017**, *18*, 615–623. [CrossRef]
41. Radzina, M.; Cantisani, V.; Rauda, M.; Nielsen, M.B.; Ewertsen, C.; D'Ambrosio, F.; Prieditis, P.; Sorrenti, S. Update on the role of ultrasound guided radiofrequency ablation for thyroid nodule treatment. *Int. J. Surg.* **2017**, *41* (Suppl. S1), S82–S93. [CrossRef]
42. Baek, J.H.; Ha, E.J.; Choi, Y.J.; Sung, J.Y.; Kim, J.K.; Shong, Y.K. Radiofrequency versus Ethanol Ablation for Treating Predominantly Cystic Thyroid Nodules: A Randomized Clinical Trial. *Korean J. Radiol.* **2015**, *16*, 1332–1340. [CrossRef]
43. Kim, Y.J.; Baek, J.H.; Ha, E.J.; Lim, H.K.; Lee, J.H.; Sung, J.Y.; Kim, J.K.; Kim, T.Y.; Kim, W.B.; Shong, Y.K. Cystic versus predominantly cystic thyroid nodules: Efficacy of ethanol ablation and analysis of related factors. *Eur. Radiol.* **2012**, *22*, 1573–1578. [CrossRef]
44. Sung, J.Y.; Baek, J.H.; Kim, K.S.; Lee, D.; Yoo, H.; Kim, J.K.; Park, S.H. Single-session treatment of benign cystic thyroid nodules with ethanol versus radiofrequency ablation: A prospective randomized study. *Radiology* **2013**, *269*, 293–300. [CrossRef]
45. Suh, C.H.; Baek, J.H.; Ha, E.J.; Choi, Y.J.; Lee, J.H.; Kim, J.K.; Chung, K.W.; Kim, T.Y.; Kim, W.B.; Shong, Y.K. Ethanol ablation of predominantly cystic thyroid nodules: Evaluation of recurrence rate and factors related to recurrence. *Clin. Radiol.* **2015**, *70*, 42–47. [CrossRef]
46. Lim, H.K.; Lee, J.H.; Ha, E.J.; Sung, J.Y.; Kim, J.K.; Baek, J.H. Radiofrequency ablation of benign non-functioning thyroid nodules: 4-year follow-up results for 111 patients. *Eur. Radiol.* **2013**, *23*, 1044–1049. [CrossRef]
47. Sim, J.S.; Baek, J.H.; Lee, J.; Cho, W.; Jung, S.I. Radiofrequency ablation of benign thyroid nodules: Depicting early sign of regrowth by calculating vital volume. *Int. J. Hyperth.* **2017**, *33*, 905–910. [CrossRef]
48. Baek, J.H.; Lee, J.H.; Valcavi, R.; Pacella, C.M.; Rhim, H.; Na, D.G. Thermal ablation for benign thyroid nodules: Radiofrequency and laser. *Korean J. Radiol.* **2011**, *12*, 525–540. [CrossRef]
49. Cesareo, R.; Palermo, A.; Benvenuto, D.; Cella, E.; Pasqualini, V.; Bernardi, S.; Stacul, F.; Angeletti, S.; Mauri, G.; Ciccozzi, M.; et al. Correction to: Efficacy of radiofrequency ablation in autonomous functioning thyroid nodules. A systematic review and meta-analysis. *Rev. Endocr. Metab. Disord.* **2019**, *20*, 45. [CrossRef]
50. Pacella, C.M.; Mauri, G.; Cesareo, R.; Paqualini, V.; Cianni, R.; De Feo, P.; Gambelunghe, G.; Raggiunti, B.; Tina, D.; Deandrea, M.; et al. A comparison of laser with radiofrequency ablation for the treatment of benign thyroid nodules: A propensity score matching analysis. *Int. J. Hyperth.* **2017**, *33*, 911–919. [CrossRef]
51. Ma, S.; Zhou, P.; Wu, X.; Tian, S.; Zhao, Y. Detection of the Single-Session Complete Ablation Rate by Contrast-Enhanced Ultrasound during Ultrasound-Guided Laser Ablation for Benign Thyroid Nodules: A Prospective Study. *Biomed Res. Int.* **2016**, *2016*, 9565364. [CrossRef]
52. Min, Y.; Wang, X.; Chen, H.; Chen, J.; Xiang, K.; Yin, G. Thermal Ablation for Papillary Thyroid Microcarcinoma: How Far We Have Come? *Cancer Manag. Res.* **2020**, *12*, 13369–13379. [CrossRef]
53. Zhang, M.; Tufano, R.P.; Russell, J.O.; Zhang, Y.; Zhang, Y.; Qiao, Z.; Luo, Y. Ultrasound-Guided Radiofrequency Ablation Versus Surgery for Low-Risk Papillary Thyroid Microcarcinoma: Results of Over 5 Years' Follow-Up. *Thyroid* **2020**, *30*, 408–417. [CrossRef]
54. Yue, W.; Wang, S.; Yu, S.; Wang, B. Ultrasound-guided percutaneous microwave ablation of solitary T1N0M0 papillary thyroid microcarcinoma: Initial experience. *Int. J. Hyperth.* **2014**, *30*, 150–157. [CrossRef]
55. Zhang, M.; Luo, Y.; Zhang, Y.; Tang, J. Efficacy and Safety of Ultrasound-Guided Radiofrequency Ablation for Treating Low-Risk Papillary Thyroid Microcarcinoma: A Prospective Study. *Thyroid* **2016**, *26*, 1581–1587. [CrossRef]
56. Mitchell, A.L.; Gandhi, A.; Scott-Coombes, D.; Perros, P. Management of thyroid cancer: United Kingdom National Multidisciplinary Guidelines. *J. Laryngol. Otol.* **2016**, *130*, S150–S160. [CrossRef]
57. Warren Frunzac, R.; Richards, M. Computed Tomography and Magnetic Resonance Imaging of the Thyroid and Parathyroid Glands. *Front. Horm. Res.* **2016**, *45*, 16–23. [CrossRef]
58. Baek, J.H.; Kim, Y.S.; Sung, J.Y.; Choi, H.; Lee, J.H. Locoregional control of metastatic well-differentiated thyroid cancer by ultrasound-guided radiofrequency ablation. *AJR Am. J. Roentgenol.* **2011**, *197*, W331–W336. [CrossRef]
59. Xiang, D.; Hong, Y.; Zhang, B.; Huang, P.; Li, G.; Wang, P.; Li, Z. Contrast-enhanced ultrasound (CEUS) facilitated US in detecting lateral neck lymph node metastasis of thyroid cancer patients: Diagnosis value and enhancement patterns of malignant lymph nodes. *Eur. Radiol.* **2014**, *24*, 2513–2519. [CrossRef]
60. Schleder, S.; Janke, M.; Agha, A.; Schacherer, D.; Hornung, M.; Schlitt, H.J.; Stroszczynski, C.; Schreyer, A.G.; Jung, E.M. Preoperative differentiation of thyroid adenomas and thyroid carcinomas using high resolution contrast-enhanced ultrasound (CEUS). *Clin. Hemorheol. Microcirc.* **2015**, *61*, 13–22. [CrossRef]
61. Zhao, R.N.; Zhang, B.; Yang, X.; Jiang, Y.X.; Lai, X.J.; Zhang, X.Y. Logistic Regression Analysis of Contrast-Enhanced Ultrasound and Conventional Ultrasound Characteristics of Sub-centimeter Thyroid Nodules. *Ultrasound Med. Biol.* **2015**, *41*, 3102–3108. [CrossRef]
62. Li, F.; Luo, H. Comparative study of thyroid puncture biopsy guided by contrast-enhanced ultrasonography and conventional ultrasound. *Exp. Ther. Med.* **2013**, *5*, 1381–1384. [CrossRef]

63. Zhou, X.; Zhou, P.; Hu, Z.; Tian, S.M.; Zhao, Y.; Liu, W.; Jin, Q. Diagnostic Efficiency of Quantitative Contrast-Enhanced Ultrasound Indicators for Discriminating Benign from Malignant Solid Thyroid Nodules. *J. Ultrasound Med.* **2018**, *37*, 425–437. [CrossRef]
64. Leenhardt, L.; Erdogan, M.F.; Hegedus, L.; Mandel, S.J.; Paschke, R.; Rago, T.; Russ, G. European thyroid association guidelines for cervical ultrasound scan and ultrasound-guided techniques in the postoperative management of patients with thyroid cancer. *Eur. Thyroid J.* **2013**, *2*, 147–159. [CrossRef]
65. Haugen, B.R.; Alexander, E.K.; Bible, K.C.; Doherty, G.M.; Mandel, S.J.; Nikiforov, Y.E.; Pacini, F.; Randolph, G.W.; Sawka, A.M.; Schlumberger, M.; et al. 2015 American Thyroid Association Management Guidelines for Adult Patients with Thyroid Nodules and Differentiated Thyroid Cancer: The American Thyroid Association Guidelines Task Force on Thyroid Nodules and Differentiated Thyroid Cancer. *Thyroid* **2016**, *26*, 1–133. [CrossRef]
66. Pacini, F.; Basolo, F.; Bellantone, R.; Boni, G.; Cannizzaro, M.A.; De Palma, M.; Durante, C.; Elisei, R.; Fadda, G.; Frasoldati, A.; et al. Italian consensus on diagnosis and treatment of differentiated thyroid cancer: Joint statements of six Italian societies. *J. Endocrinol. Investig.* **2018**, *41*, 849–876. [CrossRef]
67. Verburg, F.A.; Mäder, U.; Giovanella, L.; Luster, M.; Reiners, C. Low or Undetectable Basal Thyroglobulin Levels Obviate the Need for Neck Ultrasound in Differentiated Thyroid Cancer Patients After Total Thyroidectomy and 131I Ablation. *Thyroid* **2018**, *28*, 722–728. [CrossRef]
68. Lepoutre-Lussey, C.; Maddah, D.; Golmard, J.L.; Russ, G.; Tissier, F.; Trésallet, C.; Menegaux, F.; Aurengo, A.; Leenhardt, L. Post-operative neck ultrasound and risk stratification in differentiated thyroid cancer patients with initial lymph node involvement. *Eur. J. Endocrinol.* **2014**, *170*, 837–846. [CrossRef]
69. Matrone, A.; Gambale, C.; Piaggi, P.; Viola, D.; Giani, C.; Agate, L.; Bottici, V.; Bianchi, F.; Materazzi, G.; Vitti, P.; et al. Postoperative Thyroglobulin and Neck Ultrasound in the Risk Restratification and Decision to Perform 131I Ablation. *J. Clin. Endocrinol. Metab.* **2017**, *102*, 893–902. [CrossRef]
70. Rosario, P.W.; Calsolari, G.F.M.M.R. The risk of recurrence within the first five years is very low in patients with papillary thyroid carcinoma treated with radioiodine. *Arch. Head Neck Surg.* **2019**, *48*, e00092019. [CrossRef]
71. American Thyroid Association (ATA) Guidelines Taskforce on Thyroid Nodules and Differentiated Thyroid Cancer; Cooper, D.S.; Doherty, G.M.; Haugen, B.R.; Kloos, R.T.; Lee, S.L.; Mandel, S.J.; Mazzaferri, E.L.; McIver, B.; Pacini, F.; et al. Revised American Thyroid Association management guidelines for patients with thyroid nodules and differentiated thyroid cancer. *Thyroid* **2009**, *19*, 1167–1214. [CrossRef]
72. Baek, S.K.; Jung, K.Y.; Kang, S.M.; Kwon, S.Y.; Woo, J.S.; Cho, S.H.; Chung, E.J. Clinical risk factors associated with cervical lymph node recurrence in papillary thyroid carcinoma. *Thyroid* **2010**, *20*, 147–152. [CrossRef]
73. Wang, L.Y.; Ganly, I. Post-treatment surveillance of thyroid cancer. *Eur. J. Surg. Oncol.* **2018**, *44*, 357–366. [CrossRef]
74. Zhan, J.; Diao, X.H.; Chen, Y.; Wang, W.P.; Ding, H. Homogeneity Parameter in Contrast-Enhanced Ultrasound Imaging Improves the Classification of Abnormal Cervical Lymph Node after Thyroidectomy in Patients with Papillary Thyroid Carcinoma. *Biomed Res. Int.* **2019**, *2019*, 9296010. [CrossRef]
75. Zhao, H.; Li, H. Meta-analysis of ultrasound for cervical lymph nodes in papillary thyroid cancer: Diagnosis of central and lateral compartment nodal metastases. *Eur. J. Radiol.* **2019**, *112*, 14–21. [CrossRef]
76. Rubaltelli, L.; Corradin, S.; Dorigo, A.; Tregnaghi, A.; Adami, F.; Rossi, C.R.; Stramare, R. Automated quantitative evaluation of lymph node perfusion on contrast-enhanced sonography. *AJR Am. J. Roentgenol.* **2007**, *188*, 977–983. [CrossRef]
77. Hong, Y.R.; Luo, Z.Y.; Mo, G.Q.; Wang, P.; Ye, Q.; Huang, P.T. Role of Contrast-Enhanced Ultrasound in the Pre-operative Diagnosis of Cervical Lymph Node Metastasis in Patients with Papillary Thyroid Carcinoma. *Ultrasound Med. Biol.* **2017**, *43*, 2567–2575. [CrossRef]
78. Wang, Y.; Nie, F.; Wang, G.; Liu, T.; Dong, T.; Sun, Y. Value of Combining Clinical Factors, Conventional Ultrasound, and Contrast-Enhanced Ultrasound Features in Preoperative Prediction of Central Lymph Node Metastases of Different Sized Papillary Thyroid Carcinomas. *Cancer Manag. Res.* **2021**, *13*, 3403–3415. [CrossRef]
79. Chen, L.; Chen, L.; Liu, J.; Wang, B.; Zhang, H. Value of Qualitative and Quantitative Contrast-Enhanced Ultrasound Analysis in Preoperative Diagnosis of Cervical Lymph Node Metastasis from Papillary Thyroid Carcinoma. *J. Ultrasound Med.* **2020**, *39*, 73–81. [CrossRef]
80. Tao, L.; Zhou, W.; Zhan, W.; Li, W.; Wang, Y.; Fan, J. Preoperative Prediction of Cervical Lymph Node Metastasis in Papillary Thyroid Carcinoma via Conventional and Contrast-Enhanced Ultrasound. *J. Ultrasound Med.* **2020**, *39*, 2071–2080. [CrossRef]
81. Zhan, J.; Diao, X.; Chen, Y.; Wang, W.; Ding, H. Predicting cervical lymph node metastasis in patients with papillary thyroid cancer (PTC)—Why contrast-enhanced ultrasound (CEUS) was performed before thyroidectomy. *Clin. Hemorheol. Microcirc.* **2019**, *72*, 61–73. [CrossRef] [PubMed]

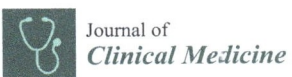

Review

Morbid Obesity and Thyroid Cancer Rate. A Review of Literature

Stefania Masone [1,*], Nunzio Velotti [2], Silvia Savastano [1], Emanuele Filice [1], Rossana Serao [2], Antonio Vitiello [2], Giovanna Berardi [2], Vincenzo Schiavone [2] and Mario Musella [2]

[1] Department of Clinical Medicine and Surgery, University of Naples "Federico II", Via Pansini n. 5, 80131 Naples, Italy; silvia.savastano@unina.it (S.S.); emanuele.filice888@gmail.com (E.F.)
[2] Department of Advanced Biomedical Sciences, University of Naples "Federico II", Via Pansini n. 5, 80131 Naples, Italy; nunzio.velotti@gmail.com (N.V.); rossyserao2@gmail.com (R.S.); AntonioVitiello_@hotmail.it (A.V.); giovannaberardi88@gmail.com (G.B.); vincenzoschiavone92@gmail.com (V.S.); mario.musella@unina.it (M.M.)
* Correspondence: stefaniamasone@yahoo.it; Tel./Fax: +39-081-7462-728

Abstract: In the past three decades, several recent studies have analyzed the alarming increase of obesity worldwide, and it has been well established that the risk of many types of malignancies is increased in obese individuals; in the same period, thyroid cancer has become the fastest growing cancer of all malignancies. We investigated the current literature to underline the presence of a connection between excess body weight or Body Mass Index (BMI) and risk of thyroid cancer. Previous studies stated that the contraposition between adipocytes and adipose-resident immune cells enhances immune cell production of multiple pro-inflammatory factors with subsequent induction of hyperlipidemia and vascular injury; these factors are all associated with oxidative stress and cancer development and/or progression. Moreover, recent studies made clear the mitogenic and tumorigenic action of insulin, carried out through the stimulation of mitogen-activated protein kinase (MAPK) and phosphoinositide-3 kinase/AKT (PI3K/AKT) pathways, which is correlated to the hyperinsulinemia and hyperglycemia found in obese population. Our findings suggest that obesity and excess body weight are related to an increased risk of thyroid cancer and that the mechanisms that combine overweight with this cancer should be searched for in the adipokine pathways and chronic inflammation onset.

Keywords: thyroid cancer; obesity; chronic inflammation; adipokines

Citation: Masone, S.; Velotti, N.; Savastano, S.; Filice, E.; Serao, R.; Vitiello, A.; Berardi, G.; Schiavone, V.; Musella, M. Morbid Obesity and Thyroid Cancer Rate. A Review of Literature. *J. Clin. Med.* **2021**, *10*, 1894. https://doi.org/10.3390/jcm10091894

Academic Editor: Giovanni Conzo

Received: 25 March 2021
Accepted: 25 April 2021
Published: 27 April 2021

Publisher's Note: MDPI stays neutral with regard to jurisdictional claims in published maps and institutional affiliations.

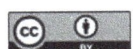

Copyright: © 2021 by the authors. Licensee MDPI, Basel, Switzerland. This article is an open access article distributed under the terms and conditions of the Creative Commons Attribution (CC BY) license (https://creativecommons.org/licenses/by/4.0/).

1. Introduction

In the past three decades, several recent studies have analyzed the alarming increase of obesity worldwide and its role as a risk factor for the onset of different metabolic disorders, such as type 2 diabetes and cardiovascular diseases [1]. Moreover, it has been well established that the risk of many types of malignancies is increased in morbid obese individuals with a body mass index (BMI) > 40 kg/m^2 or >35 kg/m^2 in the presence of obesity-related comorbidities [2]. In the same period, thyroid cancer has become the fastest growing cancer of all malignancies, with an estimated 62,450 new cases in the United States and 52,900 new thyroid cancers developed in Europe [3].

Molecular mechanisms linking excessive adiposity with the development of thyroid cancer are complex and still not completely known; furthermore, the results of several observational studies have been conflicting or inconclusive [4,5].

This review is aimed to present the current knowledge of the connection between excess body weight BMI and the risk of thyroid cancer.

2. Thyroid Cancer

Thyroid cancer accounts for only 1% of solid organ malignancies and 0.5% of all cancer deaths. Although thyroid cancer is more common overall in females, men are twice as likely as women to die from this cancer [6]. Thyroid cancers exhibit a broad range of clinical behavior that varies from indolent tumors with low mortality in most cases, to very aggressive malignancies, for example, anaplastic thyroid cancer; differentiated forms, which represent 95% of cases, are the most common category of thyroid cancer and include papillary thyroid cancer (PTC), follicular thyroid cancer (FTC), and Hurthle cell thyroid cancer [7]. Papillary thyroid cancer is the most common type with the best overall prognosis. On the other hand, follicular thyroid cancer, Hurthle cell thyroid cancer, and poorly differentiated thyroid cancers are high-risk tumors characterized by hematogenous metastasis to distant sites (lungs and bones) [8]. PTC is the most common endocrine malignancy, accounting for 96.0% of total new endocrine cancers and 66.8% of deaths due to endocrine cancers [9].

Findings from DNA sequencing studies of thyroid cancer have revealed the genetic basis for most thyroid cancers: non-overlapping mutations of the RET, TRKA, RAS, and BRAF genes are found in about 70% of PTCs, and it is well known that these genes encode activators of the mitogen-activated protein kinase (MAPK) cascade [10]. The most frequent mutation in non-medullary thyroid cancer is the BRAF^{T1799A} mutation, which is exclusive to papillary thyroid cancer and papillary-thyroid-cancer-derived anaplastic thyroid cancer. Similarly, mutations in the RAS family of oncogenes also occur most frequently in follicular thyroid cancer and follicular-variant papillary thyroid cancer [11].

Considering the role of inflammation and immune response in the onset of thyroid cancer, a link between this tumor, in particular the PTC histotype, and autoimmune thyroid diseases, such as Hashimoto's thyroiditis and Grave's disease, has already been demonstrated, although the precise mechanism is still unclear [12]. It has been proposed that inflammation might facilitate the rearrangement of the RET/PTC genomic complex through the production of free radicals, cytokine secretion, and cellular proliferation [13]. In detail, it is possible that cytokines and chemokines released by the inflammatory tumoral stroma determine the survival of those thyroid cells in which RET/PTC rearrangements randomly occur, promoting the selection of clones that acquire additional genetic lesions and thus become resistant to oncogene-induced apoptosis [14].

Another consideration regards the evidence of immune-inflammatory cell infiltrates in thyroid cancer: carcinomas are often present with a remarkable lymphocytic infiltrate in the absence of the typical signs of autoimmune thyroiditis. This phenomenon is characterized by a lymphocytic infiltrate and is generally significantly higher in patients with PTC than in patients with benign lesions [15]. Moreover, Ryder et al. found that an infiltration of macrophages and immature dendritic cells in PTC is correlated with capsule invasion and extrathyroidal extension [16].

Described findings suggest that the interaction between inflammation and genetic factors can represent a fundamental moment in the alteration of the molecular mechanisms that drive thyroid tumorigenesis.

3. Obesity, Inflammation and Cancer Development

Obesity is a chronic, low-grade inflammatory, and non-transmissible disease that affects all ages with a worldwide prevalence of 13% (11% of men and 15% of women). More than 1.9 billion adults aged 18 years and older were overweight and of these over 650 million adults were obese. In 2016, 39% of adults aged 18 years and over (39% of men and 40% of women) were overweight. The worldwide prevalence of obesity nearly tripled between 1975 and 2016 [17]. Comorbidities in patients with obesity may be due to extra body weight on the musculoskeletal system or by increased secretion of free fatty acids, peptides, and adipocytokines produced by adipocytes. More common comorbidities include depression; biliary lithiasis; hepatic steatosis; dyslipidemia; arterial hypertension; coagulopathies; endothelial dysfunction; thyroid alterations; type 2 diabetes mellitus; polycystic ovarian syndrome and hypogonadism; breast, esophagus, pancreas, and colon neoplasms; and sleep apnea [18,19].

As the definition of obesity can vary between different countries, the WHO stated a standard classification according to patients' BMI: 18.5–24.9 healthy weight; >25.0 overweight; >30 obese; >40 morbid obese [20].

Obesity is often accompanied by a low-grade chronic inflammatory state characterized by an increase in systemic markers of inflammation with a non-specific activation of the immune system, which is believed to contribute to the development of these obesity-associated pathologies [21].

In detail, contraposition between adipocytes and adipose-resident immune cells enhance immune cell production of multiple pro-inflammatory factors with subsequent induction of insulin resistance and hyperinsulinemia, hyperglycemia, hyperlipidemia, and vascular injury; these factors are all associated with oxidative stress and cancer development and/or progression [22,23].

This hypothesis is also supported by the observation that chronic infections are associated with 18% of cancer cases worldwide, as in the well-known mechanics of Helicobacter pylori infection role in gastric cancer onset, in which the intervention of immune response in the course of chronic infection determines the production of inflammatory cell mediators that sustain proliferative signaling, induce cell migration and metastasis, and promote angiogenesis [24].

For the first time in 1863, Virchow linked chronic inflammation and cancer development, observing an abundance of leukocytes in neoplastic tissue [25]. Analyzing mechanisms leading to different tumors, such as breast and colorectal cancer [26,27], it is nowadays clear that chronic inflammation produces the activation and transcription of factors such as nuclear factor kappa-light-chain-enhancer of activated B cells (NF-κB), STAT3, and activator protein 1 in pre-malignant cells; at the same time, obese white adipose tissue tends to have an increase in the production of leptin, which is pro-inflammatory, pro-angiogenic, and pro-proliferative, and a decrease in adiponectin, which is anti-inflammatory, anti-angiogenic, and anti-proliferative [28]. Moreover, obesity leads to increased endoplasmic reticulum stress, resulting in the activation of the unfolded protein response, with an increased oxidative stress, and in turn the upregulation of inflammatory cytokines [29]. All these pathways enhance cell proliferation and survival and promotes angiogenesis in conjunction with hypoxia [30].

Finally, recent studies have focused attention on the role of obese white adipose tissue in the activation of the inflammasome: multiprotein complexes that activate IL-1β and IL-18 pathways in response to pathogen-associated molecular patterns (PAMPs) and danger-associated molecular patterns (DAMPs) [31]. Inflammasomes have been shown to play a complex role in cancer through IL-1β, which promotes proliferation and invasion of tumors, and although there is no evidence for the role of inflammasome activation in obesity-associated cancer, it has been demonstrated that the inflammatory effect of leptin is dependent on IL-1β [32,33].

In such a scenario, recent evidence, primarily from bariatric surgery studies, indicates that substantial weight loss reduces cancer risk, most likely by attenuating adipose-related inflammatory mechanisms that can regulate tumor development and progression [34].

4. Obesity and Thyroid Cancer

Recent studies and metanalyses have investigated the relationship between obesity and the development of thyroid cancer.

Zhao et al. [35] first studied this field with a review of seven cohort studies for a total of 5154 thyroid cancer cases; the pooled results demonstrated that there was a statistically significant association between BMI and cancer risk. Authors also performed a stratified analysis according to sex, finding a statistically more significant association between BMI and thyroid cancer risk for males than for women.

Schmid and colleagues [36], pooling together data from 21 studies and 12,199 thyroid cancer cases, found a statistically significant 25% greater risk of thyroid cancer in overweight individuals and a 55% greater thyroid cancer risk in obese individuals; their analysis revealed that an increase of 5-unit in body mass index (BMI), 5 kg in weight, 5 cm in waist or hip circumference, and 0.1-unit in waist-to-hip ratio were associated with 30%, 5%, 5%, and 14% greater risks of thyroid cancer, respectively. Authors also evaluated histologic type, demonstrating that obesity was significantly positively related to papillary, follicular, and anaplastic thyroid cancers, whereas there was an inverse association with medullary thyroid cancer. Another important aspect is represented by the relation between obesity and the risk of cancer progression. Recently, Wang et al. [37] analyzed data from 1579 patients with PTC, clustering sample size based on BMI: underweight patients (BMI < 18.5 kg/m^2), normal body patients (18.5 < BMI < 24.0 kg/m^2), overweight patients (24.0 < BMI < 28.0 kg/m^2), and obese patients (BMI > 28.0 kg/m^2). They found a higher risk for extrathyroidal extension, advanced T stage (T III/IV), and advanced tumor-node-metastasis stage (TNM III/IV) in the overweight and obese patients' groups, concluding that obesity is closely related to the risk of PTC and, particularly, that BMI is positively associated with the invasiveness of PTC.

The complex interplay among genetic variants of thyroid cancer and dietary intake has been recently investigated [38]: it is now clear that carbohydrate intake, such as alcohol and coffee consumption, are positively associated with thyroid cancer. Considering a stratification based on demographic characteristics, Ma et al. [39] presented a metanalysis on 32 studies in which they assessed that obese women have a higher risk of thyroid cancer onset when compared with obese men (RR = 1.43 vs. RR = 1.26); moreover, significantly elevated risk was observed in obese Caucasians and Asians and in the obese population >50 years-old as opposed to the young obese population (RR = 1.28 vs. RR = 1.23).

It is worth mentioning, on the other hand, that the results published in some recent studies reveal ongoing debate over the relationship between thyroid cancer and obesity. Rotondi retrospectively analyzed 4849 fine-needle aspiration cytology (FNAC) for thyroid nodules, concluding that a significant lower rate of Thy4/5 was observed in female obese patients [40]; Farfel et al. [41], on 760 incidence cases of thyroid cancer, proposed a multivariate analysis that demonstrated that BMI was not associated with cancer incidence.

5. Studies in Animal Models

Animal studies have elucidated the complex role between obesity and thyroid cancer, helping to interpret the pathogenetic mechanisms behind this complex correlation. Kim et al. [42] evaluated the role of diet-induced obesity on the development of thyroid cancer in a mouse model that spontaneously develops thyroid cancer, finding that a high-fat diet (HFD) increases thyroid tumor cell proliferation by increasing the protein levels of cyclin D1, phosphorylated retinoblastoma protein, serum leptin levels, and STAT3 target gene expression. The same results were found by Park [43], who demonstrated the effect of S3I-201, an inhibitor of STAT3 activity, on HFD-induced thyroid cancer progression in a murine model; the authors found decreased protein levels of cyclins D1 and B1, cyclin dependent kinase 4 (CDK4), CDK6, and phosphorylated retinoblastoma protein led to the inhibition of tumor cell proliferation.

6. Molecular Mechanisms

The role of Adiponectin (APN) in endocrine cancer risk has been widely studied, but there are still controversies on the exact mechanics that rule their anti-neoplastic function: it has been proposed that low APN levels could be associated with cancers due to an excess of fat mass and sex-steroid hormones with high levels of inflammation, but there is a lack of evidence on the pathway involved.

As stated by previous research, APN's protective role on endocrine cancer cells is the activation of adenosine monophosphate-activated protein kinase (AMPK), which negatively influences cancer cells growth through p53 and p21- induced apoptosis [44,45]; moreover, it has been demonstrated that APN is able to down-regulate leptin-induced STAT3 phosphorylation, reducing tumor cell growth [46].

Despite some discrepancies, scientific research has amply demonstrated an inverse correlation between APN levels and the risk of endocrine neoplasms [47]. Considering that obesity frequently results in hypoadiponectinemia, it is very likely that the increased risk of cancer found in obese patients is at least partially attributable to the loss of the immunosuppressive effects induced by this hormone. Indeed, AFN exerts its tumor suppressor effect both directly, through the interaction with its specific receptors, and indirectly, through the regulation of the immune response, angiogenesis, and insulin sensitivity. Through the activation of its receptors and the consequent activation of the adenosine monophosphate-activated protein kinase (AMPK), APN is able to determine both a reduction of the anabolic and proliferative pathways and an increased expression of important factors involved in the arrest of cell cycle and apoptosis, such as p21 and p53 [45]. Furthermore, AMPK activation determines an indirect inhibition of both MAPK and PI3K/AKTt/mTOR pathways, with an effect of downregulation of cell proliferation [48]. Regarding indirect anti-neoplastic effects, it has been shown that APN levels are inversely related to the degree of insulin resistance and to insulin levels [49]. Furthermore, the APN effect on insulin signaling seems to be also present at the post-receptor level. In addition, through interaction with the NF-kB pathway and its capacity of inhibiting myelomonocytic progenitor's growth and macrophage phagocytic activity, APN is able to exert a real anti-inflammatory and immunomodulating effect [50]. Finally, it seems that APN may play a key role in angiogenesis regulation, but the studies currently available have provided conflicting results. In fact, some studies have shown that this adipokine is able to cause a conspicuous reduction in angiogenesis, while other studies conducted on mouse models of breast cancer suggest that adiponectin has a powerful pro-angiogenic effect [51]. Regarding the link between APN and thyroid cancer, some studies have shown an inverse relationship between APN levels and thyroid cancer [52]; however, further studies are required to confirm these findings.

Considering thyroid cancer, Mitsiades et al. [53] found lower levels of circulating APN in patients with any form of thyroid cancer compared to the control population; similarly, Warakomski et al., in a large prospective study, found that upper tertiles of IL-6 and leptin were associated with a higher clinical stage of PTC. The same results were found in the multicenter "EPIC" study from Dossus et al. [52] on 475 primary thyroid cancer cases: the authors underlined that adiponectin was inversely associated with cancer risk among women, whereas a positive association was revealed with IL-10. Supporting this interesting hypothesis, Cheng et al. [54] have shown that papillary thyroid carcinoma cell lines express a significantly lower number of AdipoR1 and AdipoR2 receptors than normal thyrocytes.

At the same time, APN may also express its anti-neoplastic role through insulin-sensitizing and angiogenesis-related effects. Considering that APN levels are inversely related to fasting insulin concentrations due to its significant effect on insulin post-receptor signaling, and considering that insulin supports tumor cell proliferation, it was proposed that APN is able to reduce tumor cell growth induced by insulin pathway [55,56].

Recently, some studies also highlighted the pro-carcinogenic role of leptin: Hedayati et al. [57] found Leptin levels were higher in thyroid cancer patients compared to healthy subjects, and Uddin and colleagues [58] demonstrated that leptin acts via its receptor to induce PTC cell proliferation and inhibit apoptosis.

Finally, it has been shown that the state of chronic hyperinsulinemia is associated with the development of different types of malignancies, such as lung, prostate, and breast cancer [59,60]. The mitogenic and tumorigenic action of insulin would seem to be carried out through the stimulation of mitogen-activated protein kinase (MAPK) and phosphoinositide-3 kinase/AKT (PI3K/AKT) pathways [61]. Of interest, several indirect mechanisms seem to underlie the link between insulin resistance and thyroid cancer. First, the condition of hyperinsulinemia and insulin resistance, typical of subjects with obesity, is associated with an increase in TSH levels, with a consequent enhancement of thyrocyte proliferation [62]. The increase in thyrocyte proliferation could lead to a mutational accumulation capable of triggering neoplastic transformation. The increase of TSH levels in the obese population probably represents an adaptive response aimed at increasing energy expenditure [63]. Furthermore, insulin receptor overexpression often occurs in DTC cells. In fact, the relative abundance of IR-A is around 40% in normal thyrocytes, while it increases to over 70% in DTC cells [64]. In addition, hyperinsulinemia determines an increase in the bioavailability of insulin-like growth factor 1 (IGF-1) through the inhibition of the synthesis of IGF binding protein 1-2 (IGFBP1-2) and the stimulation of the production of IGF-1 by the liver. The increased bioavailability of IGF-1 may contribute to tumor progression through the stimulation of IGF-1R [65]. More recently, it was demonstrated that insulin resistance may influence the evolution of thyroid nodules through an enhancement of angiogenesis and intranodular vascularization [66]. This phenomenon is probably caused by vascular endothelial growth factor (VEGF) overexpression and the consequent promotion of endothelial cell proliferation. Thus, in the condition of insulin resistance, the concomitance of hyperinsulinemia, hyperthyrotropinemia, increased bioavailability of IGF-1, and increased angiogenesis in thyroid nodules may represent important risk factors for DTC in overweight and obese patients (Figure 1).

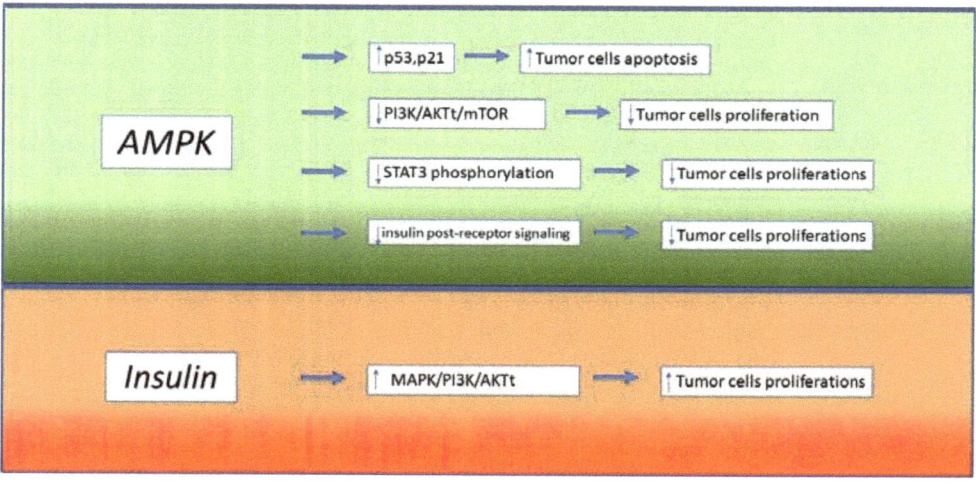

Figure 1. Molecular Mechanisms supporting the relation between obesity and thyroid cancer onset. AMPK: 5′ AMP-activated protein kinase; MAPK: mitogen-activated protein kinase; PI3K: Phosphoinositide 3-kinases; mTOR: mammalian target of rapamycin; STAT3: Signal transducer and activator of transcription 3; AKT: serine/threonine kinase.

7. Conclusions

In the last three decades, the incidence of thyroid cancer has increased simultaneously with the increase of obesity rates. Analyzing previous literature, growing interest has been focused on the adipocyte-secreted mediators as a sprouting factor in cancer pathophysiology. The most recent meta-analyses and reviews have demonstrated the causal role of APN and have reconstructed the signaling pathway that this and other molecules induce in obese patients with thyroid cancer [67]. The review conducted by Kim in 2017 confirmed that obesity accelerates the growth and progression of thyroid cancer, determining a shorter survival and promoting anaplastic transformation through elevated leptin level and the JAK2-STAT3 pathway [68]. Similarly, Averginos in 2019 stated that there was convincing evidence that excess body weight is associated with an increased cancer risk of at least 13 anatomic sites, including the thyroid; authors focused attention on insulin receptor role and chronic inflammation as major causes of cancer development [23].

However, Kim and colleagues [69], in a large retrospective study on 1579 cases, emphasized that, at present, the relationship between obesity and the pathological features of PTC remains controversial and there is still not agreement over many factors that could lead to interpretation bias. From this point of view, demographic characteristics such as age, sex, ethnicity, as well as smoking habits were analyzed on relatively small samples size in order to be able to identify their incidence on the obesity-tumor development relationship. Moreover, it is worth noting that BMI cannot be used as an exclusive criterion for assessing obesity, especially when it reflects the lack of specificity in centripetal obesity [70].

Finally, some authors have investigated the possible role of obesity on the outcomes of thyroid surgery; apart from a longer operative time and an increased risk of wound complications than patients with low BMI, obesity seems not to be associated with worse surgical outcomes. Pooling data from more than 18,000 patients, it is reasonable to perform thyroidectomy safely in obese patients, without expecting to manage major complications [71,72].

In conclusion, despite some contrasting results, the findings of this review suggested that obesity and excess body weight were related to an increased risk of thyroid cancer and the mechanisms that combine overweight with this cancer should be searched in the adipokines pathways, chronic inflammation onset, insulin-resistance development, and oxidative stress processes. Further studies, with a randomized and controlled design and large sample size, are needed to better address this interesting relation and overcome the confounding factors bias.

Funding: This research received no external funding.

Institutional Review Board Statement: Not applicable.

Informed Consent Statement: Not applicable.

Data Availability Statement: No new data were created or analyzed in this study. Data sharing is not applicable to this article.

Conflicts of Interest: The authors declare no conflict of interest.

References

1. NCD Risk Factor Collaboration (NCD-RisC). Trends in adult body-mass index in 200 countries from 1975 to 2014: A pooled analysis of 1698 population-based measurement studies with 19.2 million participants. *Lancet* **2016**, *387*, 1377–1396. [CrossRef]
2. Renehan, A.G.; Tyson, M.; Egger, M.; Heller, R.F.; Zwahlen, M. Body-mass index and incidence of cancer: A systematic review and meta-analysis of prospective observational studies. *Lancet* **2008**, *371*, 569–578. [CrossRef]
3. Ferlay, J.; Steliarova-Foucher, E.; Lortet-Tieulent, J.; Rosso, S.; Coebergh, J.W.W.; Comber, H.; Forman, D.; Bray, F. Cancer incidence and mortality patterns in Europe: Estimates for 40 countries in 2012. *Eur. J. Cancer* **2013**, *49*, 1374–1403. [CrossRef]
4. Guignard, R.; Truong, T.; Rougier, Y.; Baron-Dubourdieu, D.; Guénel, P. Alcohol drinking, tobacco smoking, and anthropometric characteristics as risk factors for thyroid cancer: A countrywide case-control study in New Caledonia. *Am. J. Epidemiol.* **2007**, *166*, 1140–1149. [CrossRef]
5. Song, Y.M.; Sung, J.; Ha, M. Obesity and risk of cancer in postmenopausal Korean women. *J. Clin. Oncol.* **2008**, *26*, 3395–3402. [CrossRef]
6. Jemal, A.; Bray, F.; Center, M.M.; Ferlay, J.; Ward, E.; Forman, D. Global cancer statistics. *CA Cancer J. Clin.* **2011**, *61*, 69–90. [CrossRef]
7. Howlader, N.; Noone, A.M.; Krapcho, M.; Miller, D.; Bishop, K.; Altekruse, S.F.; Kosary, C.L.; Yu, M.; Ruhl, J.; Tatalovich, Z.; et al. SEER Cancer Statistics Review, 1975-2018, National Cancer Institute. Bethesda. 2016. Available online: http://seer.cancer.gov/csr/1975_2013/ (accessed on 28 November 2020).
8. Cabanillas, M.E.; McFadden, D.G.; Durante, C. Thyroid cancer. *Lancet* **2016**, *388*, 2783–2795. [CrossRef]
9. Siegel, R.; Naishadham, D.; Jemal, A. Cancer statistics, 2013. *CA Cancer J Clin.* **2013**, *63*, 11–30. [CrossRef]
10. Manié, S.; Santoro, M.; Fusco, A.; Billaud, M. The RET receptor: Function in development and dysfunction in congenital malformation. *Trends Genet.* **2001**, *17*, 580–589. [CrossRef]
11. Nikiforov, Y.E.; Nikiforova, M.N. Molecular genetics and diagnosis of thyroid cancer. *Nat. Rev. Endocrinol.* **2011**, *7*, 569–580. [CrossRef] [PubMed]
12. Weetman, A.P. Cellular immune responses in autoimmune thyroid disease. *Clin. Endocrinol.* **2004**, *61*, 405–413. [CrossRef]
13. Castellone, M.D.; Cirafici, A.M.; Vita, G.D.; Falco, V.D.; Malorni, L.; Tallini, G.; Fagin, J.A.; Fusco, A.; Melillo, R.M.; Santoro, M. Ras-mediated apoptosis of PC CL 3 rat thyroid cells induced by RET/PTC oncogenes. *Oncogene* **2003**, *22*, 246–255. [CrossRef]

14. Guarino, V.; Castellone, M.D.; Avilla, E.; Melillo, R.M. Thyroid cancer and inflammation. *Mol. Cell Endocrinol.* **2010**, *321*, 94–102. [CrossRef]
15. Okayasu, I. The Relationship of Lymphocytic Thyroiditis to the Development of Thyroid Carcinoma. *Endocr. Pathol.* **1997**, *8*, 225–230. [CrossRef]
16. Ryder, M.; Ghossein, R.A.; Ricarte-Filho, J.C.; Knauf, J.A.; Fagin, J.A. Increased density of tumor-associated macrophages is associated with decreased survival in advanced thyroid cancer. *Endocr. Relat. Cancer* **2008**, *15*, 1069–1074. [CrossRef]
17. WHO. Obesity and Overweight. 2017. Available online: http://www.who.int (accessed on 27 November 2020).
18. Gallagher, E.J.; LeRoith, D. Obesity and Diabetes: The Increased Risk of Cancer and Cancer-Related Mortality. *Physiol. Rev.* **2015**, *95*, 727–748. [CrossRef] [PubMed]
19. Swinburn, B.A.; Sacks, G.; Hall, K.D.; McPherson, K.; Finegood, D.T.; Moodie, M.L.; Gortmaker, S.L. The global obesity pandemic: Shaped by global drivers and local environments. *Lancet* **2011**, *378*, 804–814. [CrossRef]
20. Available online: https://www.euro.who.int/en/health-topics/disease-prevention/nutrition/a-healthy-lifestyle/body-mass-index-bmi (accessed on 23 April 2021).
21. Olefsky, J.M.; Glass, C.K. Macrophages, inflammation and insulin resistance. *Annu. Rev. Physiol.* **2010**, *72*, 219–246. [CrossRef] [PubMed]
22. Deng, T.; Lyon, C.J.; Bergin, S.; Caligiuri, M.A.; Hsueh, W.A. Obesity, Inflammation, and Cancer. *Annu. Rev. Pathol.* **2016**, *11*, 421–449. [CrossRef]
23. Avgerinos, K.I.; Spyrou, N.; Mantzoros, C.S.; Dalamaga, M. Obesity and cancer risk: Emerging biological mechanisms and perspectives. *Metabolism* **2019**, *92*, 121–135. [CrossRef]
24. Hanahan, D.; Coussens, L.M. Accessories to the crime: Functions of cells recruited to the tumor microenvironment. *Cancer Cell.* **2012**, *21*, 309–322. [CrossRef] [PubMed]
25. Balkwill, F.; Mantovani, A. Inflammation and cancer: Back to Virchow? *Lancet* **2001**, *357*, 539–545. [CrossRef]
26. Chan, D.S.; Vieira, A.R.; Aune, D.; Bandera, E.V.; Greenwood, D.C.; McTiernan, A.; Rosenblatt, D.N.; Thune, I.; Vieira, R.; Norat, T. Body mass index and survival in women with breast cancer-systematic literature review and meta-analysis of 82 follow-up studies. *Ann. Oncol.* **2014**, *25*, 1901–1914. [CrossRef]
27. Ngo, H.T.; Hetland, R.B.; Nygaard, U.C.; Steffensen, I.L. Genetic and Diet-Induced Obesity Increased Intestinal Tumorigenesis in the Double Mutant Mouse Model Multiple Intestinal Neoplasia X Obese via Disturbed Glucose Regulation and Inflammation. *J. Obes.* **2015**, *2015*, 343479. [CrossRef]
28. Kolb, R.; Sutterwala, F.S.; Zhang, W. Obesity and cancer: Inflammation bridges the two. *Curr. Opin. Pharmacol.* **2016**, *29*, 77–89. [CrossRef]
29. Cnop, M.; Foufelle, F.; Velloso, L.A. Endoplasmic reticulum stress, obesity and diabetes. *Trends. Mol. Med.* **2012**, *18*, 59–68. [CrossRef]
30. Grivennikov, S.I.; Greten, F.R.; Karin, M. Immunity, inflammation, and cancer. *Cell* **2010**, *140*, 883–899. [CrossRef]
31. Kolb, R.; Liu, G.H.; Janowski, A.M.; Sutterwala, F.S.; Zhang, W. Inflammasomes in cancer: A double-edged sword. *Protein. Cell.* **2014**, *5*, 12–20. [CrossRef]
32. Faggioni, R.; Fantuzzi, G.; Fuller, J.; Dinarello, C.A.; Feingold, K.R.; Grunfeld, C. IL-1 beta mediates leptin induction during inflammation. *Am. J. Physiol.* **1998**, *274*, R204–R208.
33. Rustgi, V.K.; Li, Y.; Gupta, K.; Minacapelli, C.D.; Bhurwal, A.; Catalano, C.; Elsaid, M.I. Bariatric Surgery Reduces Cancer Risk in Adults with Nonalcoholic Fatty Liver Disease and Severe Obesity. *Gastroenterology* **2021**. [CrossRef] [PubMed]
34. Schauer, D.P.; Feigelson, H.S.; Koebnick, C.; Caan, B.; Weinmann, S.; Leonard, A.C.; Powers, J.D.; Yenumula, P.R.; Arterburn, D.E. Bariatric Surgery and the Risk of Cancer in a Large Multisite Cohort. *Ann. Surg.* **2019**, *269*, 95–101. [CrossRef] [PubMed]
35. Zhao, Z.G.; Guo, X.G.; Ba, C.X.; Wang, W.; Yang, Y.Y.; Wang, J.; Cao, H.Y. Overweight, obesity and thyroid cancer risk: A meta-analysis of cohort studies. *J. Int. Med. Res.* **2012**, *40*, 2041–2050. [CrossRef] [PubMed]
36. Schmid, D.; Ricci, C.; Behrens, G.; Leitzmann, M.F. Adiposity and risk of thyroid cancer: A systematic review and meta-analysis. *Obes. Rev.* **2015**, *16*, 1042–1054. [CrossRef]
37. Wang, H.; Wang, P.; Wu, Y.; Hou, X.; Peng, Z.; Yang, W.; Guan, L.; Hu, L.; Zhi, J.; Gao, M.; et al. Correlation between obesity and clinicopathological characteristics in patients with papillary thyroid cancer: A study of 1579 cases: A retrospective study. *PeerJ* **2020**, *8*, e9675. [CrossRef]
38. Song, S.S.; Huang, S.; Park, S. Association of Polygenetic Risk Scores Related to Cell Differentiation and Inflammation with Thyroid Cancer Risk and Genetic Interaction with Dietary Intake. *Cancers* **2021**, *13*, 1510. [CrossRef] [PubMed]
39. Ma, J.; Huang, M.; Wang, L.; Ye, W.; Tong, Y.; Wang, H. Obesity and risk of thyroid cancer: Evidence from a meta-analysis of 21 observational studies. *Med. Sci. Monit.* **2015**, *21*, 283–291.
40. Rotondi, M.; Castagna, M.G.; Cappelli, C.; Ciuoli, C.; Coperchini, F.; Chiofalo, F.; Maino, F.; Palmitesta, P.; Chiovato, L.; Pacini, F. Obesity Does Not Modify the Risk of Differentiated Thyroid Cancer in a Cytological Series of Thyroid Nodules. *Eur. Thyroid. J.* **2016**, *5*, 125–131. [CrossRef]
41. Farfel, A.; Kark, J.D.; Derazne, E.; Tzur, D.; Barchana, M.; Lazar, L.; Afek, A.; Shamiss, A. Predictors for thyroid carcinoma in Israel: A national cohort of 1,624,310 adolescents followed for up to 40 years. *Thyroid* **2014**, *24*, 987–993. [CrossRef]
42. Kim, W.G.; Park, J.W.; Willingham, M.C.; Cheng, S.Y. Diet-induced obesity increases tumor growth and promotes anaplastic change in thyroid cancer in a mouse model. *Endocrinology* **2013**, *154*, 2936–2947. [CrossRef]

43. Park, J.W.; Han, C.R.; Zhao, L.; Willingham, M.C.; Cheng, S.Y. Inhibition of STAT3 activity delays obesity-induced thyroid carcinogenesis in a mouse model. *Endocr. Relat. Cancer* **2016**, *23*, 53–63. [CrossRef]
44. Luo, Z.; Saha, A.K.; Xiang, X.; Ruderman, N.B. AMPK, the metabolic syndrome and cancer. *Trends. Pharmacol. Sci.* **2005**, *26*, 69–76. [CrossRef]
45. Steinberg, G.R.; Kemp, B.E. AMPK in Health and Disease. *Physiol. Rev.* **2009**, *89*, 1025–1078. [CrossRef] [PubMed]
46. Bowman, T.; Garcia, R.; Turkson, J.; Jove, R. STATs in oncogenesis. *Oncogene* **2000**, *19*, 2474–2488. [CrossRef] [PubMed]
47. Izadi, V.; Farabad, E.; Azadbakht, L. Serum Adiponectin level and different kind of cancers: A review of recent evidence. *ISRN Oncol.* **2012**, *2012*, 982769. [CrossRef]
48. Hall, J.; Roberts, R.; Vora, N. Energy homoeostasis: The roles of adipose tissue-derived hormones, peptide YY and Ghrelin. *Obes. Facts* **2009**, *2*, 117–125. [CrossRef] [PubMed]
49. Weyer, C.; Funanashi, T.; Tanaka, S.; Hotta, K.; Matsuzawa, Y.; Pratley, R.E.; Tataranni, P.A. Hypoadipoactinemia in obesity and type 2 diabetes: Close association with insulin-resistance and hyperinsulinemia. *J. Clin. Endocrinol. Metab.* **2001**, *86*, 1930–1935. [CrossRef]
50. Obeid, S.; Hebbard, L. Role of adiponectin and its receptors in cancer. *Cancer Biol. Med.* **2012**, *9*, 213–220.
51. Hebbard, L.W.; Galatti, M.; Young, L.J.T.; Cardiff, R.D.; Oshima Robert, G.; Ranscht, B. T-cadherin supports angiogenesis and adiponectin association with the vasculature in a mouse mammary tumor model. *Cancer Res.* **2008**, *68*, 1407–1416. [CrossRef] [PubMed]
52. Dossus, L.; Franceschi, S.; Biessy, C.; Navionis, A.S.; Travis, R.C.; Weiderpass, E.; Scalbert, A.; Romieu, I.; Tjønneland, A.; Olsen, A.; et al. Adipokines and inflammation markers and risk of differentiated thyroid carcinoma: The EPIC study. *Int. J. Cancer* **2018**, *142*, 1332–1342. [CrossRef]
53. Mitsiades, N.; Pazaitou-Panayotou, K.; Aronis, K.N.; Moon, H.S.; Chamberland, J.P.; Liu, X.; Diakopoulos, K.N.; Kyttaris, V.; Panagiotou, V.; Mylvaganam, G.; et al. Circulating adiponectin is inversely associated with risk of thyroid cancer: In vivo and in vitro studies. *J. Clin. Endocrinol Metab.* **2011**, *96*, E2023–E2028. [CrossRef] [PubMed]
54. Cheng, S.P.; Liu, C.L.; Hsu, Y.C.; Chang, Y.C.; Huang, S.Y.; Lee, J.J. Expression and biologic significance of adiponectin receptors in papillary thyroid carcinoma. *Cell Biochem. Biophys.* **2013**, *65*, 203–210. [CrossRef]
55. Sciacca, L.; Vella, V.; Frittitta, L.; Tumminia, A.; Manzella, L.; Squatrito, S.; Belfiore, A.; Vigneri, R. Long-acting insulin analogs and cancer. *Nutr. Metab. Cardiovasc. Dis.* **2018**, *28*, 436–443. [CrossRef]
56. Pollak, M. Insulin and insulin-like growth factor signalling in neoplasia. *Nat. Rev. Cancer* **2008**, *8*, 915–923. [CrossRef]
57. Hedayati, M.; Yaghmaei, P.; Pooyamanesh, Z.; Yeganeh, M.Z.; Rad, L.H. Leptin: A correlated Peptide to papillary thyroid carcinoma? *J. Thyroid. Res.* **2011**, *2011*, 832163. [CrossRef]
58. Uddin, S.; Bavi, P.; Siraj, A.K.; Ahmed, M.; Al-Rasheed, M.; Hussain, A.R.; Ahmed, M.; Amin, T.; Alzahrani, A.; Al-Dayel, F.; et al. Leptin-R and its association with PI3K/AKT signaling pathway in papillary thyroid carcinoma. *Endocr. Relat. Cancer* **2010**, *17*, 191–202. [CrossRef]
59. Nam, S.; Park, S.; Park, H.S.; Kim, S.; Kim, J.Y.; Kim, S.I. Association between insulin resistance and luminal B subtype breast cancer in postmenopausal women. *Medicine* **2016**, *95*, e2825. [CrossRef]
60. Argirion, I.; Weinstein, S.J.; Mannisto, S.; Albanes, D.; Mondul, A.M. Serum insulin, glucose, indices of insulin resistance, and risk of lung cancer. *Cancer Epidemiol. Biomark. Prev.* **2017**, *26*, 1519–1524. [CrossRef] [PubMed]
61. Braun, S.; Worms, K.B.; LeRoith, D. The link between the metabolic syndrome and cancer. *Int. J. Biol. Sci.* **2011**, *7*, 1003–1015. [CrossRef]
62. Biondi, B. Thyroid and obesity: An intriguing relationship. *J. Clin. Endocrinol. Metab.* **2010**, *95*, 3614–3617. [CrossRef] [PubMed]
63. Fontenelle, L.C.; Feitosa, M.M.; Severo, J.S.; Freitas, T.E.C.; Morais, J.B.S.; Torres-Leal, F.L.; Henriques, G.S.; Marreiro, D.D.N. Thyroid function in human obesity: Underlying mechanisms. *Horm. Metab. Res.* **2016**, *48*, 787–794. [CrossRef]
64. Malaguarnera, R.; Frasca, F.; Garozzo, A.; Giani, F.; Pandini, G.; Vella, V.; Vigneri, R.; Belfiore, A. Insulin receptor isoforms and insulin-like growth factor receptor in human follicular cell precursors from papillary thyroid cancer and normal thyroid. *J. Clin. Endocrinol. Metab.* **2011**, *96*, 766–774. [CrossRef]
65. Belfiore, A.; Malaguarnera, R. Insulin receptor and cancer. *Endocr. Relat. Cancer* **2011**, *18*, R125–R147. [CrossRef]
66. Wang, K.; Yang, Y.; Wu, Y.; Chen, J.; Zhang, D.; Mao, X.; Wu, X.; Long, X.; Liu, C. The association between insulin re-sistance and vascularization of thyroid nodules. *J. Clin. Endocrinol. Metab.* **2015**, *100*, 184–192. [CrossRef]
67. Pappa, T.; Alevizaki, M. Obesity and thyroid cancer: A clinical update. *Thyroid* **2014**, *24*, 190–199. [CrossRef]
68. Kim, W.G.; Cheng, S.Y. Mechanisms Linking Obesity and Thyroid Cancer Development and Progression in Mouse Models. *Horm. Cancer.* **2018**, *9*, 108–116. [CrossRef]
69. Kim, S.K.; Woo, J.W.; Park, I.; Lee, J.H.; Choe, J.H.; Kim, J.H.; Kim, J.S. Influence of Body Mass Index and Body Surface Area on the Behavior of Papillary Thyroid Carcinoma. *Thyroid* **2016**, *26*, 657–666. [CrossRef] [PubMed]
70. Rosen, E.D.; Spiegelman, B.M. What we talk about when we talk about fat. *Cell* **2014**, *156*, 20–44. [CrossRef] [PubMed]
71. Canu, G.L.; Medas, F.; Cappellacci, F.; Podda, M.G.; Romano, G.; Erdas, E.; Calò, P.G. Can thyroidectomy be considered safe in obese patients? A retrospective cohort study. *BMC Surg.* **2020**, *20*, 275. [CrossRef] [PubMed]
72. Buerba, R.; Romar, S.A.; Sosa, J.A. Thyroidectomy and parathyroidectomy in patients with high body mass index are safe overall: Analysis of 26,864 patients. *Surgery* **2011**, *150*, 950–958. [CrossRef]

MDPI
St. Alban-Anlage 66
4052 Basel
Switzerland
Tel. +41 61 683 77 34
Fax +41 61 302 89 18
www.mdpi.com

Journal of Clinical Medicine Editorial Office
E-mail: jcm@mdpi.com
www.mdpi.com/journal/jcm

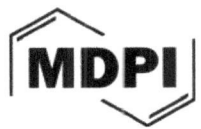